Death and Dying

Death and Dying

Theory/Research/Practice

Larry A. Bugen

St. Edwards University,
Austin, Texas

ꭐꞔꞎ Wm. C. Brown Company Publishers
Dubuque, Iowa

wcb   **Wm. C. Brown**   Chairman of the Board
       Larry W. Brown   President, WCB Group

Book Team

Marilyn A. Phelps   Designer
Elizabeth Munger   Production
    Editor

Wm. C. Brown Company Publishers, College Division

Lawrence E. Cremer   President
Raymond C. Deveaux   Executive Director of Product Development
David Wm. Smith   National Sales Manager
David A. Corona   Director of Production Development and Design
Ruth Richard   Production Editorial Manager
Marilyn A. Phelps   Manager of Design

Cover photo   Chris Grajczyk

To Mom, Dad, Bobby, and Paul

. . . being to timelessness as it's to time,
love did no more begin than love will end;

e.e. cummings

To Jack
with best wishes
from: John Scholl
November 18/08.

Contributors

David Aderman, Ph.D. Associate Professor, Department of Psychology, Duke University

Ignacio Aguilar, M.S.W. Director, XIPE-Totec Clinica de Salud Mental, Metropolitan State Hospital, Norwalk, California

Zorena S. Bolton, M.S.W. Field Supervisor, School of Social Work, University of Texas-Austin

Larry A. Bugen, Ph.D. Assistant Professor, College of Education, University of Texas-Austin; Director of Psychological Services, St. Edward's University, Austin, Texas

Eric J. Cassell, M.D. Clinical Professor, School of Public Health, Cornell University Medical College

John Clancy, M.D., F.R.C.P. Professor, Department of Psychiatry, University of Iowa

Rachel Ogren Clark Co-director, The SHANTI Project, Berkeley, California

Joseph A. Durlak, Ph.D. Associate Professor, Department of Psychology, Southern Illinois University

Charles Edgley, Ph.D. Associate Professor, Oklahoma State University, Stillwater, Oklahoma

Gerald Epstein, M.A. Graduate Student, Department of Psychology, George Peabody College

Charles A. Garfield, Ph.D. Director, SHANTI Project, Berkeley, California; Research Psychologist, Cancer Research Institute, University of California Medical Center

Stephen P. Hersh, M.D. Assistant Director for Children and Youth, National Institute of Mental Health

Albert R. Hollenbeck, Ph.D. Staff Fellow, Laboratory of Developmental Psychology, National Institute of Mental Health

Sharon H. Imbus, R.N., M.Sc. Department of Surgery, Los Angeles County, University of Southern California Medical Center

Richard A. Kalish, Ph.D. Professor of Behavioral Sciences, Graduate Theological Union, Berkeley, California

Frederic T. Kapp, Ph.D. Assistant Professor, College of Nursing and Health, University of Cincinnati

Orville E. Kelly Founder, Make Today Count, Burlington, Iowa

Gerald Koocher, Ph.D. Chief Psychologist, Sidney Farber Cancer Institute, Boston, Massachusetts

Pamela Ennis Koza, Ph.D. Scientist, Addiction Research Foundation, Toronto, Ontario

Elisabeth Kübler-Ross, M.D. Co-director, Ross Medical Associates; Medical Director, Family Service and Mental Health Center, South Cook County, Illinois

Arthur S. Levine, M.D. Chief, Pediatric Branch, National Cancer Institute

Erich Lindemann, M.D. (deceased) Professor, Department of Diseases of the Nervous System, Harvard Medical School

Helena Znaniecki Lopata, Ph.D. Professor of Sociology, Center for the Comparative Study of Social Roles, Loyola University

Patrick M. McGrady, Jr. Free-lance writer; President, American Society of Journalists and Authors

Embry McKee, M.D. Assistant Professor of Psychiatry, Vanderbilt University School of Medicine

Ellen D. Nannis, M.S.W. Social Science Analyst, Laboratory of Developmental Psychology, National Institute of Mental Health

Russell Noyes, Jr., M.D. Associate Professor, Department of Psychiatry, University of Iowa

Ashton Pitre, B.A. Communications Specialist, School of Communications, University of Texas-Austin

Phillip A. Pizzo, M.D. Senior Investigator, Pediatric Branch, National Cancer Institute

David K. Reynolds, Ph.D. Professor, Department of Human Behavior, School of Medicine, University of Southern California

Howard Roback, Ph.D. Associate Professor of Psychiatry, Vanderbilt University School of Medicine

Diane M. Ross, B.A. Graduate Student, School of Public Health, University of California, Los Angeles, California

Kay F. Rowland, Ph.D. Psychologist, Neuropsychiatric Institute, University of California, Los Angeles

Claire F. Ryder, M.D., M.P.H. Director, Division of Policy Development, Public Health Services, Rockville, Maryland

Benjamin Schlesinger, Ph.D. Professor, Faculty of Social Work, University of Toronto

Richard Schulz, Ph.D. Associate Professor, Department of Psychology, Carnegie Mellon University

O. Carl Simonton, M.D. Medical Director, Cancer Counseling and Research Center, Fort Worth, Texas

Stephanie Simonton Director of Counseling, Cancer Counseling and Research Center, Fort Worth, Texas

Barbara E. Strope, B.S. Social Science Analyst, Laboratory of Developmental Psychology, National Institute of Mental Health

Elizabeth J. Susman, R.N., Ph.D. Visiting Fellow, Laboratory of Developmental Psychology, National Institute of Mental Health

Sally Tullos, B.A. (deceased) Humanitarian and Public Speaker, Austin, Texas

Ronny E. Turner, Ph.D. Associate Professor, Colorado State University, Fort Collins, Colorado

Vamik Volkan, M.D. Associate Professor of Psychiatry, University of Virginia School of Medicine, Charlottesville, Virginia

Lawrence Weitz, Ph.D. Associate Professor of Psychology, George Peabody College

Carolyn Winget, Ph.D. Department of Psychiatry, College of Medicine, University of Cincinnati

Virginia N. Wood, Ph.D. Special Consultant, XIPE-Totec, Clinica de Salud Mental, Metropolitan State Hospital, Norwalk, California

Rosalee C. Yeaworth, Ph.D. College of Nursing and Health, University of Cincinnati

Bruce E. Zawacki, M.D. Department of Surgery, Los Angeles County/University of Southern California Medical Center

Contents

Part

3

Preface

I began teaching a course on Death and Dying at The University of Texas at Austin in January 1976. The course was offered there for the first time only one year before. While many colleges and universities offer this elective within the disciplines of psychology or sociology, we offer it through our health education department. The course thereby embodies a multidisciplinary richness. My students represent a broad cross section of undergraduate and graduate specialities—medicine, law, nursing, psychology, sociology, education, health, and anthropology—which makes for a remarkably fertile learning environment.

From interaction with my students I have discovered that they are as frightened, as hesitant, as curious, and as opinionated about death and dying as I am! I have discovered that we share a strong need to understand current theories and thought on the subject. And I have discovered that we share an appreciation of how research contributes to a "new" knowledge base. I have discovered that their desire to understand how people mobilize resources to face death is as strong as mine! Finally, I have discovered that they feel as great a need to share their personal fears, attitudes, and concerns with one another as I do. This book is about these discoveries.

I would be remiss not to mention my strong personal motivations for editing this text. My own professional training and experience have been wide-ranging. I have been a fourth-grade teacher, counseling psychologist, community psychologist, and health educator, and learned from the inside how deeply ingrained is the ethnocentrism of each of these professions. Each discipline believes its perspective is the answer to the world's problems. I believe strength must come from all. This text is thoroughly interdisciplinary in that it presents perspectives from a variety of disciplines.

I, like other people, have experienced the deaths of persons very close to me. My experiences have been dismally depressing and frustrating. A silent and frightened world confronts both the dying and the bereaved. My experiences so far suggest that there is great need—at the individual, institutional, and societal levels—for education about death. This book is an attempt to help us move from lonely vigils to compassionate involvement.

Features of the Text

This volume is intended to serve as a basic text for courses relating to death and dying. The selected readings are broad enough to satisfy the requirements of an introductory survey course. The research articles identify some important issues at the forefront as well as the core of the field and thereby make the book useful for instruction at the graduate level. The articles included in the "Practice" subsections of the book will appeal to a wide range of professional schools that are concerned about applications and interventions characterizing the field.

The unique feature of the book is its integration of *levels of study,* i.e., theory, research, and practice. Students will be able to recognize the impact of death and dying on the entire fabric of our lives with this organization.

The one-third of the book devoted to "Practice" shows us what is happening in the field and in our lives *now!* It includes innovative programs in the United States and around the world. So often the subject of death and dying is treated as if it were intellectually petrified. It is not! Things are happening—with individuals, institutions, and the whole society.

Sixteen structured experiential exercises in the Appendix are cross-referenced to appropriate chapters in the book. These exercises allow students to explore their personal feelings and attitudes regarding death and dying.

Articles focus on the entire developmental life span so that students will understand how death is viewed, caused, and responded to differently—depending upon age.

An introduction to each of the three major sections of the book summarizes the chapters of that section.

A brief introduction to each chapter then poses stimulus questions and sometimes case studies intended to motivate students to seek answers to difficult issues.

Acknowledgments

This project owes so much to my loving wife, Claire, whose emotional and intellectual support helps to nourish me when I seem to need it the most. I would also like to acknowledge the influence of my precious Erik Sean, whose unyielding demands at the age of two provided numerous enjoyable respites from my work. To my students, I thank you all for your wonderful ideas and emotional risk-takings. To friends and colleagues, I thank you for your words of encouragement. And to David Smith, Mavis Oeth, and Elizabeth Munger, of William C. Brown Company, I would like to extend warm regards for your support and conviction that this project could be transformed from an idea into a reality.

One person merits special acknowledgment. Sally Tullos, a friend, colleague, and "professional dying person" (as she described herself), has taught me much about living, loving, and quality of life. Your influence in my life, Sally, shall always be felt and shared in this volume which you so willingly helped to shape.

Larry A. Bugen

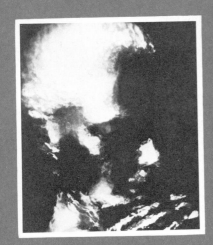

Part 1

Individual Dynamics

A premise of this book is that death must be understood at many different levels. It is therefore organized into three parts to coincide with the three main levels that impinge on everyone's life. Part 1 is concerned with individual dynamics in response to death. The individual may be facing his or her own death as a terminally ill patient. Or, as a bereaved child, husband, wife, or friend, he or she may be confronted by the death of someone else. Part 2 views death and its ramifications from the perspective of the family, group, and organization. Part 3 sees death from the level of the community and whole society. Of course, individual dynamics are not separate from the dynamics of the organizational and community levels. Each level of analysis is symbiotically related to the other levels.

The chapters of part 1 address such questions as: What were the early theoretical notions regarding human grief and how have they affected intervention practices today? What is the course of human grief? Do terminally ill persons die in stages, and if so, what are the stages? Do some people grieve more intensely and for a longer time than others? What factors may be important in determining the intensity and prolongation of human grief? Do children understand death differently from the way adults understand it? What must an individual do in order to "work through" the grief process? Are there different methods of helping someone through the grief process? What are the effects of culture in understanding and intervening in grief work?

To understand these and other questions, we must examine theory, research, and practice. Each of the three parts has, accordingly, been divided into sections to discuss, in turn, theory, research, and practice.

In chapter 1, "Symptomatology and Management of Acute Grief," Erich Lindemann lays a theoretical foundation for understanding human grief and crisis intervention. His early pioneering work is considered "biblical" even today. Lindemann offers us observations from a variety of patients while distinguishing between normal and abnormal (morbid) grief reactions. He suggests that normal grief is typified by somatic distress, preoccupation with the image of the deceased, guilt, hostile reactions, and loss of patterns of conduct. Morbid grief is characterized by delayed and distorted reactions.

Two concepts discussed by Lindemann—"anticipatory grief" and "grief work"—recur as pivotal points in chapters of other contributors. Anticipatory grief is a genuine grief reaction *prior* to an actual loss. Lindemann first noticed this response in family members sending loved ones overseas during World War II. They were in effect preparing themselves for the "possible death" of significant others. The concept is certainly useful in helping us understand our emotional responses to a variety of potential losses, including symbolic ones, such as loss of status. But Lindemann's conception of grief work was perhaps his most significant contribution. Successful grief work consisted on three steps: (a) emancipation from bondage to the deceased, (b) readjustment to an environment without the deceased, and (c) formation of new relationships. By successfully doing one's grief work, a person's grief is likely to be of much shorter duration. The "practice" section of part 1 shows that the concept of grief work is very much alive and well.

In chapter 2, "The Stages of Dying," Elisabeth Kübler-Ross suggests that persons with terminal illness progress through five stages of dying: (a) denial, (b) anger, (c) bargaining, (d) depression, and (e) acceptance. They are in effect mourning their own deaths in a process much the same as anticipatory grief. Kübler-Ross is perhaps the most renowned student of death and dying. She broke through the conspiracy of silence regarding death by writing *On Death and Dying* for the general public, published in 1969. Since then there has been a proliferation of writings and electronic media presentations that describe humanistically this previously forbidden subject.

The work of Kübler-Ross is not without controversy, however, as Bugen points out in chapter 3, "Human Grief: A Model for Prediction and Intervention." Bugen critically analyzes the stages-of-dying concept proposed by Kübler-Ross and Kavanaugh and concludes that it has a number of weaknesses. (a) The stages are not separate entities. (b) They are not necessarily successive. (c) Certain stages are not necessarily experienced. (d) Certain stages will vary in duration and intensity from person to person. (e) Little empirical evidence exists that substantiates the notion of stages.

Bugen hypothesizes that degree of grief is best predicted by a combination of two factors: how close the relationship to the deceased was, and how preventable the death is perceived to have been. Four predictions are possible from this model. (a) A mourner who considered the deceased a central person in his or her life and also believes that the death was preventable would experience intense and prolonged grief. (b) A mourner who considered the deceased a peripheral person in his/her life and believes that the death was preventable would experience mild but prolonged grief. (c) A mourner who considered the deceased a central person and believes that the death was not preventable would experience intense grief but for a short time. (d) A mourner who considered the deceased a peripheral person and believes that the death was unpreventable would experience mild grief and for a short time. Implications for intervention in bereavement are discussed in relation to these factors.

In the final chapter of the "theory" section, "Death Encounters of the Close Kind—The Realities of Transition," Ashton Pitre provides us with a personal view of the out-of-body experience popularized by Moody.[1] Pitre highlights some of the events that characterize the experience: high-pitched hums, a bright light, a dark tunnel, and a definite sense of actually leaving one's body. Pitre describes his frustration at being unable to explain his experiences for many years to a very skeptical society. Changing perspectives and increased acceptance of such phenomena allow not only present discussion of the subject but also description of means for achieving similar states, which Pitre describes at the conclusion of his chapter.

Research findings that underscore the impact of bereavement in our lives are selectively and critically reviewed by Epstein, Weitz, Roback, and McKee in chapter 5. They begin by recognizing the significance of Lindemann's early work but mention a number of shortcomings. They point out that Lindemann (1) neglected to take account of the interrelationships between symptoms described and their variability over time; (2) presented minimal data on the frequency of reported symptoms; and (3) provided no information on how soon after bereavement the interviews were conducted.

Epstein et al. suggest that response to bereavement can be viewed psychologically, physiologically, and behaviorally. Their review discusses these reactions in relation to parental loss and conjugal loss and as predictors of unfavorable bereavement outcome. They document well the tremendous impact of death, and detail a number of methodological concerns that frustrate our efforts to profile normal bereavement. They also take note of the high mortality rates of widows and widowers and offer a number of hypotheses that might promote our understanding of this impact.

The impact of death is felt not only at the time of a bereavement, but also during the course of our daily lives. Death is a powerful force that creates fear and anxiety in many of us and yet can serve as a motivating factor in our lives. In his review article entitled "Death Anxiety: Intuitive and Empirical Perspectives," Richard Schulz guides us through an array of studies dealing with death anxiety. Schulz helps us understand that the negative aspects of death and dying can be categorized as either psychological or physical suffering. Methods for investigating death anxiety are reviewed and critically analyzed. We learn, for instance, that many sex and age differences thought to characterize death anxiety are artifacts of the measuring instruments. Schulz concludes by suggesting that "death anxiety

1. Raymond A. Moody, Jr., *Life after Life* (New York: Bantam, 1976).

does not appear to be a unidimensional concept." Instead, it appears to be a dynamic force in our lives, with many components, each of which can be assessed at different levels.

Our responses to death depend upon a variety of factors. The two explored by Koocher in his article "Talking with Children about Death" are age and cognitive functioning. Koocher questions the assumption that children respond to death as adults do or that age alone is a good predictor of a child's understanding of death. Previous descriptive studies by Nagy[2] and by Anthony[3] had suggested that children between the ages of five and nine personify death. Their work also suggested that a child would not fully grasp the inevitability and universality of death until at least the age of ten. Not a single child in Koocher's study personified death. Neither did age alone predict what a child's response to death-related questions would be. The child's level of cognitive development was a crucial factor. Children at lower levels of cognitive functioning were found to be egocentric, magical in their thoughts, and highly concrete. Children at higher levels of cognitive functioning produced more mature and higher-order responses. Based on these differences, Koocher offers suggestions for discussing death with a child who has experienced a loss.

How are individuals experiencing the throes of loss and grief helped? The last four chapters of this part provide a perspective on current approaches to bereavement intervention.

Bugen's "Fundamentals of Bereavement Intervention" opens this "practice" section of "part 1—Individual Dynamics." He provides a framework in which death is viewed as a life crisis. Individuals attempting to help others in crisis must understand the characteristics of crisis and the bereaved person's perception of the crisis and reactions to it. The concepts of incremental and decremental crises are introduced. Incremental crises are deliberately chosen transitions which require an emotional or behavioral time commitment and which allow us to enhance our lives. Decremental crises are viewed as unavoidable loss which threatens our preferred way of living in relation to others, ourselves, or the environment. Death is usually understood to be a decremental crisis. Bugen suggests that we need both internal and external resources to manage death as a life crisis. Internal resources are the abilities, desires, resourcefulness, and problem-solving skills that help each of us to cope with change. External resources are the people, agencies, customs, religions, and other situational supports that facilitate our passage through a life crisis. Both sets of resources are important constructs in the following chapters.

Volkan's "Study of a Patient's Re-Grief Work" distinguishes between uncomplicated and complicated grieving. Volkan studied fifty patients and developed re-grief work as a method of brief psychotherapy with complicated grieving. Re-grief work is defined as resolving the conflicts of separation and consists of three phases: (a) demarcation, in which the griever seeks a reunion with the deceased in order to determine "what belongs to each"; (b) externalization, during which feelings are expressed;

2. M. Nagy, "The Child's Theories Concerning Death," *J. Genet. Psychol.* 73 (1948): 3–27.
3. S. Anthony, *The Child's Discovery of Death* (New York: Harcourt, Brace, 1940).

and (c) reorganization, during which time the griever is encouraged to direct psychic energies to new objects. Volkan also introduces us to the concept of "linking objects," which are memorabilia introduced during the demarcation phase in order to promote externalization later on.

The application of concepts proposed by other contributors found in this volume can be seen in the Volkan article. Lindemann's concepts of emancipation and reestablishment appear throughout Volkan's study of re-grieving. In addition, Kübler-Ross's urgings to accept the full array of emotions characterizing grief are evident in the externalization phase. Bugen's emphasis on external and internal resources in managing grief is also found in Volkan's study.

In their article "Therapy through a Death Ritual," Aguilar and Wood address the needs of Spanish-speaking people who find themselves marginal members of the American culture. The authors point out that death affects Mexicans differently from Anglos. Recognition of these varying needs has led to the development of a special bereavement intervention program at the Xipe-Totec Clinica de Salud Mental. Essentially, mourning is viewed as a two-stage process in which there are activities connected with burial and honoring the dead and activities reaffirming the survivors' position in the world of the living. In the clinic itself, a three-step death ritual for grievers is set in motion: (a) the scene is set; (b) emotional catharsis is encouraged; and (c) reestablishment of daily activities is then resumed. Lindemann's notions of emancipation from the deceased as well as reestablishment appear quite clearly in the above process. The importance of internal and external resources, as stressed by Bugen, is also noteworthy.

The final chapter of this section describes an innovative technique: "Belief Systems and Management of the Emotional Aspects of Malignancy." The Simontons suggest that the loss of a serious love object, when associated with feelings of helplessness and hopelessness, may predispose certain persons to cancer six to eighteen months later. Evidence is reported that links certain personality types with a variety of cancers and heart disease. Cancer patients are found to (a) hold resentments, (b) possess self-pity, (c) be inadequate in forming meaningful, long-term relationships, and (d) possess very poor self-images. The Simontons believe that personality is subject to change, however, and that it is crucial to change belief systems in patients, family members, and physicians. They believe that combining psychotherapy with radiation therapy/chemotherapy, spontaneous remissions from cancer have been achieved. They use both relaxation and visualization as integral processes. Central to their approach is the notion that we participate actively in the disease concept: that we are capable of participating in the creation of disease and also in the cure of it. More than any other contributors in this section, the Simontons believe that internal resources are the critical variable in coping with dying as a life crisis.

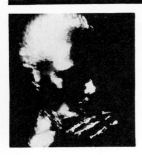

1

Theory

A terrible fire raged through an Ohio night club in 1977 just prior to the engagement of John Davidson. Many people were trapped and consequently died. Imagine being a surviving relative in this catastrophe. How are you feeling? What kind of grief reaction are you having? Erich Lindemann attempted to answer such questions in 1944 when he interviewed victims of a similar fire in Boston, Massachusetts. When you have completed the chapter, the following Appendix exercises are recommended:

    C.   Awareness of Grief Process

    D.   Awareness of Losses

    E.   Confronting the Realization of Death

    H.   Fantasizing Grief Reaction of Significant Others

    M.   Saying Good-bye to a Loved One

Symptomatology and Management of Acute Grief

Erich Lindemann

Introduction

At first glance, acute grief would not seem to be a medical or psychiatric disorder in the strict sense of the word but rather a normal reaction to a distressing situation. However, the understanding of reactions to traumatic experiences whether or not they represent clear-cut neuroses has become of ever-increasing importance to the psychiatrist. Bereavement or the sudden cessation of social interaction seems to be of special interest because it is often cited among the alleged psychogenic factors in psychosomatic disorders. The enormous increase in grief reactions due to war casualties, furthermore, demands an evaluation of their probable effect on the mental and physical health of our population.

The points to be made in this paper are as follows:

1. Acute grief is a definite syndrome with psychological and somatic symptomatology.

2. This syndrome may appear immediately after a crisis; it may be delayed; it may be exaggerated or apparently absent.

3. In place of the typical syndrome there may appear distorted pictures, each of which represents one special aspect of the grief syndrome.

4. By appropriate techniques these distorted pictures can be successfully transformed into a normal grief reaction with resolution.

Our observations comprise 101 patients. Included are (1) psychoneurotic patients who lost a relative during the course of treatment, (2) relatives of patients who died in the hospital, (3) bereaved disaster victims (Cocoanut Grove Fire) and their close relatives, (4) relatives of members of the armed forces.

The investigation consisted of a series of psychiatric interviews. Both the timing and the content of the discussions were recorded. These records

This material was first published in the *American Journal of Psychiatry,* vol. 101, pp. 141–148, 1944. Copyright 1944, the American Psychiatric Association. Reprinted by permission.

The picture shown by persons in acute grief is remarkably uniform.

were subsequently analyzed in terms of the symptoms reported and of the changes in mental status observed progressively through a series of interviews. The psychiatrist avoided all suggestions and interpretations until the picture of symptomatology and spontaneous reaction tendencies of the patients had become clear from the records. The somatic complaints offered important leads for objective study. Careful laboratory work on spirograms, gastrointestinal functions, and metabolic studies are in progress and will be reported separately. At present we wish to present only our psychological observations.

Symptomatology of Normal Grief

The picture shown by persons in acute grief is remarkably uniform. Common to all is the following syndrome: sensations of somatic distress occurring in waves lasting from twenty minutes to an hour at a time, a feeling of tightness in the throat, choking with shortness of breath, need for sighing, and an empty feeling in the abdomen, lack of muscular power, and an intense subjective distress described as tension or mental pain. The patient soon learns that these waves of discomfort can be precipitated by visits, by mentioning the deceased, and by receiving sympathy. There is a tendency to avoid the syndrome at any cost, to refuse visits lest they should precipitate the reaction, and to keep deliberately from thought all references to the deceased.

The striking features are (1) the marked tendency to sighing respiration; this respiratory disturbance was most conspicuous when the patient was made to discuss his grief. (2) The complaint about lack of strength and exhaustion is universal and is described as follows: "It is almost impossible to climb up a stairway." "Everything I lift seems so heavy." "The slightest effort makes me feel exhausted." "I can't walk to the corner without feeling exhausted." (3) Digestive symptoms are described as follows: "The food tastes like sand." "I have no appetite at all." "I stuff food down because I have to eat." "My saliva won't flow." "My abdomen feels hollow." "Everything seems slowed up in my stomach."

The sensorium is generally somewhat altered. There is commonly a slight sense of unreality, a feeling of increased emotional distance from other people (sometimes they appear shadowy or small), and there is intense preoccupation with the image of the deceased. A patient who lost his daughter in the Cocoanut Grove disaster visualized his girl in the telephone booth calling for him and was much troubled by the loudness with which his name was called by her and was so vividly preoccupied with the scene that he became oblivious of his surroundings. A young navy pilot lost a close friend; he remained a vivid part of his imagery, not in terms of a religious survival but in terms of an imaginary companion. He ate with him and talked over problems with him, for instance, discussing with him his plan of joining the Air Corps. Up to the time of the study, six months later, he denied the fact that the boy was no longer with him. Some patients are much concerned about this aspect of their grief reaction because they feel it indicates approaching insanity.

Another strong preoccupation is with feelings of guilt. The bereaved searches the time before the death for evidence of failure to do right by the lost one. He accuses himself of negligence and exaggerates minor omissions. After the fire disaster the central topic of discussion for a young married woman was the fact that her husband died after he left her following a quarrel, and of a young man whose wife died that he fainted too soon to save her.

In addition, there is often disconcerting loss of warmth in relationship to other people, a tendency to respond with irritability and anger, a wish not to be bothered by others at a time when friends and relatives make a special effort to keep up friendly relationships.

These feelings of hostility, surprising and quite inexplicable to the patients, disturbed them and again were often taken as signs of approaching insanity. Great efforts are made to handle them, and the result is often a formalized, stiff manner of social interaction.

The activity throughout the day of the severely bereaved person shows remarkable changes. There is no retardation of action and speech; quite to the contrary, there is a push of speech, especially when talking about the deceased. There is restlessness, inability to sit still, moving about in an aimless fashion, continually searching for something to do. There is, however, at the same time, a painful lack of capacity to initiate and maintain organized patterns of activity. What is done is done with lack of zest, as though one were going through the motions. The bereaved clings to the daily routine of prescribed activities; but these activities do not proceed in the automatic, self-sustaining fashion which characterizes normal work but have to be carried on with effort, as though each fragment of the activity became a special task. The bereaved is surprised to find how large a part of his customary activity was done in some meaningful relationship to the deceased and has now lost its significance. Especially the habits of social interaction—meeting friends, making conversation, sharing enterprises with others—seem to have been lost. This loss leads to a strong dependency on anyone who will stimulate the bereaved to activity and serve as the initiating agent.

These five points—(1) somatic distress, (2) preoccupation with the image of the deceased, (3) guilt, (4) hostile reactions, and (5) loss of patterns of conduct—seem to be pathognomonic for grief. There may be added a sixth characteristic, shown by patients who border on pathological reactions, which is not so conspicuous as the others but nevertheless often striking enough to color the whole picture. This is the appearance of traits of the deceased in the behavior of the bereaved, especially symptoms shown during the last illness, or behavior which may have been shown at the time of the tragedy. A bereaved person is observed or finds himself walking in the manner of his deceased father. He looks in the mirror and believes that his face appears just like that of the deceased. He may show a change of interests in the direction of the former activities of the deceased and may start

There is . . . a painful lack of capacity to initiate and maintain organized patterns of activity.

enterprises entirely different from his former pursuits. A wife who lost her husband, an insurance agent, found herself writing to many insurance companies offering her services with somewhat exaggerated schemes. It seemed a regular observation in these patients that the painful preoccupation with the image of the deceased described above was transformed into preoccupation with symptoms or personality traits of the lost person, but now displaced to their own bodies and activities by identification.

Course of Normal Grief Reactions

The duration of a grief reaction seems to depend upon the success with which a person does the *grief work,* namely, emancipation from the bondage to the deceased, readjustment to the environment in which the deceased is missing, and the formation of new relationships. One of the big obstacles to this work seems to be the fact that many patients try to avoid the intense distress connected with the grief experience and to avoid the expression of emotion necessary for it. The men victims after the Cocoanut Grove fire appeared in the early psychiatric interviews to be in a state of tension with tightened facial musculature, unable to relax for fear they might "break down." It required considerable persuasion to yield to the grief process before they were willing to accept the discomfort of bereavement. One assumed a hostile attitude toward the psychiatrist, refusing to allow any references to the deceased and rather rudely asking him to leave. This attitude remained throughout his stay on the ward, and the prognosis for his condition is not good in the light of other observations. Hostility of this sort was encountered on only occasional visits with the other patients. They became willing to accept the grief process and to embark on a program of dealing in memory with the deceased person. As soon as this became possible there seemed to be a rapid relief of tension and the subsequent interviews were rather animated conversations in which the deceased was idealized and in which misgivings about the future adjustment were worked through.

Examples of the psychiatrist's role in assisting patients in their readjustment after bereavement are contained in the following case histories. The first shows a very successful readjustment.

A woman, aged 40, lost her husband in the fire. She had a history of good adjustment previously. One child, ten years old. When she heard about her husband's death she was extremely depressed, cried bitterly, did not want to live, and for three days showed a state of utter dejection.

When seen by the psychiatrist, she was glad to have assistance and described her painful preoccupation with memories of her husband and her fear that she might lose her mind. She had a vivid visual image of his presence, picturing him as going to work in the morning and herself as wondering whether he would return in the evening, whether she could stand his not returning, then, describing to herself how he does return, plays with the dog, receives his child, and gradually tried to accept the fact that he is not there any more. It was only after ten days that she succeeded in accepting his loss and then only after having described in detail the remarkable qualities of her husband, the tragedy of his having to stop his activities at the pinnacle of his success, and his deep devotion to her.

In the subsequent interviews she explained with some distress that she had become very much attached to the examiner and that she waited for the hour of his coming. This reaction she considered disloyal to her husband but at the same time she could accept the fact that it was a hopeful sign of her ability to fill the gap he had left in her life. She then showed a marked drive for activity, making plans for supporting herself and her little girl, mapping out the preliminary steps for resuming her old profession as secretary, and making efforts to secure help from the occupational therapy department in reviewing her knowledge of French.

Her convalescence, both emotional and somatic, progressed smoothly, and she made a good adjustment immediately on her return home.

A man of 52, successful in business, lost his wife, with whom he had lived in happy marriage. The information given him about his wife's death confirmed his suspicions of several days. He responded with a severe grief reaction, with which he was unable to cope. He did not want to see visitors, was ashamed of breaking down, and asked to be permitted to stay in the hospital on the psychiatric service, when his physical condition would have permitted his discharge, because he wanted further assistance. Any mention of his wife produced a severe wave of depressive reaction, but with psychiatric assistance he gradually became willing to go through this painful process, and after three days on the psychiatric service he seemed well enough to go home.

He showed a high rate of verbal activity, was restless, needed to be occupied continually, and felt that the experience had whipped him into a state of restless overactivity.

As soon as he returned home he took an active part in his business, assuming a post in which he had a great many telephone calls. He also took over the role of amateur psychiatrist to another bereaved person, spending time with him and comforting him for his loss. In his eagerness to start anew, he developed a plan to sell all his former holdings, including his house, his furniture, and giving away anything which could remind him of his wife. Only after considerable discussion was he able to see that this would mean avoiding immediate grief at the price of an act of poor judgment. Again he had to be encouraged to deal with his grief reactions in a more direct manner. He has made a good adjustment.

With eight to ten interviews in which the psychiatrist shares the grief work, and with a period of from four to six weeks, it was ordinarily possible to settle an uncomplicated and undistorted grief reaction. This was the case in all but one of the thirteen Cocoanut Grove fire victims.

Morbid Grief Reactions

Morbid grief reactions represent distortions of normal grief. The conditions mentioned here were transformed into "normal reactions" and then found their resolution.

a. *Delay of Reaction.* The most striking and most frequent reaction of this sort is *delay* or *postponement*. If the bereavement occurs at a time when the patient is confronted with important tasks and when there is necessity for maintaining the morale of others, he may show little or no reaction for weeks or even much longer. A brief delay is described in the following example.

A girl of 17 lost both parents and her boy friend in the fire and was herself burned severely, with marked involvement of the lungs. Throughout her stay in the hospital her attitude was that of cheerful acceptance without any sign of adequate distress. When she was discharged at the end of three weeks she appeared cheerful, talked rapidly, with a considerable flow of ideas, seemed eager to return home and to assume the role of parent for her two younger siblings. Except for slight feelings of "lonesomeness" she complained of no distress.

This period of griefless acceptance continued for the next two months, even when the household was dispersed and her younger siblings were placed in other homes. Not until the end of the tenth week did she begin to show a true state of grief with marked feelings of depression, intestinal emptiness, tightness in her throat, frequent crying, and vivid preoccupation with her deceased parents.

That this delay may involve years became obvious first by the fact that patients in acute bereavement about a recent death may soon upon exploration be found preoccupied with grief about a person who died many years ago. In this manner a woman of 38, whose mother had died recently and who had responded to the mother's death with a surprisingly severe reaction, was found to be but mildly concerned with her mother's death but deeply engrossed with unhappy and perplexing fantasies concerning the death of her brother, who died twenty years ago under dramatic circumstances from metastasizing carcinoma after amputation of his arm had been postponed too long. The discovery that a former unresolved grief reaction may be precipitated in the course of the discussion of another recent event was soon demonstrated in psychiatric interviews by patients who showed all the traits of a true grief reaction when the topic of a former loss arose.

The precipitating factor for the delayed reaction may be a deliberate recall of circumstances surrounding the death or may be a spontaneous occurrence in the patient's life. A peculiar form of this is the circumstance that a patient develops the grief reaction at the time when he himself is as old as the person who died. For instance, a railroad worker, aged 42, appeared in the psychiatric clinic with a picture which was undoubtedly a grief reaction for which he had no explanation. It turned out that when he was 22, his mother, then 42, had committed suicide.

b. *Distorted Reactions.* The delayed reactions may occur after an interval which was not marked by any abnormal behavior or distress, but in which there developed an *alteration* in the patient's *conduct* perhaps not conspicuous or serious enough to lead him to a psychiatrist. These alterations may be considered as the surface manifestations of an unresolved grief reaction, which may respond to fairly simple and quick psychiatric management if recognized. They may be classified as follows: (1) *overactivity without a sense of loss,* rather with a sense of well-being and zest, the activities being of an expansive and adventurous nature and bearing semblance to the activities formerly carried out by the deceased, as described above; (2) *the acquisition of symptoms belonging to the last illness of the deceased.* This type of patient appears in medical clinics and is often labeled hypochondriasis or hysteria. To what extent actual alterations of physiological functions occur under these circumstances will have to be a field of further careful inquiry. I owe to Dr. Chester Jones a report about a patient whose electrocardiogram showed a definite change during a period of three weeks, which started two weeks after the time her father died of heart disease.

While this sort of symptom formation "by identification" may still be considered as conversion symptoms such as we know from hysteria, there is another type of disorder doubtlessly presenting (3) a recognized *medical disease,* namely, a group of psychosomatic conditions, predominantly ulcerative colitis, rheumatoid arthritis, and asthma. Extensive studies in ulcerative colitis have produced evidence that 33 out of 41 patients with ulcerative colitis developed their disease in close time relationship to the loss of an important person. Indeed, it was this observation which first gave the impetus for the present detailed study of grief. Two of the patients developed bloody diarrhea at funerals. In the others it developed within a few weeks after the loss. The course of the ulcerative colitis was strikingly benefited when this grief reaction was resolved by psychiatric technique.

At the level of social adjustment there often occurs a conspicuous (4) *alteration in relationship to friends and relatives.* The patient feels irritable, does not want to be bothered, avoids former social activities, and is afraid he might antagonize his friends by his lack of interest and his critical attitudes. Progressive social isolation follows, and the patient needs considerable encouragement in re-establishing his social relationships.

While overflowing hostility appears to be spread out over all relationships, it may also occur as (5) *furious hostility against specific persons;* the doctor or the surgeon are accused bitterly for neglect of duty and the patient may assume that foul play has led to the death. It is characteristic that while patients talk a good deal about their suspicions and their bitter feelings, they are not likely to take any action against the accused, as a truly paranoid person might do.

(6) Many bereaved persons struggled with much effort against these feelings of hostility, which to them seem absurd, representing a vicious change in their characters and to be hidden as much as possible. Some patients succeed in hiding their hostility but become wooden and formal, with affectivity and conduct *resembling schizophrenic pictures.* A typical report is this, "I go through all the motions of living. I look after my children. I do my errands. I go to social functions, but it is like being in a play; it doesn't really concern me. I can't have any warm feelings. If I were to have any feelings at all I would be angry with everybody." This patient's reaction to therapy was characterized by growing hostility against the therapist, and it required considerable skill to make her continue interviews in spite of the disconcerting hostility which she had been fighting so much. The absence of emotional display in this patient's face and actions was quite striking. Her face had a mask-like appearance, her movements were formal, stilted, robot-like, without the fine play of emotional expression.

> . . . the patient needs considerable encouragement in re-establishing his social relationships.

(7) Closely related to this picture is a *lasting loss of patterns of social interaction*. The patient cannot initiate any activity, is full of eagerness to be active—restless, can't sleep—but throughout the day he will not start any activity unless "primed" by somebody else. He will be grateful at sharing activities with others but will not be able to make up his mind to do anything alone. The picture is one of lack of decision and initiative. Organized activities along social lines occur only if a friend takes the patient along and shares the activity with him. Nothing seems to promise reward; only the ordinary activities of the day are carried on, and these in a routine manner, falling apart into small steps, each of which has to be carried out with much effort and without zest.

(8) There is, in addition, a picture in which a patient is active but in which most of his activities attain a coloring which is *detrimental to his own social and economic existence*. Such patients with uncalled for generosity, give away their belongings, are easily lured into foolish economic dealings, lose their friends and professional standing by a series of "stupid acts," and find themselves finally without family, friends, social status, or money, This protracted self-punitive behavior seems to take place without any awareness of excessive feelings of guilt. It is a particularly distressing grief picture because it is likely to hurt other members of the family and drag down friends and business associates.

(9) This leads finally to the picture in which the grief reaction takes the form of a straight *agitated depression* with tension, agitation, insomnia, feelings of worthlessness, bitter self-accusation, and obvious need for punishment. Such patients may be dangerously suicidal.

A young man aged 32 had received only minor burns and left the hospital apparently well on the road to recovery just before the psychiatric survey of the disaster victims took place. On the fifth day he had learned that his wife had died. He seemed somewhat relieved of his worry about her fate; impressed the surgeon as being unusually well-controlled during the following short period of his stay in the hospital.

On January 1st he was returned to the hospital by his family. Shortly after his return home he had become restless, did not want to stay at home, had taken a trip to relatives trying to find rest, had not succeeded, and had returned home in a state of marked agitation, appearing preoccupied, frightened, and unable to concentrate on any organized activity. The mental status presented a somewhat unusual picture. He was restless, could not sit still or participate in any activity on the ward. He would try to read, drop it after a few minutes, or try to play pingpong, give it up after a short time. He would try to start conversations, break them off abruptly, and then fall into repeated murmured utterances: "Nobody can help me. When is it going to happen? I am doomed, am I not?" With great effort it was possible to establish enough rapport to carry on interviews. He complained about his feeling of extreme tension, inability to breathe, generalized weakness and exhaustion, and his frantic fear that something terrible was going to happen. "I'm destined to live in insanity or I must die. I know that it is God's will. I have this awful feeling of guilt." With intense morbid guilt feelings, he reviewed incessantly the events of the fire. His wife had stayed behind. When he tried to pull her out, he had fainted and was shoved out by the crowd. She was burned while he was saved. "I should have saved her or I should have died too." He complained about being filled with an incredible violence and did not know what to do about it. The rapport established with him lasted for only brief periods of time. He then would fall back into his state of intense agitation and muttering. He slept poorly even with large sedation. In the course of four days he became somewhat more composed, had longer periods of contact with the psychiatrist, and seemed to feel that he was being understood and might be able to cope with his morbid feelings of guilt and violent impulses. On the sixth day of his hospital stay, however, after skillfully distracting the attention of his special nurse, he jumped through a closed window to a violent death.

. . . to a certain extent the type and severity of the grief reaction can be predicted.

If the patient is not conspicuously suicidal, it may nevertheless be true that he has a strong desire for painful experiences, and such patients are likely to desire shock treatment of some sort, which they picture as a cruel experience, such as electrocution might be.

A 28-year-old woman, whose 20 months-old son was accidentally smothered developed a state of severe agitated depression with self-accusation, inability to enjoy anything, hopelessness about the future, overflow of hostility against the husband and his parents, also with excessive hostility against the psychiatrist. She insisted upon electric-shock treatment and was finally referred to another physician who treated her. She responded to the shock treatments very well and felt relieved of her sense of guilt.

It is remarkable that agitated depressions of this sort represent only a small fraction of the pictures of grief in our series.

Prognostic Evaluation

Our observations indicate that to a certain extent the type and severity of the grief reaction can be predicted. Patients with obsessive personality make-up and with a history of former depressions are likely to develop an agitated depression. Severe reactions seem to occur in mothers who have lost young children. The intensity of interaction with the deceased before his death seems to be significant. It is important to realize that such interaction does not have to be of the affectionate type; on the contrary, the death of a person who invited much hostility, especially hostility which could not well be expressed because of his status and claim to loyalty, may be followed by a severe grief reaction in which hostile impulses are the most conspicuous feature. Not infrequently the person who passed away represented a key person in a social system, his death being followed by disintegration of this social system and by a profound alteration of the living and social conditions for the bereaved. In such cases readjustment presents a severe task quite apart from the reaction to the loss incurred. All these factors seem to be more important than a tendency to react with neurotic symptoms in previous life. In this way the most conspicuous forms of morbid identification were found in persons who had no former history of a tendency to psychoneurotic reactions.

. . . psychiatric
management of
grief reactions
may prevent
prolonged and
serious alterations
in the patient's
social
adjustment. . . .

Management

Proper psychiatric management of grief reactions may prevent prolonged and serious alterations in the patient's social adjustment, as well as potential medical disease. The essential task facing the psychiatrist is that of sharing the patient's grief work, namely, his efforts at extricating himself from the bondage to the deceased and at finding new patterns of rewarding interaction. It is of the greatest importance to notice that not only overreaction but underreaction of the bereaved must be given attention, because delayed responses may occur at unpredictable moments and the dangerous distortions of the grief reaction, not conspicuous at first, be quite destructive later and these may be prevented.

Religious agencies have led in dealing with the bereaved. They have provided comfort by giving the backing of dogma to the patient's wish for continued interaction with the deceased, have developed rituals which maintain the patient's interaction with others, and have counteracted the morbid guilt feelings of the patient by Divine Grace and by promising an opportunity for "making up" to the deceased at the time of a later reunion. While these measures have helped countless mourners, comfort alone does not provide adequate assistance in the patient's grief work. He has to accept the pain of the bereavement. He has to review his relationships with the deceased, and has to become acquainted with the alterations in his own modes of emotional reaction. His fear of insanity, his fear of accepting the surprising changes in his feelings, especially the overflow of hostility, have to be worked through. He will have to express his sorrow and sense of loss. He will have to find an acceptable formulation of his future relationship to the deceased. He will have to verbalize his feelings of guilt, and he will have to find persons around him whom he can use as "primers" for the acquisition of new patterns of conduct. All this can be done in eight to ten interviews.

Special techniques are needed if hostility is the most marked feature of the grief reaction. The hostility may be directed against the psychiatrist, and the patient will have such guilt over his hostility that he will avoid further interviews. The help of a social worker or a minister, or if these are not available, a member of the family, to urge the patient to continue coming to see the psychiatrist may be indispensable. . . .

Since it is obvious that not all bereaved persons, especially those suffering because of war casualties, can have the benefit of expert psychiatric help, much of this knowledge will have to be passed on to auxiliary workers. Social workers and ministers will have to be on the look-out for the more ominous pictures, referring these to the psychiatrist while assisting the more normal reactions themselves.

Anticipatory Grief Reactions

While our studies were at first limited to reactions to actual death, it must be understood that grief reactions are just one form of separation reactions.

Separation by death is characterized by its irreversibility and finality. Separation may, of course, occur for other reasons. We were at first surprised to find genuine grief reactions in patients who had not experienced a bereavement but who had experienced separation, for instance with the departure of a member of the family into the armed forces. Separation in this case is not due to death but is under the threat of death. A common picture hitherto not appreciated is a syndrome which we have designated *anticipatory grief*. The patient is so concerned with her adjustment after the potential death of father or son that she goes through all the phases of grief—depression, heightened preoccupation with the departed, a review of all the forms of death which might befall him, and anticipation of the modes of readjustment which might be necessitated by it. While this reaction may well form a safeguard against the impact of a sudden death notice, it can turn out to be of a disadvantage at the occasion of reunion. Several instances of this sort came to our attention when a soldier just returned from the battlefront complained that his wife did not love him anymore and demanded immediate divorce. In such situations apparently the grief work had been done so effectively that the patient has emancipated herself and the readjustment must now be directed toward new interaction. It is important to know this because many family disasters of this sort may be avoided through prophylactic measures.

Bibliography

Many of the observations are, of course, not entirely new. Delayed reactions were described by Helene Deutsch (1). Shock treatment in agitated depressions due to bereavement has recently been advocated by Myerson (2). Morbid identification has been stressed at many points in the psychoanalytic literature and recently by H. A. Murray (3). The relation of mourning and depressive psychoses has been discussed by Freud (4), Melanie Klein (5), and Abraham (6). Bereavement reactions in war time were discussed by Wilson (7). The reactions after the Cocoanut Grove fire were described in some detail in a chapter of the monograph on this civilian disaster (8). The effect of wartime separations was reported by Rosenbaum (9). The incidence of grief reactions among the psychogenic factors in asthma and rheumatoid arthritis has been mentioned by Cobb, *et al.* (10, 11)

1. Deutsch, Helene. Absence of grief. *Psychoanalyt. Quart.*, 6:12, 1937.
2. Myerson, Abraham. The use of shock therapy in prolonged grief reactions. *New England J. Med.*, 230:9, Mar. 2, 1944.
3. Murray, H. A. Visual manifestations of personality. *Jr. Abn. & Social Psychol.*, 32:161–184, 1937.
4. Freud, Sigmund. Mourning and melancholia. *Collected Papers* IV, 288–317; 152–170.
5. Klein, Melanie. Mourning and its relation to manic-depressive states. *Internat. J. Psychoan.*, 21:125–153, 1940.
6. Abraham, C. Notes on the psycho-analytical investigation and treatment of the libido, viewed in the light of mental disorder. *Selected Papers*.
7. Wilson, A. T. M. Reactive emotional disorders. *Practitioner*, 146:254–258.
8. Cobb, S., & Lindemann, E. Neuropsychiatric observations after the Cocoanut Grove fire. *Ann. Surg.*, June 1943.
9. Rosenbaum, Milton. Emotional aspects of wartime separations. *Family*, 24:337–341, 1944.
10. Cobb, S., Bauer, W., and Whiting, I. Environmental factors in rheumatoid arthritis. *J. A. M. A.*, 113:668–670, 1939.
11. McDermott, M., and Cobb, S. Psychogenic factors in asthma. *Psychosom. Med.*, 1:204–234, 1939.
12. Lindemann, Erich. *Psychiatric factors in the treatment of ulcerative colitis*. In press.

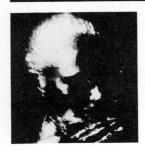

2
Theory

M ost people, when asked, prefer a quick painless way to die. Many people, however, experience the process of dying over time. In this chapter, Elisabeth Kübler-Ross suggests that we die in successive stages. Before beginning the chapter you might take a moment to think of someone you know who experienced a prolonged death. What was the process of dying like? When you have completed the chapter, the following Appendix exercises are suggested:

A. Announcing One's Own Death

B. Appropriate Death Fantasy

K. Planning for Living

N. The Final Rite of Passage: A Technological Update

The Stages of Dying

Elisabeth Kübler-Ross

First Stage: Denial and Isolation

Among the over two hundred dying patients we have interviewed, most reacted to the awareness of a terminal illness at first with the statement, "No, not me, it cannot be true," This *initial* denial was as true for those patients who were told outright at the beginning of their illness as it was true for those who were not told explicitly and who came to this conclusion on their own a bit later on. One of our patients described a long and expensive ritual, as she called it, to support her denial. She was convinced that the X-rays were "mixed up"; she asked for reassurance that her pathology report could not possibly be back so soon and that another patient's report must have been marked with her name. When none of this could be confirmed, she quickly asked to leave the hospital, looking for another physician in the vain hope "to get a better explanation for my troubles." This patient went "shopping around" for many doctors, some of whom gave her reassuring answers, others of whom confirmed the previous suspicion. Whether confirmed or not, she reacted in the same manner; she asked for examination and re-examination, partially knowing that the original diagnosis was correct, but also seeking further evaluations in the hope that the first conclusion was indeed an error, at the same time keeping in contact with a physician in order to have help available "at all times" as she said.

This anxious denial following the presentation of a diagnosis is more typical of the patient who is informed prematurely or abruptly by someone who does not know the patient well or does it quickly "to get it over with" without taking the patient's readiness into consideration. Denial, at least partial denial, is used by almost all patients, not only during the first stages of illness or following confrontation, but also later on from time to time. Who was it who said, "We cannot look at the sun all the time, we cannot

Man barracades against himself.
Tagore,
from *Stray Birds,*
LXXIX

This material was first published in *On Death and Dying,* pp. 38–42, 50–56, 82–84, 85–88, 112–114, Macmillan Publishing Co., Inc., 1970. Copyright 1969 by Elisabeth Kübler-Ross. It is printed here in slightly modified form by permission.

> **Denial is usually a temporary defense and will soon be replaced by partial acceptance.**

face death all the time"? These patients can consider the possibility of their own death for a while but then have to put this consideration away in order to pursue life.

I emphasize this strongly since I regard it a healthy way of dealing with the uncomfortable and painful situation with which some of these patients have to live for a long time. Denial functions as a buffer after unexpected shocking news, allows the patient to collect himself and, with time, mobilize other, less radical defenses. This does not mean, however, that the same patient later on will not be willing or even happy and relieved if he can sit and talk with someone about his impending death. Such a dialogue will and must take place at the convenience of the patient, when he (not the listener!) is ready to face it. The dialogue also has to be terminated when the patient can no longer face the facts and resumes his previous denial. It is irrelevant when this dialogue takes place. We are often accused of talking with very sick patients about death when the doctor feels—very rightly so—that they are not dying. I favor talking about death and dying with patients long before it actually happens if the patient indicates that he wants to. A healthier, stronger individual can deal with it better and is less frightened by oncoming death when it is still "miles away" than when it "is right in front of the door," as one of our patients put it so appropriately. It is also easier for the family to discuss such matters in times of relative health and well-being and arrange for financial security for the children and others while the head of the household is still functioning. To postpone such talks is often not in the service of the patient but serves our own defensiveness.

Denial is usually a temporary defense and will soon be replaced by partial acceptance. Maintained denial does not always bring increased distress if it holds out until the end, which I still consider a rarity. Among our two hundred terminally ill patients, I have encountered only three who attempted to deny its approach to the very last. Two of these women talked about dying briefly but only referred to it as "an inevitable nuisance which hopefully comes during sleep" and said "I hope it comes without pain." After these statements they resumed their previous denial of their illness.

The third patient, also a middle-aged spinster, apparently had used denial during most of her life. She had a visible, large ulcerative type of cancer of the breast but refused treatment until briefly before she died. She had great faith in Christian Science and held onto this belief to the last day. In spite of her denial, one part of her must have faced the reality of her illness since she did finally accept hospitalization and at least some of the treatments offered to her. When I visited her prior to planned surgery, she referred to the operation as "cutting part of the wound out so it can heal better." She also made it clear that she wished only to know details regarding her hospitalization "which have nothing to do with my wound." Repeated visits made it obvious that she feared any communications from staff members, who might possibly break down her denial, i.e., talk about her advanced cancer. As she grew weaker, her makeup became more grotesque. Originally rather discreetly applied red lipstick and rouge, the makeup became brighter and redder until she resembled a clown. Her clothing became equally brighter and more colorful as her end approached. During the last few days she avoided looking in a mirror, but continued to apply the masquerade in an attempt to cover up her increasing depression and her rapidly deteriorating looks. When asked if there was anything we could do for her, she replied, "Come tomorrow." She did not say, "Leave me alone," or "Don't bother me," but left the possibility open that tomorrow might be the day that her defenses would not hold up any longer, thus making help mandatory. Her last statement was, "I guess I cannot make it anymore." She died less than an hour later.

Most patients do not use denial so extensively. They may briefly talk about the reality of their situation, and suddenly indicate their inability to look at it realistically any longer. How do we know, then, when a patient does not wish to face it anymore? He may talk about relevant issues as far as his life is concerned, he may share some important fantasies about death itself or life after death (a denial in itself), only to change the topic after a few minutes, almost contradicting what he said earlier. Listening to him at this point may seem like listening to a patient with a minor ailment, nothing as serious as a life-threatening condition. This is when we try to pick up the cues and acknowledge (to ourselves) that this is the moment at which the patient prefers to look at brighter, more cheery things. We then allow the patient to daydream about happier things, no matter how improbable they may be. (We have had several patients who daydreamed about seemingly impossible situations which—much to our surprise—became true.) What I am trying to emphasize is that the need for denial exists in every patient at times, at the very beginning of a serious illness more so than toward the end of life. Later on the need comes and goes, and the sensitive and perceptive listener will acknowledge this and allow the patient his defenses without making him aware of the contradictions. It is much later, usually, that the patient uses isolation more than denial. He can then talk about his health and his illness, his mortality and his immortality as if they were twin brothers permitted to exist side by side, thus facing death and still maintaining hope.

In summary, then, the patient's first reaction may be a temporary state of shock from which he recuperates gradually. When his initial feeling of numbness begins to disappear and he can collect himself again, man's usual response is "No, it cannot be me." Since in our unconscious mind we are all immortal, it is almost inconceivable for us to acknowledge that we too have to face death. Depending very much on how a patient is told, how much time he has to gradually acknowledge the inevitable happening, and how he has been prepared throughout life to cope with successful situations, he will gradually drop his denial and use less radical defense mechanisms.

We have also found that many of our patients have used denial when faced with hospital staff members who had to use this form of coping for their own reasons. Such patients can be quite elective in choosing different people among family members or staff with whom they discuss matters of

> . . . the sensitive and perceptive listener will . . . allow the patient his defenses without making him aware of the contradictions.

their illness or impending death while pretending to get well with those who cannot tolerate the thought of their demise. It is possible that this is the reason for the discrepancy of opinions in regard of the patient's needs to know about a fatal illness. . . .

Second Stage: Anger

We read the world wrong and say that it deceives us.

Tagore,
from *Stray Birds,*
LXXV

If our first reaction to catastrophic news is, "No it's not true, no, it cannot involve me," this has to give way to a new reaction, when it finally dawns on us: "Oh, yes, it is me, it was not a mistake." Fortunately or unfortunately very few patients are able to maintain a make-believe world in which they are healthy and well until they die.

When the first stage of denial cannot be maintained any longer, it is replaced by feelings of anger, rage, envy, and resentment. The logical next question becomes: *"Why me?"* As one of our patients, Dr. G., puts it, "I suppose most anybody in my position would look at somebody else and say, 'Well, why couldn't it have been him?' and this has crossed my mind several times. . . . An old man whom I have known ever since I was a little kid came down the street. He was eighty-two years old, and he is of no earthly use as far as we mortals can tell. He's rheumatic, he's a cripple, he's dirty, just not the type of a person you would like to be. And the thought hit me strongly, now why couldn't it have been old George instead of me?" (extract from interview of Dr. G.).

In contrast to the stage of denial, this stage of anger is very difficult to cope with from the point of view of family and staff. The reason for this is the fact that this anger is displaced in all directions and projected onto the environment at times almost at random. The doctors are just no good, they don't know what tests to require and what diet to prescribe. They keep the patients too long in the hospital or don't respect their wishes in regards to special privileges. They allow a miserably sick roommate to be brought into their room when they pay so much money for some privacy and rest, etc. The nurses are even more often a target of their anger. Whatever they touch is not right. The moment they have left the room, the bell rings. The light is on the very minute they start their report for the next shifts of nurses. When they do shake the pillows and straighten out the bed, they are blamed for never leaving the patients alone. When they do leave the patients alone, the light goes on with the request to have the bed arranged more comfortably. The visiting family is received with little cheerfulness and anticipation, which makes the encounter a painful event. They then either respond with grief and tears, guilt or shame, or avoid future visits, which only increases the patient's discomfort and anger.

The problem here is that few people place themselves in the patient's position and wonder where this anger might come from. Maybe we too would be angry if all our life activities were interrupted so prematurely; if all the buildings we started were to go unfinished, to be completed by someone else; if we had put some hard-earned money aside to enjoy a few years of rest and enjoyment, for travel and pursuing hobbies, only to be confronted with the fact that "this is not for me." What else would we do with our anger, but let it out on the people who are most likely to enjoy all these things? People who rush busily around only to remind us that we cannot even stand on our two feet anymore. People who order unpleasant tests and prolonged hospitalization with all its limitations, restrictions, and costs, while at the end of the day they can go home and enjoy life. People who tell us to lie still so that the infusion or transfusion does not have to be restarted, when we feel like jumping out of our skin to be doing something in order to know that we are still functioning on some level!

Wherever the patient looks at this time, he will find grievances. He may put the television on only to find a group of young jolly people doing some of the modern dances, which irritates him when every move of his is painful or limited. He may see a movie western in which people are shot in cold blood with indifferent onlookers continuing to drink their beer. He will compare them with his family or the attending staff. He may listen to the news full of reports of destruction, war, fires, and tragedies—far away from him, unconcerned about the fight and plight of an individual who will soon be forgotten. So this patient makes sure that he is not forgotten. He will raise his voice, he will make demands, he will complain and ask to be given attention, perhaps as the last loud cry, "I am alive, don't forget that. You can hear my voice, I am not dead yet!"

A patient who is respected and understood, who is given attention and a little time, will soon lower his voice and reduce his angry demands. He will know that he is a valuable human being, cared for, allowed to function at the highest possible level as long as he can. He will be listened to without the need for a temper tantrum, he will be visited without ringing the bell every so often because dropping in on him is not a necessary duty but a pleasure.

The tragedy is perhaps that we do not think of the reasons for patients' anger and take it personally, when it has originally nothing or little to do with the people who become the target of the anger. As the staff or family reacts personally to this anger, however, they respond with increasing anger on their part, only feeding into the patient's hostile behavior. They may use avoidance and shorten the visits or the rounds or they may get into unnecessary arguments by defending their stand, not knowing that the issue is often totally irrelevant.

An example of a rational anger provoked by the reaction of a nurse was the case of Mr. X. He had been flat in bed for several months and had just been allowed to come off the respirator for a few hours during the daytime. He had led a life of many activities and had taken it hard to be so utterly restricted. He was quite aware that his days were numbered, and his greatest wish was to be moved into different positions (he was paralyzed to his neck). He begged the nurse never to put the siderails up as it reminded him of being in a casket. The nurse, who was very hostile to this patient, agreed

> **The tragedy is . . . that we do not think of the reasons for patients' anger. . . .**

We have to learn to listen to our patients and at times even to accept some irrational anger. . . .

that she would leave them down at all times. This private duty nurse was very angry when she was disturbed in her reading, and she knew that he would keep quiet as long as she fulfilled this wish.

During my last visit to Mr. X., I saw that this usually dignified man was furious. He said over and over again to his nurse, "You lied to me," staring at her in angry disbelief. I asked him the reason for this outburst. He tried to tell me that she had put the siderails up as soon as he asked to be put in an upright position so that he could put his legs out of bed "once more." This communication was interrupted several times by the nurse, who, equally angry, stated her side of the story, namely, that she had to put the siderails up in order to get help to fulfill his demands. A loud argument ensued during which the nurse's anger was perhaps best expressed in her statement: "If I had left them down, you would have fallen out of bed and cracked your head open." If we look at this incident again in an attempt to understand the reactions rather than to judge them, we must realize that this nurse also used avoidance by sitting in a corner reading paperbacks and "at all costs" tried to keep the patient quiet. She was deeply uncomfortable in taking care of a terminally ill patient and never faced him voluntarily or attempted to have a dialogue with him. She did her "duty" by sitting in the same room, but emotionally she was as far detached from him as possible. This was the only way this woman was able to do this job. She wished him dead ("crack your head open") and made explicit demands on him to lie still and quiet on his back (as if he were already in a casket). She was indignant when he asked to be moved, which for him was a sign of still being alive and which she wanted to deny. She was obviously so terrified by the closeness of death that she had to defend herself against it with avoidance and isolation. Her wish to have him quiet and not move only reinforced the patient's fear of immobility and death. He was deprived of communication, lonely and isolated as well as utterly helpless in his agony and increasing anger. When his last demand was met with an initially increased restriction (the symbolic locking him up with the siderails raised), his previously unexpressed rage gave way to this unfortunate incident. If the nurse had not felt so guilty about her own destructive wishes, she probably would have been less defensive and argumentative, thus preventing the incident from happening in the first place and allowing the patient to express his feelings and to die a bit more comfortably a few hours later.

I use these examples to emphasize the importance of our tolerance of the patient's rational or irrational anger. Needless to say, we can do this only if we are not afraid and therefore not so defensive. We have to learn to listen to our patients and at times even to accept some irrational anger, knowing that the relief in expressing it will help them toward a better acceptance of the final hours. We can do this only when we have faced our own fears of death, our own destructive wishes, and have become aware of our own defenses which may interfere with our patient care.

Another problem patient is the man who has been in control all his life and who reacts with rage and anger when he is forced to give up these controls. I am reminded of Mr. O. who was hospitalized with Hodgkin's disease which, he claimed, was caused by his poor eating habits. He was a rich and successful businessman who had never had any problems in eating, and had never been obliged to diet to lose weight. His account was totally unrealistic, yet he insisted that he, and only he, caused "this weakness." This denial was maintained in spite of the radiotherapy and his superior knowledge and intelligence. He claimed that it was in his hands to get up and walk out of the hospital the moment he made up his mind to eat more.

His wife came one day to my office with tears in her eyes. It was hard for her to bear it any longer, she said. He had always been a tyrant and kept strict control over his business and his home life. Now that he was in the hospital, he refused to let anybody know what business transactions had to take place. He was angry with her when she visited and overreacted when she asked questions of him or tried to give him any advice. Mrs. O. asked for help in the management of a domineering, demanding, controlling man, who was unable to accept his limits and unwilling to communicate some of the realities that had to be shared.

We showed her—in the example of his need to blame himself for "his weakness"—that he had to be in control of all situations and wondered if she could give him more of a feeling of being in control, at a time when he had lost control of so much of his environment. She did that by continuing her daily visits but she telephoned him first, asking him each time for the most convenient time and duration of the visit. As soon as it was up to him to set the time and length of the visits, they became brief but pleasant encounters. Also, she stopped giving him advice as to what to eat and how often to get up, but rather rephrased it into statements like, "I bet only you can decide when to start eating this and that." He was able to eat again, but only after all staff and relatives stopped telling him what to do.

The nursing staff used the same approach by allowing him to control certain times for infusions, changing bed sheets, etc., and—not surprising perhaps—he chose approximately the same times for these procedures as they had been previously done, with no anger and struggles involved. His wife and daughter enjoyed their visits more and also felt less angry and guilty about their own reactions to this very sick husband and father, who had been difficult to live with when he was well, but who became almost unbearable when he was in the process of losing his controlling grasp on his environment.

For a counselor, psychiatrist, chaplain, or other staff member, such patients are especially difficult as our time is usually limited and our workload great. When we finally have a free moment to visit patients like Mr. O., we are told, "Not now, come later." It is very easy then to forget such patients, to just leave them out; after all, they did it to themselves. They had their chance and our time is limited. It is the patient like Mr. O., however, who is the most lonely, not only because he is hard to take but because he rejects first and can only accept when it is on his terms. In that respect, the rich and successful, the controlling VIP is perhaps the poorest under these circumstances, as he is to lose the very things that made life so comfortable for him. In the end, we are all the same, but the Mr. O.s cannot

> . . . the rich and successful, the controlling VIP is perhaps the poorest under these circumstances. . . .

admit that. They fight it to the end and often miss an opportunity for reaching a humble acceptance of death as a final outcome. They provoke rejection and anger, and are yet the most desperate of them all. . . .

The woodcutter's axe begged for its handle from the tree. The tree gave it.

Tagore,
from *Stray Birds,*
LXXI

Third Stage: Bargaining

The third stage, the stage of bargaining, is less well known but equally helpful to the patient, though only for brief periods of time. If we have been unable to face the sad facts in the first period and have been angry at people and God in the second phase, maybe we can succeed in entering into some sort of an agreement which may postpone the inevitable happening: "If God has decided to take us from this earth and he did not respond to my angry pleas, he may be more favorable if I ask nicely." We are all familiar with this reaction when we observe our children first demanding, then asking for a favor. They may not accept our "No" when they want to spend a night in a friend's house. They may be angry and stamp their foot. They may lock themselves in their bedroom and temporarily express their anger by rejecting us. But they will also have second thoughts. They may consider another approach. They will come out eventually, volunteer to do some tasks around the house, which under normal circumstances we never succeeded in getting them to do, and then tell us, "If I am very good all week and wash the dishes every evening, then will you let me go?" There is a slight chance naturally that we will accept the bargain and the child will get what was previously denied.

The terminally ill patient uses the same maneuvers. He knows, from past experiences, that there is a slim chance that he may be rewarded for good behavior and be granted a wish for special services. His wish is most always an extension of life, followed by the wish for a few days without pain or physical discomfort. A patient who was an opera singer, with a distorting malignancy of her jaw and face who could no longer perform on the stage, asked "to perform just one more time." When she became aware that this was impossible, she gave the most touching performance perhaps of her lifetime. She asked to come to the seminar and to speak in front of the audience, not behind a one-way mirror. She unfolded her life story, her success, and her tragedy in front of the class until a telephone call summoned her to return to her room. Doctor and dentist were ready to pull all her teeth in order to proceed with the radiation treatment. She had asked to sing once more—to us—before she had to hide her face forever.

Another patient was in utmost pain and discomfort, unable to go home because of her dependence on injections for pain relief. She had a son who proceeded with his plans to get married, as the patient had wished. She was very sad to think that she would be unable to attend this big day, for he was her oldest and favorite child. With combined efforts, we were able to teach her self-hypnosis which enabled her to be quite comfortable for several hours. She had made all sorts of promises if she could only live long enough to attend this marriage. The day preceding the wedding she left the hospital as an elegant lady. Nobody would have believed her real condition. She was "the happiest person in the whole world" and looked radiant. I wondered what her reaction would be when the time was up for which she had bargained.

I will never forget the moment when she returned to the hospital. She looked tired and somewhat exhausted and—before I could say hello—said, "Now don't forget I have another son!"

The bargaining is really an attempt to postpone; it has to include a prize offered "for good behavior," it also sets a self-imposed "deadline" (e.g., one more performance, the son's wedding), and it includes an implicit promise that the patient will not ask for more if this one postponement is granted. None of our patients have "kept their promise"; in other words, they are like children who say, "I will never fight my sister again if you let me go." Needless to add, the little boy will fight his sister again, just as the opera singer will try to perform once more. She could not live without further performances and left the hospital before her teeth were extracted. The patient just described was unwilling to face us again unless we acknowledged the fact that she had another son whose wedding she also wanted to witness.

Most bargains are made with God and are usually kept a secret or mentioned between the lines or in a chaplain's private office. In our individual interviews without an audience we have been impressed by the number of patients who promise "a life dedicated to God" or "a life in the service of the church" in exchange for some additional time. Many of our patients also promised to give parts of or their whole body "to science" (if the doctors use their knowledge of science to extend their life).

Psychologically, promises may be associated with quiet guilt, and it would therefore be helpful if such remarks by patients were not just brushed aside by the staff. If a sensitive chaplain or physician elicits such statements, he may well wish to find out if the patient feels indeed guilty for not attending church more regularly or if there are deeper, unconscious hostile wishes which precipitated such guilt. It is for this reason that we found it so helpful to have an interdisciplinary approach in our patient care, as the chaplain often was the first one to hear about such concerns. We then pursued them until the patient was relieved of irrational fears or the wish for punishment because of excessive guilt, which was only enforced by further bargaining and more unkept promises when the "deadline" was past.

Fourth Stage: Depression

When the terminally ill patient can no longer deny his illness, when he is forced to undergo more surgery or hospitalization, when he begins to have more symptoms or becomes weaker and thinner, he cannot smile it off anymore. His numbness or stoicism, his anger and rage will soon be replaced with a sense of great loss. This loss may have many facets: a woman with a breast cancer may react to the loss of her figure; a woman with a

The world rushes on over the strings of the lingering heart making the music of sadness.
Tagore,
from *Stray Birds,*
XLIV

. . . two kinds of
depressions, . . .
the first one a
reactive
depression, the
second one a
preparatory
depression.

cancer of the uterus may feel that she is no longer a woman. Our opera singer responded to the required surgery of her face and the removal of her teeth with shock, dismay, and the deepest depression. But this is only one of the many losses that such a patient has to endure.

With the extensive treatment and hospitalization, financial burdens are added; little luxuries at first and necessities later on may not be afforded anymore. The immense sums that such treatments and hospitalizations cost in recent years have forced many patients to sell the only possessions they had; they were unable to keep a house which they built for their old age, unable to send a child through college, and unable perhaps to make many dreams come true.

There may be the added loss of a job due to many absences or the inability to function, and mothers and wives may have to become the breadwinners, thus depriving the children of the attention they previously had. When mothers are sick, the little ones may have to be boarded out, adding to the sadness and guilt of the patient.

All these reasons for depressions are well known to everybody who deals with patients. What we often tend to forget, however, is the preparatory grief that the terminally ill patient has to undergo in order to prepare himself for his final separation from this world. If I were to attempt to differentiate these two kinds of depressions, I would regard the first one a reactive depression, the second one a preparatory depression. The first one is different in nature and should be dealt with quite differently from the latter.

An understanding person will have no difficulty in eliciting the cause of the depression and in alleviating some of the unrealistic guilt or shame which often accompanies the depression. A woman who is worried about no longer being a woman can be complimented for some especially feminine feature; she can be reassured that she is still as much a woman as she was before surgery. Breast prosthesis has added much to the breast cancer patient's self-esteem. Social worker, physician, or chaplain may discuss the patient's concerns with the husband in order to obtain his help in supporting the patient's self-esteem. Social workers and chaplains can be of great help during this time in assisting in the reorganization of a household, especially when children or lonely old people are involved for whom eventual placement has to be considered. We are always impressed by how quickly a patient's depression is lifted when these vital issues are taken care of. . . .

The second type of depression is one which does not occur as a result of a past loss but is taking into account impending losses. Our initial reaction to sad people is usually to try to cheer them up, to tell them not to look at things so grimly or so hopelessly. We encourage them to look at the bright side of life, at all the colorful, positive things around them. This is often an expression of our own needs, our own inability to tolerate a long face over any extended period of time. This can be a useful approach when dealing with the first type of depression in terminally ill patients. It will help such a mother to know that the children play quite happily in the neighbor's garden since they stay there while their father is at work. It may help a mother to know that they continue to laugh and joke, go to parties, and bring good report cards home from school—all expressions that they function in spite of mother's absence.

When the depression is a tool to prepare for the impending loss of all the love objects, in order to facilitate the state of acceptance, then encouragements and reassurances are not as meaningful. The patient should not be encouraged to look at the sunny side of things, as this would mean he should not contemplate his impending death. It would be contraindicated to tell him not to be sad, since all of us are tremendously sad when we lose one beloved person. The patient is in the process of losing everything and everybody he loves. If he is allowed to express his sorrow he will find a final acceptance much easier, and he will be grateful to those who can sit with him during this stage of depression without constantly telling him not to be sad. This second type of depression is usually a silent one in contrast to the first type, during which the patient has much to share and requires many verbal interactions and often active interventions on the part of people in many disciplines. In the preparatory grief there is no or little need for words. It is much more a feeling that can be mutually expressed and is often done better with a touch of a hand, a stroking of the hair, or just a silent sitting together. This is the time when the patient may just ask for a prayer, when he begins to occupy himself with things ahead rather than behind. It is a time when too much interference from visitors who try to cheer him up hinders his emotional preparation rather than enhances it.

The example of Mr. H. will illustrate the stage of depression which worsened because of the lack of awareness and understanding of this patient's needs on the part of those in his environment, especially his immediate family. He illustrates both types of depression as he expressed many regrets for his "failures" when he was well, for lost opportunities while there was still time to be with his family, and sorrow at being unable to provide more for them. His depression paralleled his increasing weakness and inability to function as a man and provider. A chance for additional promising treatment did not cheer him up. Our interviews revealed his readiness to separate himself from this life. He was sad that he was forced to struggle for life when he was ready to prepare himself to die. It is this discrepancy between the patient's wish and readiness and the expectation of those in his environment which causes the greatest grief and turmoil in our patients.

If the members of the helping professions could be made more aware of the discrepancy or conflict between the patient and his environment, they could share their awareness with their patient's families and be of great assistance to them and to the patients. They should know that this type of depression is necessary and beneficial if the patient is to die in a stage of acceptance and peace. Only patients who have been able to work through their anguish and anxieties are able to achieve this stage. If this reassurance could be shared with their families, they too could be spared much unnecessary anguish. . . .

When the depression is a tool to prepare for the impending loss of all the love objects, . . . encouragements and reassurances are not as meaningful.

I have got my leave.
Bid me farewell, my
brothers! I bow to you
all and take my depar-
ture.

Here I give back the
keys of my door—and I
give up all claims to my
house. I only ask for
last kind words from
you.

We were neighbours
for long, but I received
more than I could give.
Now the day has dawn-
ed and the lamp that lit
my dark corner is out.
A summons has come
and I am ready for my
journey.

Tagore,
from *Gitanjali,*
XCIII

Fifth Stage: Acceptance

If a patient has had enough time (i.e., not a sudden, unexpected death) and has been given some help in working through the previously described stages, he will reach a stage during which he is neither depressed nor angry about his "fate." He will have been able to express his previous feelings, his envy for the living and the healthy, his anger at those who do not have to face their end so soon. He will have mourned the impending loss of so many meaningful people and places and he will contemplate his coming end with a certain degree of quiet expectation. He will be tired and, in most cases, quite weak. He will also have a need to doze off to sleep often and in brief inter- vals, which is different from the need to sleep during the times of depres- sion. This is not a sleep of avoidance or a period of rest to get relief from pain, discomfort, or itching. It is a gradually increasing need to extend the hours of sleep very similar to that of the newborn child but in reverse order. It is not a resigned and hopeless "giving up," a sense of "what's the use" or "I just cannot fight it any longer," though we hear such statements too. (They also indicate the beginning of the end of the struggle, but the latter are not indications of acceptance.)

Acceptance should not be mistaken for a happy stage. It is almost void of feelings. It is as if the pain had gone, the struggle is over, and there comes a time for "the final rest before the long journey" as one patient phrased it. This is also the time during which the family needs usually more help, understanding, and support than the patient himself. While the dying pa- tient has found some peace and acceptance, his circle of interest diminishes. He wishes to be left alone or at least not stirred up by news and problems of the outside world. Visitors are often not desired and if they come, the pa- tient is no longer in a talkative mood. He often requests limitation on the number of people and prefers short visits. This is the time when the televi- sion is off. Our communications then become more nonverbal than verbal. The patient may just make a gesture of the hand to invite us to sit down for a while. He may just hold our hand and ask us to sit in silence. Such moments of silence may be the most meaningful communications for people who are not uncomfortable in the presence of a dying person. We may together listen to the song of a bird from the outside. Our presence may just confirm that we are going to be around until the end. We may just let him know that it is all right to say nothing when the important things are taken care of and it is only a question of time until he can close his eyes forever. It may reassure him that he is not left alone when he is no longer talking and a pressure of the hand, a look, a leaning back in the pillows may say more than many "noisy" words.

A visit in the evening may lend itself best to such an encounter as it is the end of the day both for the visitor and the patient. It is the time when the hospital's page system does not interrupt such a moment, when the nurse does not come in to take the temperature, and the cleaning woman is not mopping the floor—it is this little private moment that can complete the day at the end of the rounds for the physician, when he is not interrupted by anyone. It takes just a little time but it is comforting for the patient to know that he is not forgotten when nothing else can be done for him. It is gratifying for the visitor as well, as it will show him that dying is not such a frightening, horrible thing that so many want to avoid.

There are a few patients who fight to the end, who struggle and keep a hope that makes it almost impossible to reach this stage of acceptance. They are the ones who will say one day, "I just cannot make it anymore," the day they stop fighting, the fight is over. In other words, the harder they struggle to avoid the inevitable death, the more they try to deny it, the more difficult it will be for them to reach this final stage of acceptance with peace and dignity. The family and staff may consider these patients tough and strong, they may encourage the fight for life to the end, and they may implicitly communicate that accepting one's end is regarded as a cowardly giving up, as a deceit or, worse yet, a rejection of the family.

How, then, do we know when a patient is giving up "too early" when we feel that a little fight on his part combined with the help of the medical profession could give him a chance to live longer? How can we differentiate this from the stage of acceptance, when our wish to prolong his life often contradicts his wish to rest and die in peace? If we are unable to differentiate these two stages we do more harm than good to our patients; we will be frustrated in our efforts, and will make his dying a painful last experience.

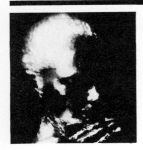

3

Theory

Take a moment to recollect an important loss you have experienced. How intense was your grief reaction? How prolonged was it? Are you still grieving sometimes? In this chapter Larry Bugen explores two factors that may help explain why we grieve the way we do. After you complete the reading, one of the following Appendix exercises may be illuminating:

      C.   Awareness of Grief Process

      D.   Awareness of Losses

      H.   Fantasizing Grief Reaction of Significant Others

      P.   Warm-up Exercise

Human Grief: A Model for Prediction and Intervention

Larry A. Bugen

This paper will present a model to facilitate both prediction and understanding of grief reactions. The model is presently intended only to apply to conventional grief in response to death rather than "anticipatory grief" as formulated by Schoenberg et al. (1974). The generally accepted approach to conceptualizing grief reactions posits the existence of stages. Kavanaugh (1972) declared that seven phases can be identified in the grieving process: shock, disorganization, volatile emotions, guilt, loss and loneliness, relief, and reestablishment. Kübler-Ross (1969), emphasizing proaction, suggested five stages of "adjustment," including denial, anger, guilt, preparatory grief, and the "goodbye" stage. A separate set of stages was also proposed by Kübler-Ross to account for the grieving process of the dying themselves, in the mourning of their own incipient loss. The work of these pioneers in the study of dying and grief has led to an increasing social acceptance of the broad range of human grief response and has encouraged mourners to express their sorrow without shame or guilt.

The "stage" concepts of grieving, however, contain a number of theoretical weaknesses and inconsistencies. First, both Kavanaugh and Kübler-Ross recognized that their stages are not separate entities but subsume one another or blend dynamically. Second, the stages are not successive; any individual may experience anger, for instance, prior to denial, or perhaps disorganization before shock. Third, it is not necessary to experience every stage. Depression, or for that matter any volatile emotion, may never be a recognizable response to loss. Fourth, the intensity and duration of any one stage may vary idiosyncratically among those who grieve. For one mourner, sadness may be a short-lived experience, while anger is a more protracted stage; the duration of these two emotional stages

This material was first published in the *American Journal of Orthopsychiatry,* vol. 47, no. 2, pp. 196–206, April 1977. Copyright 1977 by the American Orthopsychiatric Association, Inc. It is printed here in slightly modified form by permission.

might be reversed for someone else. Finally, little empirical evidence is offered by proponents to substantiate the theory of stages.

These flaws in the "stage" approach to understanding human grief suggest the need for a model that will (1) link pivotal determinants with consequent grief reactions in such a way as to allow for (2) predictive value, as well as (3) guidelines for constructive intervention. The model that will be outlined in this paper identifies two dimensions—centrality-peripherality and preventability-nonpreventability—believed to contribute to both the intensity and the duration of the human grief response. Clinical illustrations of the model's formulations will be offered where possible, and the employment of the model as an aid in therapeutic interventions will be explored.

The thesis underlying the model to be presented holds that stages, in the strictest sense, do not exist in the grieving process. Instead, it will be proposed that the existence of *a variety of emotional states* is the essential point, and *not* the need to order them.

The Model

The graphic illustration of the model (Table 1) is a 2×2 matrix in which the vertical axis represents the closeness of the relationship between the mourner and the deceased and the horizontal axis represents the extent to which the mourner believes the death might have been prevented. These two dimensions interact to create four reactive states reflecting both duration and intensity. As shown in Table 1, a mourner who considered the deceased a central person in his or her life and also believes that the death was preventable would be predicted to experience both an intense and prolonged grieving process. Perhaps the dynamic opposite is the mourner who had only a peripheral relationship with the deceased, and believes that the death could not have been prevented; here, the grieving

Table 1 Interaction of closeness of relationship and perception of preventability as predictors of grief

	Preventable	Unpreventable
Central relationship	Intense and Prolonged	Intense and Brief
Peripheral relationship	Mild and Prolonged	Mild and Brief

process would be predicted to be both mild and brief. Dimensions of the model will be defined, and examples presented, below.

A person whose very existence serves as a . . . symbol . . . may be a central figure.

Centrality

The closeness of the relationship between the mourner and the deceased is directly related to the intensity of the grief reaction. If the relationship to the deceased is seen as central, the grief reaction will be intense. If the relationship is considered peripheral, the grief reaction will be mild. Any one, or some combination, of the following criteria may help define a central relationship.

Centrality refers to a person whose presence and importance is so profound that "I feel I have no life without him." This is perhaps the most powerful of all conditions, and the most likely to sustain a sense of hopelessness. The mourner typically feels as though his or her life is meaningless or senseless without the loved one. Expressions such as "What am I going to do now?" "It's not worth going on," or "I wish I were dead too" are very common. Age offers little protection from these feelings. The author recalls rather painfully a recent letter from a longtime friend of the family who was 76 years old. Two years had elapsed since the death of her husband, and little change could be found in her mood. Her despair and utter despondency were evidenced most vividly when she confided, "Well, another Christmas has passed. That means one less that I have to bear alone."

Centrality may refer, at a lesser intensity, to a person whose love is experienced as being a needed element in one's own life. For the dead to be considered central, it is not enough for the mourner merely to have loved the deceased. Mourners must see the nurturance and love of the dead as having been a vital source of daily support (a father's reassuring smile from the grandstand, for example, at the start of a teenage athlete's race), the loss of which is felt deeply and constantly.

Centrality may also refer to a person to whom the survivor had become behaviorally committed through daily activities. The most obvious example is the death of a child for whom a parent had daily set the alarm for school, made breakfast, washed dishes and clothes, gone out to meet after school, helped with homework, etc. But even an old cantankerous grandmother may be sorely missed when her close survivors realize in retrospect that delivering hot water bottles to a "storming old biddie" was one of the more vital moments in the day.

A person whose very existence serves as a reminder and symbol for our hope and beliefs may be a central figure. Thousands of individuals mourned President Kennedy's assassination with incredible intensity. It is striking that most of these mourners had never even met the President, yet experienced profound loss.

Peripherality

The other pole of this dimension is meant to describe distance and minimally important relationships. There may, in fact, be no relationship at all, as with neighbors who rarely speak to one another although living in close proximity. It is suggested that any grief reaction will be mild in the case of peripheral relationships.

Peripherality refers, at one extreme, to a person whose presence is both felt and respected, but whose loss is not viewed or experienced as irreplaceable. This may well fit the case of a coworker's death, in which the survivor had recognized the contributions of the deceased but had not extended the working relationship into the social arena. Peripherality could also refer to a person whose presence is not recognized or necessarily respected. Such "strangers," in effect, elicit minimal grief reactions.

Peripherality may also denote the behavioral view that our rewards and pleasures are not contingent upon the behavior or presence of the deceased. The obverse of this would also be true. In this case, the mourner recognizes that significant aspects of his or her life will not be affected by the death at hand—the loss will not affect the usual ways which the mourner obtains love, attention, etc. that give meaning to his or her life. Seligman (1975) described in some detail the situation just opposite to this, in which mourners believe that outcomes are independent of their responses; this will be discussed more fully below.

Preventability

Establishing whether the mourner *believes* the cause of death was preventable or unpreventable is essential, since this dimension directly relates to the duration of a grief reaction. If the cause of death is believed to have been preventable, the grieving process will likely be prolonged. If the cause of death is considered to have been unpreventable, the grieving process will be relatively brief. To summarize:

Preventability refers to the *general belief* that the factors contributing to the death may have been sufficiently controlled so that the death might have been avoided. Whether or not the factors could actually have been controlled, it is the mourner's obsession that they *should* have been; the commitment, therefore, is to an idea rather than a fact. The use of "general" in the above definition is meant to connote all causative factors other than the mourner himself. Lambasting the hospital staff for their delay in using a respirator would be an example of this.

Preventability also refers to the specific "belief" of survivors that they themselves contributed to the death either directly or indirectly. A mother giving her daughter permission to attend a dance may "never forgive herself" if her daughter is killed in an automobile accident on the way home.

Unpreventability

Unpreventability refers to the belief that nothing could have been done by any mortal to divert the forces contributing to the death.

Unpreventability refers to the belief that everything was done to divert the forces contributing to the death.

Unpreventability is demonstrated by attributions to, for example, God, fate, inevitability, luck, or misfortune.

In effect, the locus of control is believed to lie outside the realm of human influence. This belief absolves the mourner of both responsibility and guilt.

Intense Grief Reaction

An intense grief response may include the following physical symptoms: tightness in the throat, shortness of breath, sighing, loss of appetite, loss of sleep, and emotional waves lasting from twenty minutes to one hour (Lindemann 1944). Psychologically, mourners may manifest general subjective distress, depression, uncontrolled crying, and debilitating anxiety leading to nightmares. The intensity of a mourner's grief may be so formidable that, Kavanaugh (1972, p. 107) concluded, "few tasks in life cause more anxiety than consoling the bereaved!" In relation to intensity, this author hypothesizes that:

A relationship exists between the intensity of our grief reaction and the extent to which we actually grieve for ourselves as compared to the deceased. With the death of a loved one, we certainly lose a part of ourselves. When we begin to recognize this lost part, this new void, we may begin to grieve for ourselves. As grief intensifies, an egocentric concern with oneself may be assumed on the part of the mourner. In fact, the psychoanalytic notions of narcissism will probably be associated with the most pathological cases of severe grief response. In most cases, then, what appears to be deep concern for the deceased is actually deep concern for the bereaved.

Experientially, the intensity of our grieving is directly related to a personal feeling of depression and a profound belief that our lives have been *hopelessly* altered. This conviction of helplessness and utter despair may be so severe that death of the mourner results. Examples are available in the realm of "voodoo" death (Cannon 1942), spouse death at the loss of a loved one (Engel 1971), and institutionalized helplessness (Ferrari 1962; Schulz and Aderman 1973). When a

. . . person is placed in a situation where a particular outcome is—or *appears* to be—independent of his responses, he learns that his responses are ineffective. The affected individual may conclude that any responses he makes will be powerless to affect the outcome. The number of responses decreases; a "what's the use" syndrome develops; and helplessness becomes a self-fulfilling prophecy. If the outcome

Mourning is partly a belief in helplessness.

is a traumatic event—if it involves physical or emotional pain—the helpless subject may progress through successive stages of fear and anxiety to a deep depression, and, in some instances, death [Seligman 1975, back cover].

Mild Grief Reaction

Mild grief reactions may be characterized by an absence or mildness of physical symptoms. A loss is perceived by the mourner without significant physiological stress or acute psychological distress. Psychological symptoms such as sadness, loneliness, or irritability may well be experienced; severe despair and hopelessness, however, would not be present.

Prolonged Duration

Predicting the length of an appropriate grief reaction is an extremely difficult task. On the one hand, crisis theory suggests that most depressions will lift within a two-month period and an individual will find himself or herself beginning a process of reestablishment. . . . On the other hand, some clinicians maintain that the mourner must experience a full year of activities without the deceased in order to work through the grieving process. Christmas, New Year, and birthdays are seen as necessary transition periods in this case. For the purpose of this paper, prolonged grief will be defined as extending beyond a six-month period subsequent to the death. More specifically:

Prolonged grief exists when medical diseases such as ulcerative colitis, rheumatoid arthritis, or asthma are manifest in the mourner beyond the six-month interval following the death. Other symptoms, such as sleeplessness, oversleeping, or loss of appetite beyond the six-month interval may also connote prolonged grief.

Prolonged grief exists when the bereaved fail to separate themselves from the deceased, while maintaining a relationship only with memorabilia symbolic of the death. A mother may lock a child's room, preserving it "as it was," and perhaps even sit in the room for hours each day. More common examples would include the need to retain the clothing of the dead, the need to frequently visit the graveside, or even to aspire toward the occupation of the deceased. It is interesting to note that most religions provide some ceremonial occasion for special interactions with the deceased. Such occasions represent opportunities to cherish sensitive and time-honored moments of recollection and would not be characteristic, by themselves, of a prolonged grief response.

Prolonged grief may be considered to exist in the special case of *helplessness proliferation.* Mourning is partly a belief in helplessness. The bereaved is, in a sense, saying, "I won't be able to go on without the deceased." The longer this "belief" is held on to, the longer the grieving process. This dynamism is very similar to what Seligman described as transfer of helplessness. Helplessness proliferation may be seen in the individual who first decides that he or she just can't make it to the Christmas party. This feeling soon proliferates to not needing friends, and eventually to being unable to maintain a job. By the end of the six-month period, this mourner may be ready for hospitalization or perhaps suicide.

Prolonged grief exists when the bereaved fails to find new, or to re-establish old, patterns of rewarding interaction within the environment. In order to move beyond grieving, the bereaved must review the relationship to the deceased, accept the hurt in not having its pleasures any longer, and finally be willing to explore and establish new networks among the rich supply of resources still available to them.

. . . when the anticipatory grief period was of sufficient duration . . . a prolonged conventional grieving period is not necessary.

Brief Grief Reactions

A brief grief reaction may exist when the anticipatory grief period was of sufficient duration to allow for a "working through process," so that a prolonged conventional grieving period is not necessary. In cases in which cancer has been the slow, deteriorating cause of death, most mourners have had opportunities to experience the full impact of the anticipated loss of a loved one prior to the death.

At one extreme, brief grief may reflect the intense process of painfully separating oneself from the deceased and finding new patterns of rewarding interaction. This process may well occur within a two to six month period, and is usually facilitated by societal support groups or sanctions. The traditional Irish wake serves such a function by encouraging full grief expression on the part of the mourners.

At the other extreme, brief grief may reflect the *absence* of an emotional bond between bereaved and deceased. In such a case, little remains to work through. Instead, the death may stimulate pensivity regarding existential questions such as: "Is hard work worth the effort?" "What does exist after life?" and "How much in control of my life am I?"

Employing the Model

As described above, four possible outcomes may be expected, given the interaction of the two sets of determinants: (1) Given a central relationship between bereaved and deceased and the belief that the death was preventable, we would expect the grieving process to be both intense and prolonged. (2) Given a central relationship between bereaved and deceased and the belief that the death was unpreventable, we would expect the grieving process to be intense but brief. (3) Given a peripheral relationship between bereaved and deceased and the belief that the death was preventable, we would expect the grieving process to be mild but prolonged. (4) Given a peripheral relationship between bereaved and deceased and the belief that

The *belief* that a death might have been prevented is the single most influential factor contributing to . . . prolongation of . . . grief. . . .

the death was unpreventable, we would expect the grieving process to be both mild and brief.

Four abbreviated case studies may help to further clarify each of the above grief reactions. The first two are from Lindemann (1944), the latter two from the author's own clinical experience.

Intense and Prolonged

[After the Cocoanut Grove fire] a young man aged 32 [who] had received only minor burns and left the hospital apparently well on the road to recovery . . . learned that his wife had died. . . . On January 1st he was returned to the hospital by his family. Shortly after his return home he had become restless, did not want to stay at home, had taken a trip to relatives trying to find rest, had not succeeded, and had returned home in a state of marked agitation, appearing preoccupied, frightened, and unable to concentrate on any organized activity. . . . He could not sit still or participate in any activity on the ward . . . [and fell] into repeated murmured utterances: "Nobody can help me. When is it going to happen? I am doomed, am I not?" . . . He complained about his feeling of extreme tension, inability to breathe, . . . and exhaustion. . . . "I'm destined to live in insanity or I must die. I know that it is God's will. I have this awful feeling of guilt." With intense morbid guilt feelings, he reviewed incessantly the events of the fire. . . . When he tried to pull [his wife] out, he had fainted and was shoved out by the crowd. She was burned while he was saved. "I should have saved her or I should have died too." . . . On the sixth day of his hospital stay . . . he jumped through a closed window to a violent death. [Lindemann 1944, p. 146].

By definition, centrality refers to those whose presence and importance is so profound that "I feel I have no life without them." The apparent meaninglessness of this man's life suggests the strong likelihood of a central relationship with his wife. The power and intensity of this condition is amplified many times over by the belief that he personally might have prevented her death. The interaction of these two determinants lends substance to a prediction that the grieving process would be both intense and prolonged. The intensity of this man's grief was certainly apparent. The severity of his despair and guilt also strongly suggest that his grief response would be quite prolonged. It was perhaps the hopelessness of assuaging such an incapacitating and prolonged grieving process which led to the suicide.

The *belief* that a death might have been prevented is the single most influential factor contributing to the prolongation of the human grief response. Preventability may be presumed to be a factor when any cause of death is unknown or when the mourner was present at the time of death. An example of profound significance is crib death. Which parents have not shuddered at the approach of their child's third month of life and subsequently breathed a deep sigh of relief in welcoming the twelfth month. The combination of proximity and unknown etiology suggests both an intense and prolonged grief response for parents of any crib death.

Intense and Brief

A woman, aged 40, lost her husband in the [Cocoanut Grove] fire. She had . . . one child ten years old. When she heard about her husband's death she was extremely depressed, cried bitterly, did not want to live, and for three days showed a state of utter dejection.

When seen by the psychiatrist, she was glad to have assistance and described her painful preoccupation with memories of her husband. . . . She had a vivid visual image of his presence, picturing him as going to work in the morning and herself as wondering whether he would return in the evening . . . [to play] with the dog [and] . . . his child. . . . It was only after ten days that she succeeded in accepting his loss and then only after having described in detail the remarkable qualities of her husband . . . and his deep devotion to her.

In subsequent interviews she explained with some distress that she had become very much attached to the examiner and that she waited for . . . his coming. . . . [She came to see] that it was a hopeful sign of her ability to fill the gap he had left in her life. She then showed a marked drive for activity, making plans for supporting herself and her little girl, . . . resuming her old profession as secretary, and making efforts to secure help from the occupational therapy department . . . [Lindemann 1944, p. 143].

This woman's vivid recollections of her husband's behavioral commitments each day (i.e., going to work, playing with dog and child) suggest a central relationship. Her belief that his love was a needed element in her daily routine contributed to her initial wish to die, and also outlined this man's importance to her. Nowhere in this case study is there any indication that she believed that his death might have been prevented. An intense but brief grief response would be predicted given such information. Her behavior bore this out, as she painfully wrestled with the agony of detaching herself from her dead husband, while also finding new patterns of rewarding interaction. The support of her psychiatrist certainly seemed to facilitate her coping with the process of reestablishment.

Mild and Prolonged

A relatively young doctor, aged 36, had just completed his residency and was working in a large metropolitan hospital. On a particular day he had to perform abdominal surgery on a 21-year-old female whose stomach had ulcerated to such an extent that immediate removal of half of the tissue appeared necessary. During the course of the operation, the patient began to hemorrhage and died within five minutes on the table. The final few minutes of agonized effort in this irreversible condition left the young doctor distraught. Believing that more expeditious use of clamps and diagnostic workups might have prevented the rapid deterioration of the patient's status, the doctor felt very much to blame and repeatedly muttered on his way out of the operating room, "Why did my first one have to be like this." During the next seven months irritability was an apparent beacon warning other hospital personnel that this doctor was about to operate on a "young woman." Supportive counseling by colleagues eventually helped this man work through the lingering doubts and preoccupations which accompanied him in these special circumstances.

. . . belief that one is responsible for another's death may certainly trigger a prolonged reaction. . . .

Of the four reactions suggested in this paper, this condition is perhaps the most difficult to define. Most grief reactions which do linger are likely to be more intense than mild, or at least to begin as more intense states. As portrayed above, however, a personal belief that one is responsible for another's death may certainly trigger a prolonged reaction of this nature. The irritability mentioned in the narrative, though quite noticeable to hospital support staff, was not debilitating. The mildness of this doctor's response in part reflects the nature of his relationship to the deceased. Though her presence was both felt and respected, the doctor's usual daily rewards and pleasures were not contingent upon the behavior or presence of the deceased. Perhaps even more contributory to the mildness of this brief reaction is the notion that many doctors either deny or are reluctant to share their feelings. As Kasper (1965, p. 268) strongly pointed out: "While touched by pain and saddened by each patient's death, [doctors] often contrive to show their feelings in devious and distorted ways."

Mild and Brief

> While walking down a busy street in New York, an adolescent boy notices an elderly man staggering 30 feet ahead of him. Before he knows what happened the man has collapsed and a crowd has formed around him. Stunned, the boy rushes to the packed crowd quite aware that his own heart is pumping rapidly and his face is flushed. He is aware of being pushed by the crowd, someone screaming, "Get an ambulance," while someone utters, "It's too late." The lad is aware that the old man is dead, and that he has witnessed his first death. Slowly walking away, he takes time to stop in front of a store window a block away from the frightening scene he has just witnessed. Peering at himself with unknown intensity, he again becomes aware of his beating heart, his own flushed face, and sweating palms. Sensing the contrast between these sensations and their absence in the old man, the boy swallows hard and understands that for the first time he has feared his own dying. Then, as though a breeze propels him, he runs off very quickly. He knows that he has a baseball game to make and must concentrate on winning.

The adolescent boy in this vignette experienced both a mild and brief grief reaction, as would be expected on the basis of the known determinants. The relationship between the boy and old man is clearly peripheral, and the old man's loss is in no way seen as irreplaceable. In addition, there were no indications that the boy "believed" that the death was preventable. Given these factors, the boy's brief encounter with his own inevitable death is as predictable as is its quick denial. This scene, in fact, may capture the American way of life and death. We are forever being bombarded with images, scenes, and news of death through both electronic and paper media. The peripherality and anonymity of the countless victims allow us to escape from death and experience minimal pain.

The Intervention Process

The grief model presented is a dynamic model. Not only can movement be monitored by the model, but actual interventions are suggested. Positive movement essentially occurs in two ways: (1) an individual may move from a belief in preventability to a belief in unpreventability, or (2) an individual may shift a relationship with the deceased from centrality to peripherality.

The belief that a death was preventable suggests an intense grief reaction, according to the model. In order to mollify the intensity to a more mild and manageable state, a shift in belief toward unpreventability must occur. Traditional methods of grief work may succeed in encouraging a shift in belief or reduction of guilt. Such methods usually include empathic listening, unconditional positive regard, reassurance, physical presence and contact, and general acceptance. Attitude change research, however, suggests that stronger interventions must occur in order to change belief. In addition to the above effective techniques, the clinician must recognize the cognitive structure supporting the belief of preventability. Every conceivable strategy that can contradict this belief should be used to dissuade the mourner, particularly when he or she feels personally responsible for the death.

The first case study presented the situation of a young man who was overwhelmed with guilt regarding the death of his wife. Recognizing that the alleviation of his intense grieving was dependent upon an attitude change toward unpreventability, every credible source should have been consulted. These might have included: (1) a doctor who would stress the physical incapability of the mourner to save his wife due to smoke inhalation and subsequent fainting; (2) a priest who might argue against the patient's belief that it was God's will that he die; (3) an engineer who might enumerate various elements of the physical structure at the scene of the fire which made the survivor a victim of that particular environment; and (4) other widows and widowers who might have experienced guilt feelings of their own and were willing to track their own movement toward unpreventability.

Where a mourner does not know the cause of death, a belief that the death was preventable is most likely. Every effort should be made to establish the cause of death, particularly in situations where the death occurred suddenly in the presence of the mourner. For instance, by seeking a consultation from a number of pathologists, a sufficient understanding of an autopsy report may reveal biological causes and dispel the notion that prompter action by the mourner may have saved the victim's life.

The belief that a death might have been prevented is such a powerful dynamic that some doctors take every conceivable precaution to ensure that such a belief never establishes itself. One rather controversial strategy is never to let relatives make life and death decisions regarding surgical tech-

> . . . to mollify
> . . . intensity. . . .
> a shift in
> belief toward
> unpreventability
> must occur.

niques. This should be the doctor's domain, particularly in cases of potential child mortality. Should the patient die, the family is thus spared the guilt of having made a "wrong" decision. Though such strategies have merit according to the model, the trend of the times is to increase the decision-making prerogative of the public in cases of euthanasia, abortion, and living wills. This increases control but decreases the sense of preventability. Controversy surely lies ahead.

The second major shift in any grief reaction is a change in relationship from centrality to peripherality. In order to curtail a prolonged grieving process, this shift must occur. Individuals who believe that they now have no life of their own or who cling to symbolic vestiges of the deceased will perceive their world only through grief-colored glasses. An active helping process with such individuals can work toward two goals: (1) facilitating the needed detachment of the mourner from the deceased, and (2) facilitating the mourner's process of reconstructing new patterns of living. The first detachment step is a sensitive stage requiring the skills and patience of an understanding person. Talking through the hurt and pain, encouraging the mourner to review his or her life with the loved one, and learning to say good-bye are difficult processes that can be influenced by others. The essential key to this process requires working through the common idea that the dead, one's family, friends, society, and God will somehow disapprove if we even think of having a new life on our own. Understanding this hesitancy and guilt, it behooves family, friends, ministers, and perhaps psychologists to sanction this needed "letting go" process, while encouraging in addition the required reconstruction process.

The middle-aged woman in the second case study represents a good example of this working-through process. An unnecessarily prolonged grieving process was curtailed through the help of the "examiner," most likely a psychiatrist. The woman needed to review her relationship with her dead husband and accept his loss as a first step. Secondly, she needed assurance from someone—in this case, the examiner—that she was still respectable and lovable. She did not need to feel guilty for being attracted to the examiner. Only then was she ready to "fill the gap" and make new plans not only for herself, but also for her children.

In conclusion, it must be stressed that this model is not being presented as a panacea for either understanding or working through human grief. It is offered, however, as having potential value as a resource in working with the bereaved. Understanding that a belief in preventability will most likely lead to an intense grief reaction, for instance, may provide a pathway through the thicket of congested feelings and swirling thoughts. It is hoped that the torturous grief of the mourner may be in some measure assuaged by the application of the model.

References

Cannon, W. 1942. "Voodoo" death. *Amer. Anthropol.* 44:169–181.

Engel, G. 1971. Sudden and rapid death during psychological stress: folklore or folkwisdom? *Annals Intern. Med.* 74:771–782.

Ferrari, N. 1962. Institutionalization and attitude change in an aged population: a field study and dissidence theory. Doctoral dissertation, Western Reserve University.

Kasper, A. 1965. The doctor and death. In *The Meaning of Death,* H. Feifel, ed. New York: McGraw-Hill.

Kavanaugh, R. 1972. *Facing Death.* Baltimore: Penguin Books.

Kübler-Ross, E. 1969. *On Death and Dying.* New York: Macmillan.

Lindemann, E. 1944. Symptomatology and management of acute grief. *Amer. J. Psychiat.* 101:141–148.

Schoenberg, B. et. al. 1974. *Anticipatory Grief.* New York: Columbia University Press.

Schulz, R., and D. Aderman. 1973. Effect of residential change on the temporal distance to death of terminal cancer patients. *Omega* 2:147–162.

Seligman, M. 1975. *Helplessness: On Depression, Development, and Death.* San Francisco: Freeman and Co.

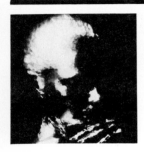

4

Theory

I magine that you are on an operating table in a large general hospital. Suddenly you realize that you are looking down at the surgeons hovering over "your" body. They appear to be excited and you hear them saying, "He's dead," "He's dead." How are you feeling? Is this a potentially real situation?

This chapter presents Ashton Pitre's personal encounter with such an "out-of-body" experience. The extraordinary nature of Pitre's experience accounts for his reluctance to report it to anyone for fifteen years. While skeptics may doubt the credibility of Pitre's story, the inquisitive may find themselves with many questions. The following Appendix exercises may help you clarify some of your thoughts.

B. Appropriate Death Fantasy

E. Confronting the Realization of Death

Death Encounters of the Close Kind: The Realities of Transition

Ashton Pitre

Common Factors of the Transition State

Advancement of medical technology saves ever more lives. Hence, more reports are filed of near-death encounters and what the experience is like. They tend to substantiate earlier reports of events associated with these encounters.

Let us assume that you are having this experience of death. First you hear someone in the room saying, "He is dead—there is nothing more to be done." This pronouncement usually comes from a doctor or a friend. You think, "Why are they saying I'm dead? I'm not dead!" You try to tell them this but you do not hear your voice speaking. You try to move your body but nothing responds. You know something strange is happening.

You hear a high-pitched hum or sound inside your head. This can be beautiful or annoying, depending on your response. The sound is G or G-sharp—the last one on the piano keyboard.

Everything in the room begins to swirl around you, followed by a brief moment of darkness. You rush through this "dark tunnel" and come out at the end of it. Here you encounter a "beautiful Being of Light." This "Being" seems to have a different identity for different persons—based on choice of religion, philosophy, etc.—but it is always friendly, loving, and peaceful. Some reports say the "Being" is just a "person." With the aid of the "Being," you review your life experience on earth. The "re-view" is like looking at a high-speed television show—and you are the star! The "Being" then says, "This is what you have learned during your lifetime on the earth." There is no condemnation, no praise, no judging—your record is just "there," like something recorded in history.

Standing before you are relatives and friends who have already made their transition from earth to "there." You experience great happiness and excitement—a feeling more beautiful than anything you have known on earth. Somehow you "know" you may go with them for a wonderful homecoming party! Then comes the disappointment! One of your loved ones will step forward and say, "No, not yet. It is not the time for you to go with us. You *must* go back." What a terrible thing to happen! Almost *no one* wants to come back to the wearisome struggle of earth's existence. You are drawn back quickly through the "tunnel" and find yourself on earth again.

Reports of the near-death encounter may vary in wording, but one unmistakable conclusion is always present—*there is no death—a part of us consciously continues.* There is only *transition* from this level of awareness to the next. In the process, the physical body is discarded and left behind like "an old overcoat that you take off and throw on the bed."

The increasing amount of research, literature, TV shows, and movies tends to obscure earlier material dealing with death and dying. There were many reports, often discarded, prior to today's interest in the topic. Anyone reporting a near-death experience was often ignored, ridiculed, or both—thus, discouraging any real investigation into the field. I was one of them.

Personal Experiences of Death Encounters

Crises such as war and terminal illness often intensify awareness of near-death encounters. My own encounter was during World War II. I was working with the Medical Corps, U.S. Naval Reserve. After a prolonged and very difficult assignment, admittance to the hospital as a patient seemed the only answer. My bodily functions reached such a low point that the real "me"—the energy field called the spirit—left my body. Everything became vague and the things in the room seemed to swim around in a whirlwind. I heard beautiful, high-pitched musical notes that sounded like a bow continuously drawn across a violin string.

After a few seconds of darkness, I passed through a "window" of some sort and found myself standing in the hospital room—looking at my physical body in the bed. The world was suddenly wonderful—no more pain—no more worry—no more care for the physical body or its needs! The best way to explain the feeling is like waking up on a spring morning after a good night's sleep. You are thoroughly rested, a gentle breeze is blowing, the birds are singing. You step outdoors and take a breath of clean, fresh air and wish that moment could last forever.

The potential in this new world was amazing. I could go anywhere I wished to go—to a symphony—to the moon—anywhere—just by wishing to be there! Thought seemed to be the fuel that moved me through an unobstructed universe.

The people in the hospital were all just as visible to me as when I had been in my physical body. I heard everything that was said—saw everything that happened. The most immediate difficulty was that the person I spoke to would not answer. The patient in the bed next to mine called the nurse, she called the doctor, and both came running down the ward to my bed. I kept telling them, "Leave my body alone! *I* am over here. I am through with it." No one would answer. They could neither hear nor see me. This was *very upsetting*. How could I stop them?

The doctor put an injection into my arm. I was drawn back immediately into my body. There was a kind of "swish-thump" sound, and I seemed to come back through the top of my head. There I was—back in my tired, worn-out body. I was so angry I could have easily "flattened" each of them—and mine is not a violent nature.

Later I reported all that had happened. I told them what I had seen and heard while out of my body. It was completely verified; still they did not believe me. After that I would tell no one what I had experienced. I thought I was the only person in the whole world to whom this had happened. I eventually found other individuals who have had the same kind of experience. I do not mind discussing it. One thing is certain—for me there is no death. I shall just step out of this physical body into the next dimension to a more wonderful existence.

Another case was reported to me by a young woman of the Buddhist faith who was severely wounded during the Vietnam conflict. She said she heard a "strange sound, not heard before," after which she passed through a "dark hole." At the end of this passage she beheld a brilliant light that temporarily blinded her. As she adjusted to the light, her eyes beheld a "magnificent Being." The "Being" she recognized as Christ, though she had never seen a picture of Him. Somehow she "knew" who He was. She refused to discuss what was said between them. "Some of the Old Master paintings of Christ that I have seen since then do resemble Him," she says. Since this unusual encounter she has followed the Christian belief.

A person occasionally reports choosing to return to earth. When this happens, the person wishes to return to help others, not for any selfish reason. Unfinished work—music, art, invention, or worldly accomplishment—do not seem to be enough motivation to prompt a return. Love and the wish to give service to others do motivate return.

An excellent case of this kind was reported to me personally. The mother of two sons who were still in her care was hospitalized in a serious condition. While in the hospital, her condition became so critical that she faced death. Here is how she told of her near-death encounter:

> While a patient at the hospital a strange thing occurred. Although I knew everything that was going on around me, I seemed to be standing on a vast plain. Everything behind me was absolutely dark. In front of me was a very narrow stream of crystal clear water. Standing across the stream was my father, who has been dead for many years. To his left was my grandmother, who was 97 years old when she died. Her appearance was that of a woman about 65, her white hair shining. She was laughing because I could not get across the narrow stream while she, being much older, had crossed the stream easily. I felt paralyzed and could not move my legs. Behind my father and grandmother was a beautiful sunrise. Father held out his hands to me, but I could not go to him because of the intense pain. I believe that if I had ever been able to touch his hand, I would have been in heaven. I was not sad at the thought of leaving the earth—in fact, it seemed quite pleasant. All of this time I

. . . for me there is no death. I shall just step out of this physical body into the next dimension to a more wonderful existence.

was conscious of the terrible pain in my body on the bed; but I felt no pain in the "me" who was seeing all of this before me. If this is the way a person dies, the Christian has nothing to fear.

Several days later, after being off the pain medication, I realized how close to death I had been. I realized I was not ready to leave my loved ones. I was ready to fight to stay here.

The next night and all of the following day, at the foot of my bed to the right stood a horrible, indefinite figure of jet black I understood to be death. At the foot of my bed to the left side stood Christ, with very definite form and features. Yet further back, behind Him, stood by father, smiling at me. Not willing to leave my loved ones, I became terrified. Each time death moved toward me, Christ would say, "You cannot have her—she is mine." This went on *all night* and *through the next day*. These forms were there continually, whether my eyes were open or shut. I was always aware of them.

Finally, late in the afternoon, I said, "All right, God, if it will serve your purpose for me to die, I am willing. I don't want to die, but so be it." My father said, "Honey, don't be afraid. When it does come, it will be all right. It will be the right time—and it will be good." Then he turned and walked away. At this moment Christ raised His left arm, in the direction of death, and lowered it, saying, "And the last thing, I conquered death." As He lowered His arm, the horrible black figure seemed to melt away.

The mother in this report is still alive and has a calm and beautiful outlook on life. She has had no further encounters of this nature.

In a more recent case, a young man known to me personally reported a close encounter with death that occurred a few weeks before his actual death. He had been operated on for cancer. During the operation he was out of his physical body and made the following report. He belonged to no religion and expressed no mystic philosophy.

As the anesthetic was being given, everything began to swirl around in the room. I heard a strange musical note being constantly played. In a few seconds everything went black and I seemed to be flying through a dark tube. I remember thinking, it must be the anesthetic. I was suddenly out of the darkness and in the hospital operating room. I could see my body on the table and see and hear everything. I was even aware of everyone who came and went through the door. At some point I seemed to "fall" from above, where I had been, back into my body. When the operation was over, I told everyone what I had seen. They said it was correct in every detail.

Somehow, I knew that there was very little time left for me on earth. I knew, also, that dying must be just this easy. It may be because I do not want to live with the pain of cancer, but I see death as nonexistent—it is just a step to something better.

Three weeks later he died without pain, in his sleep.

The last words a person speaks before leaving the earth are most revealing. Curiously, many fixed ideas change at the last minute. The dying words reflect similar visions—be the person dying king or poet. "How beautiful it all is!" "Why, it is so simple—so easy." "There is really nothing to fear. If only you could see what I see—how lovely it is." "There is nothing to it—I never realized it would be so easy!" "Well, look who is here to meet me! You told me you would."

Death always seems so hard on those left behind. It is so important for those who teach courses or comfort the terminally ill to understand the emotional aspects of death encounters. But how does one learn about death without dying?

Preparing for the Reality of Transition

Let's face the situation logically and realistically. If you were going to take a trip or move to a place where you had never been, how would you go about it? Let us suppose you are going to the island of "Kauai." You do not know where it is or how to get there. You are told that if you go in a certain direction for a given distance, you will arrive at Kauai. You would be wise to learn about life there—customs, restrictions, etc.

Much to your surprise, you learn that a neighbor down the block has been to Kauai. Being a wise person, you meet this neighbor; ask all the questions you can think to ask; discover any books or studies you may use to help you have a satisfying stay in Kauai.

How much more important it is to do the same things when you are preparing for the greatest move you will ever make! You may even hear of someone who has had the near-death encounter and talk to that person who has been "there."

There is yet another method to learn about the death experience. With enough time and effort—and the necessary method—you may learn much through meditation. Here is a brief description from someone who practices this form of meditation.

You have asked me to describe what happens when I meditate. What I do is sit on the floor or in a chair in an upright position. This must be done in a quiet place. I sit in a semi-lotus position because the Western-type body I have will not allow a full lotus. I use soft rubber ear plugs to stop out all sound and cover my eyes with a dark cloth to shut out all light. Some persons I know sit with the feet flat on the floor, without shoes on, when using a chair to meditate. There is to be no binding clothing, belts, etc. The body must be completely relaxed.

I take a few deep breaths to clear the lungs, then begin to concentrate on a spot in the darkness about twelve feet in front of my nose. I think of nothing. This is the hardest part—to clear the mind of all thought. I sit and wait quietly in the darkness and silence.

After a few minutes I hear a high-pitched sound that begins and continues throughout meditation. Then there comes a bright spot of light off to my right. By concentrating on this light, I "bring it to myself." It is on this "stream of light and sound" that the spirit leaves the body. I go through a "tunnel" at a high speed and come out at the end of it, where there is a bright light shining. I have then left the physical body behind and am in the "other level of awareness." My breath and heart beat drop to a very low state, as if I may be in a deep sleep or coma. There is no fear nor anxiety, only total elevation and elation. It is in this state that I go places and see people. I travel from place to place using my thought as energy. I talk with people who may have been relatives or friends on earth, but I prefer to be with teachers who instruct in the eternal truths and ways of life. All beings on this level have "light" bodies. When so-called death takes place, I shall merely make my transition to this level, where I shall continue until it is time to "die" there and move on to a higher awareness.

Notice the points in this report that duplicate many of the ones spoken of in the near-death experience. The sound is heard and the light is seen after going through a tunnel. The lowering of the pulse and heart rate even approach a deathlike state. "Thought" energy is used to travel. These points are in close agreement with other findings reported to be "beyond this dimension." It is evident that time and effort will be necessary if anyone wishes to use this method.

More changes have been made in this world in the last fifty years than have taken place in the past 3,000 years! Our understanding of life on earth is in such a state of change; is it not reasonable to expect that our understanding of life "beyond" is also changing?

Bibliography

Ebon, M. 1977. *The Evidence for Life after Death*. New York: Signet.
Moody, R. 1977a. *Life after Life*. New York: Bantam Books.
————. 1977b. *Reflections on Life after Life*. New York: Bantam Books.

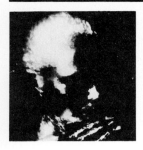

5

Research

If someone close to you died, would you imagine that *you* would begin seeing a physician more regularly, that *you* would lose weight and fear losing your mind, or that *you* might actually die much earlier than expected? This chapter explores some of the research findings that help clarify the health consequences of bereavement. The following Appendix exercises are recommended when you complete this reading:

        C.   Awareness of Grief Process

        H.   Fantasizing Grief Reaction of Significant Others

Research on Bereavement: A Selective and Critical Review

Gerald Epstein

Lawrence Weitz

Howard Roback

Embry McKee

The literature on bereavement is primarily case-historical and theoretical-conceptual in nature and scope. Bereavement refers to the complex reactions of survivors following the experience of separation by death from a significant person. Freud[1] considered grief work to involve the painful task of "decathecting" libido from a lost object and reinvesting it in a new reality situation.

Eric Lindemann[2] provided the first intensive study of bereavement reactions; his 101 subjects included: (1) psychoneurotic patients who lost a relative during the course of treatment, (2) relatives of patients who died in the hospital, (3) bereaved disaster victims (Cocoanut Grove fire) and their close relatives, and (4) relatives of members of the armed forces.

Lindemann recorded the following symptoms as common to all individuals suffering from acute grief: somatic distress occurring repeatedly and lasting from 20 minutes to an hour at a time, feelings of tightness in the throat, choking with shortness of breath, loss of muscular power, and intense subjective distress described as tension or mental pain. Psychologically, the bereaved were described as preoccupied with an image of the deceased and with guilt feelings. Behaviorally, they were often hostile toward friends and relatives, unable to complete tasks, restless, moving about in an aimless fashion and constantly searching for something to do. They also lacked the ability to maintain organized patterns of activity. Most individuals successfully worked through their grief in 4 to 6 weeks. Unfortunately, the investigator (1) failed to reveal the interrelationships between symptoms described and the variability of each over time, (2) presented minimal information on the frequency of occurrence of described reactions, and (3) provided no time perspective as to how fre-

This material was first published in *Comprehensive Psychiatry,* vol. 16, no. 6, pp. 537–546, November/December 1975. It is reprinted by permission of Grune & Stratton, Inc. and the authors.

Antisocial behavior appeared either immediately or within a few months subsequent to the death of a parent. . . .

quently or how long after bereavement the interviews were conducted. Nonetheless, Lindemann's pioneering effort is a significant one.

Since Lindemann's clinical study, a substantial number of empirical studies on behavioral and psychophysiological consequences of bereavement have been conducted. Investigations dealing with parental loss, conjugal loss, and predictors of unfavorable bereavement outcome are examined critically in this article.

Parental Loss During Childhood and Adolescence

Personality theorists[1,3-6] have postulated that parental loss by death or desertion seriously impedes the consequent socioemotional development of the child. Consistent with this assertion, delinquent acting-out behavior in previously conforming children and/or adolescents has been reported in several relevant studies.[7-10] Antisocial behavior appeared either immediately or within a few months subsequent to the death of a parent and included theft, sexual promiscuity, drinking, traffic violations, truancy, burglary, and defiance of authority figures. Brown's data[11] revealed a similar increase in violence, bullying, lying, truancy, and stealing among 2,196 London children. Kirkpatrick[12] found reduced academic achievement, social withdrawal, accident-proneness, and a propensity for running away from home in many children following a parent's death.

Fulton and Markusen[13] presented evidence suggesting that persons who lose a parent during childhood have relatively high divorce and crime rates. Other investigators[14-20] have attempted to link parental death in early childhood with subsequent mental disorders such as schizophrenia, psychotic depression, and alcoholism. These authors also discuss methodological problems common to efforts at validating hypotheses linking early bereavement and later behavior disorders. The deficiencies cited included: a tendency toward assertion of etiology based on findings of association; small samples; lack of standardization in recording data; unrepresentative samples; poor controls; and failure to take into account age at time of loss and unexpectedness of loss.

A difficulty in establishing normal bereavement rates is the lack of consensus as to which population to regard as the normal control. Other constraints on research in this area include problems in selecting psychiatric patients for comparisons with normals, deficiencies of data gathering (e.g., interviews are heavily dependent upon selective memory and the good will of the subject), failure to consider demographic factors (e.g., ethnicity, socioeconomic class, religion, marital status, or residences), failure to consider intervening variables that could affect the cause-effect relationship (e.g., nature of prebereavement and postbereavement home environment, circumstances of death, and emotional characteristics of the surviving parent), and appropriate use of statistical tests of significance and fallacious deduction in interpretation. Thus determination of the precise relationship between childhood bereavement and later behavioral pathology awaits the application of more sophisticated research methodology to the field.

Conjugal Loss

Among the somatic illnesses sometimes thought to be precipitated by bereavement are ulcerative colitis and rheumatoid arthritis,[21-23] asthma,[24] hyperthyroidism,[25] and osteoarthritis.[26] Such potentially fatal conditions as coronary thrombosis, blood cancers, and cancer of the neck of the womb may be precipitated or aggravated by major losses.[27-30]

The nonpsychiatric clinical morbidity of widowhood has been the focus of three major studies.[26,30,31] Only the Maddison study[31] included a nonbereaved control group. Parkes[26] found that among widows under 65, general practitioners' consultation rates for psychological symptoms (anxiety, depression, insomnia) more than tripled during the first 6 months of bereavement. The amount of sedation prescribed to widows under 65 was seven times greater during the 18-month period after the death than in the control period. No such changes were observed among widows over 65, and consultation rates for physical symptoms did not increase in the younger age group but did among the older women. The most common consultation for physical symptoms was that of arthritis and rheumatic conditions. Parkes conjectured that the increase in visits to family doctors might reflect heightened dependency resulting from loss of the husband's support.

Maddison[31] studied 132 widows from Boston and 221 from Sydney, Australia, and compared them with matched controls of married women. Data were collected by means of a postal questionnaire. The following results were reported: Of the total sample of widows, all under age 60, 28 percent obtained scores indicating marked health deterioration, as compared to 4.5 percent of the married women. Symptoms more common among the bereaved were nervousness, depression, fears of nervous breakdown, feelings of panic, persistent fears, nightmares, insomnia, trembling, loss of appetite, loss of weight, reduced working capacity, and fatigue. Such symptoms are frequently encountered in grief reactions and are therefore not unexpected among newly bereaved widows. However, other symptoms that were less obviously features of grieving were also frequently observed among the bereaved sample: headaches, dizziness, fainting spells, blurred vision, skin rashes, excessive sweating, indigestion, difficulty in swallowing, vomiting, heavy menstrual periods, chest pains, palpitations, shortness of breath, frequent infections, and general aching. In addition, 12.8% of the bereaved compared to 1.0% of controls consulted a physician for treatment of depression during the previous 12 months.

The essence of Maddison's findings were replicated in the study of Parkes and Brown[32] of 49 widows and 19 widowers under 45 who had been

. . . somatic illnesses sometimes thought to be precipitated by bereavement. . . .

bereaved 14 months previously. Sixty-eight matched male and female controls provided comparison data. The bereaved sample showed greater evidence of depression and general emotional difficulty, as reflected by recent disturbance of sleep, appetite and weight fluctuation, loneliness, restlessness, indecisiveness, poor memory, and an increased consumption of tranquilizers, alcohol, and tobacco. Survivors were four times as likely as controls to have been hospitalized (general medical and psychiatric) in the preceding year. There was no distinction between the bereaved and control groups obtained with regard to chronic physical symptoms, although there was a significant difference between the groups with respect to psychological symptoms and somatic symptoms associated with anxiety (primarily those of the autonomic system, i.e., dizziness, fainting, trembling, twitching, nervousness, chest pains, sweating without cause, palpitations, and lump in throat). Members of the widowed group more often than controls sought advice for emotional problems from physicians and clergy (and sometimes psychiatrists, social workers, or psychologists).

Long-term follow-up revealed a steady decline in depression and autonomic symptoms, so that by the third year of bereavement little difference remained between the groups. Moreover, the bereaved were slightly more likely than the married controls to avoid new relationships, to feel apart or remote even among friends, to prefer going out alone, and to avoid worrying about problems that were seen as insuperable. However, widowers remained more depressed than married men.

The work of Pugh and MacMahon,[33] Parkes,[26] and Stein and Susser[34] suggests a higher incidence of hospitalized mental illness among widowed than married persons. At every age, widowed males and females experience a higher risk for psychiatric institutionalization than married persons of corresponding sex and age. The excess in risk seems greater for widowers than for widows, especially at the under-30 age range. Once hospitalized, widowed individuals stay institutionalized longer than married persons of the same age and sex. Here, too, the finding is more salient for widowers than for widows, and more striking at the younger ages for both sexes. Parkes's main findings revealed that bereaved patients suffer from various psychiatric illnesses, with reactive depression the most common.[26]

In evaluating these findings it must be noted that the data pertain only to risk of mental hospitalization; appropriate evidence is not available as to the relative risk by marital status of emotional disorders treated outside the psychiatric hospital or simply untreated in the community at large. The excess risk reported could be a consequence of other than poor coping. For example, the stress of living without a mate could entail sufficient deprivation, hardship, and loss of care to cause the increased risk. (It should be noted that the excess risk of mental hospitalization for single persons in comparison with the married is even higher than that for the widowed in comparison with the married. Poor mental health may operate as a selective factor in the choice of single status). Excess risk may also arise spuriously from systematic differences between widowed and the married. One serious difference may be that the widowed group in comparison with the married contains a significantly higher percentage of lower social class individuals. Hollingshead and Redlich[35] have already established an association between mental illness (as defined by hospitalization) and social class. The apparent risk among surviving spouses may thus be generated by this systematic difference between the widowed and the married groups. The self-selective factor of widowhood may also be a compelling consideration, i.e., those who stay widowed may have poorer mental health than those who remarry.

Clayton[36] summarized the most prominent findings with respect to morbidity of the first year of bereavement among the widowed as follows: (1) There is an increase in the number of physician visits in the first year.[30,31] (2) Widowed consult physicians (internists, general practitioners, *not* psychiatrists or psychologists) for psychological symptoms and receive increased numbers of tranquilizers and sedatives.[30,34,37] (3) Consultations for nonpsychiatric symptoms are similar to those of controls.[30,31] (4) The question of whether consultations with physicians are due to the bereavement per se or the loss of support resulting from bereavement is still uncertain. (5) The cardinal symptoms of the bereavement reactions appear to be crying, depressed moods, and sleep disturbances.[37] (6) Loss of interest in television, news, friends, and clubs, difficulty in concentrating, poor memory, anorexia, and weight loss are also common among widows and widowers in the first six months of bereavement, while suicidal ideas and fears of losing one's mind are less common.[37,38] (7) Although treatment for the widowed centers primarily on psychophysiological symptoms, the responsibility of taking care of the bereaved does not typically fall to the mental health professionals but to other caretakers such as physicians and clergymen. (8) In analyzing the validity of the data presented, the methodological issues and problems discussed earlier must also be taken into consideration here.

Death in the family produces an increased postbereavement mortality rate among close relatives. . . .

Adult Mortality Studies

Epidemiological data concerning the mortality of widowhood have been well documented.[39-42] Several interesting facts abstracted are as follows:

1. At every age, widowed males and females experience a higher risk of dying than married persons of corresponding sex and age.[39] At the younger ages, below 34, even single and divorced individuals have lower mortality rates than the widowed.

2. The excess in risk is greater for widowers than widows, and for each sex in turn the excess is greater at the younger ages.[39]

3. Death in the family produces an increased postbereavement mortality rate among close relatives, with the greatest increase in mortality risk occurring among surviving spouses.[28]

. . . widows who
remarry do so
after the first two
years.

4. The highest death rates occur in the first six months of bereavement as compared to later periods.[40] Among 4,486 widowers over the age of 54, a 40 percent increase in death rate was found.

5. Records of 903 relatives dying in semirural areas of Wales over a six-year period showed that within the first year of bereavement there is a seven times higher mortality rate among relatives than among controls (4.76 percent vs. 1.2 percent). After the first year of bereavement, mortality rates fell sharply and were no longer significantly higher than among matched controls. The suddenness of death also proved to be a factor in the risk of death among relatives. The risk of a bereaved relative dying within one year was more than twice as high if the relative died suddenly in a hospital, as opposed to slowly at home.[28]

6. In reanalyzing the data of Young et al.,[40] Parkes et al.[29] found that the increased mortality rate in the widowed sample of 4,486 was not only confined to the first months of bereavement but that the predominant cause of death (three-fourths of the increased death rate) was coronary thrombosis or other arteriosclerotic or degenerative heart diseases.

7. In general, the data among the replicated studies in both England and the United States showed that the risk of dying is at least twice as great for widows and widowers at all age levels for a great variety of diseases.

It is possible to view the aforementioned studies collectively and assess the validity of a variety of explanations proposed to account for the high mortality rates of widows and widowers.

The *selection hypothesis* states that the mortality rates reported in most studies are considered to be artifactual, because the widowed that are in good health tend to remarry quickly and select themselves out, thus leaving the widowed population with higher mortality rates. Evidence contradicting the explanation has been presented by Kraus and Lilienfeld[39] and others.[40,41] Firstly, the deleterious impact of widowhood is greatest in the first six months. Secondly, after two years of widowhood the mortality rates among the widowed decline to a level equal to that of married persons. Thirdly, on the average, those widows who remarry do so after the first two years. For the selection hypothesis to be valid, these individuals would have had to select themselves out within six months after becoming widowed.

The *homogamy* or *mutual choice of poor-risk mates hypothesis* points out that individuals with a short survival potential tend knowingly or unknowingly to choose mates with a similar potential. Both Kraus and Lilienfeld[39] and Young et al.[40] reported evidence that there is a tendency for the fit to marry the fit and the unfit to marry the unfit. Individuals with apparent disabilities of sense organs or limbs tend to marry persons with similar disabilities. Kraus and Lilienfeld went on to point out that if psychological characteristics are important in the etiology of certain diseases then it is not implausible that mates choosing each other on similar traits may die at about the same time and of the same disease. The only study partially supporting the tendency for married couples to die of the same disease is that of Ciocco.[43] There was a nonsignificant tendency for husbands and wives to die from the same cause when either tuberculosis, influenza and pneumonia, heart disease, or cancer was the cause of death, with the strongest relationship involving the first two causes. The relationship can probably be better explained by the presence of a joint unfavorable infectious environment.

The *joint unfavorable environment hypothesis* points out that the widowed and their deceased spouses may have shared common unfavorable environmental factors that not only led to the death of the one spouse but also resulted in an excessive risk for the surviving spouse. Although this hypothesis may account for some of the early deaths among the bereaved, it does not account for (1) the greater impact of sudden death as compared to a prolonged death and (2) the relatively rare occurrences of couples dying of the same disease.

The *non-grief-related behavior-change hypothesis* posits that high-risk behavior in the survivor may be less a consequence of bereavement over the death of a spouse and more a consequence of non-grief-related behavior. The survivor may not eat properly, take his medicines regularly, or visit the doctor when ill—not because he is grief-stricken but simply because the deceased spouse is no longer around to encourage and support these adaptive behaviors.

The *desolation-effects hypothesis* states that the event and new conditions of widowhood may have a deleterious effect that results in the increased death rate. The effects include grief, new worries and responsibilities, alterations in diet, work, or recreational activities, a difficult economic situation, general feelings of hopelessness, or the broken-heart syndrome.[29] The suggested state of hopelessness may result in direct physiological changes such as lowered resistance to diseases and/or in behavioral changes detrimental to the individual's well-being.

Epidemiological data have been offered to emphasize the negative consequences of bereavement. Five alternative hypotheses were presented to account for the high mortality rates of survivors. Three of the five hypotheses (*joint unfavorable environment, non-grief-related behavior changes,* and *desolation effects*) were able to account for the data presented more adequately than the *selection hypothesis* or the *homogamy hypothesis.* The *desolation hypothesis* with its emphasis on psychophysiological and sociological explanations seems to be cited most frequently in the literature and is probably the most convincing of the alternatives offered.

At this time a description will be presented of some of the physiological reactions possibly induced by the general feelings of hopelessness and desolation associated with the stress of bereavement.

Bereaved individuals have often reported a sense of hopelessness, despair, and general loss of environmental control, i.e., perceiving their environmental support system including clergy, friends, relatives, and neighbors as minimally helpful.[44] Richter[45] and other investigators[46-50] studying the effects of prolonged stress on animals have depicted concomitant changes in endocrine functioning. They have found an association be-

> . . . hopelessness may result in direct physiological changes such as lowered resistance to diseases. . . .

. . . inability to cope alters neural biochemistry, which further accentuates depression. . . .

tween catecholamine levels in the central nervous system and the psychological state. Helpless rats unable to avoid or escape shock showed a decrease in the brain level of norepinephrine. Depletion of norepinephrine has been viewed by Schildkraut and Kety[51] and Coppen[52] as instrumental in mitigating assertive active responses and bringing about depression in humans. As Weiss[48] has speculated, the sequence leading from helplessness to behavioral depression may depend on biochemical changes, such as norepinephrine in the central nervous system. The implication for the bereaved individual seems as follows: "Depressed behavior can be perpetuated in a vicious circle: the inability to cope alters neural biochemistry, which further accentuates depression, increasing the inability to cope, which further alters neural biochemistry and so on" (page 113).

Parkes,[30] speculating on his finding of 1969 (i.e., three-fourths of the increased death rate among survivors during the first six months was attributable to heart disease), stated that it is very possible that the stress of bereavement may produce changes in the blood pressure and heart rate, in the flow of blood through the coronary arteries, and in the chemical constituents of the blood. Any of these changes could play a part in precipitating clotting within a coronary artery, leading to a thrombosis. He went on to say that bereavement probably does not originate a heart condition but aggravates one that is already present.

The bereaved individual's lowered resistance to disease (changes in catecholamine and corticosteroid levels and the lack of immunological state of readiness) may be aggravated by behavior detrimental to physical well-being. The bereaved person may not get enough sleep, may neglect taking medication, ignore medical problems, and eat poorly due to a loss of appetite (Parkes[30]).

Rushing[53] and Bunch[54] have reported higher suicide rates for widows than for their married counterparts. These studies further reveal that the death of one or both parents in childhood is common among attempted and actual suicide victims and that the incidence of suicide among such persons when they reach adulthood is much greater than that for comparable groups in the general population. In comparing bereaved individuals who commit suicide versus bereaved individuals who do not (within two years following death), Bunch[54] found that the suicide victims' severe emotional states were in response to less support from relatives or family members and more social disruption; they were more likely to be living alone and were more likely to have had a prior history of emotional difficulties (before death of spouse).

Predictors of Unfavorable Bereavement Outcome

Maddison[31,44] attempted to determine parameters predictive of an unfavorable resolution (defined by the presence of physical and emotional difficulties that precipitate a deterioration in health) of the bereavement crisis.

The evidence available thus far comes predominantly from studies of bereaved women rather than bereaved men.

The widow who turned out to be a bad-outcome subject was dissatisfied with the help available to her during the crisis. She perceived a high frequency of unhelpful interactions with persons within her social network during the first 3 months following the death of her spouse. She considered persons around her to be actively or passively opposing her wish to review past memories and experiences with the deceased spouse. Not only were significant others (including family, friends, clergy, and physicians) minimally helpful in assisting the widow in ventilating her feelings, but the people often encouraged development of new activities and new romantic relationships at times when the widow was not prepared emotionally for such suggestions. Such attempts were met with great anger and bitterness.

Other significant factors (other than inadequate and ineffectual environmental support) contributing to bad outcome were: (1) age of widow less than 45 with dependent children; (2) evidence of preexisting marital difficulties; (3) protracted death (associated with severe suffering and disfigurement) maximizing preexisting ambivalence, leading to feelings of guilt and inadequacy; (4) prior history of severe reaction to death of another family member; (5) additional stresses or crises in close temporal relationship to bereavement; (6) deliberate avoidance of affective expression, especially controlling hostile and angry feelings; (7) continued reaction formation against dependence; (8) poor interpersonal relationship with own mother or husband's family.

No relationship was found between outcome and length of time for which death had been anticipated. Contrary to popular belief, Maddison[31] found that sudden death or death with minimal warning does not necessarily lead to a worse outcome. Proximity to protracted death with its overlay of constant pain and suffering seems to create greater intensity of intrapsychic and physical strain than does sudden unexpected death. The work of Clayton et al.,[36,38] supported Maddison's findings, i.e., the duration of illness was unrelated to prevalence of symptoms in widows and widowers.

With respect to factor 1 above, it appears that in those widows under 45, bereavement was more traumatic because of the intensity of sexual involvement with the deceased, i.e., the person was highly cathected. Although the presence of dependent children might have been highly valued in terms of distracting the widow from her own problems of grief and giving meaning to her existence, additional problems were created such as trying to give social emotional support to the children while hiding one's own grief reactions. These widows have reported difficulty in filling the children's dependency needs when their own were unfulfilled and in filling a paternal role for which they were unprepared.

With respect to conjugal bereavement, good-outcome subjects are differentiated from bad-outcome subjects in their perception of the supportiveness of interpersonal relationships during crisis, i.e., dissatisfaction with available environmental resources. Good-outcome subjects tend to

Proximity to protracted death . . . seems to create greater . . . strain than does sudden unexpected death.

perceive permissive support as helpful, while bad-outcome subjects tend to appreciate more active encouragement from the milieu. Bad-outcome subjects also tend to perceive the environment as actively unhelpful, the relevant interchanges usually involving either the blocking of a widow's expression of affect or overt or covert hostility directed toward her in response to expressing her grief. Attempts to focus her attention on the future and to dissuade her thinking of the past tend also to be found unhelpful by bad-outcome subjects. A high-risk case tends to be a young widow with children living at home and no close relatives living nearby. Cultural and familial norms prevent her from expressing feelings of anger, ambivalence, and guilt. Other stresses occurring before or after the bereavement, such as loss of income, change in residence, and difficulties with children increase the widow's burdens.

It is important to keep in mind that predictors of outcome are only in terms of probability and that a person may fit all of these predictors and still successfully weather the hazard of bereavement, while another person may fit none of these categories and still have an unfavorable outcome.

References

1. Freud, S. Mourning and melancholia (1917), in *Collected Papers,* vol. 4. New York: Basic Books, 1959.
2. Lindemann, E. Symptomatology and management of acute grief. *Am. J. Psychiatry* 101:141–148, 1944.
3. Deutsch, H. Absence of grief. *Psychoanal. Q.* 6:12–22, 1937.
4. Klein, M. A contribution to the theory of anxiety and guilt. *Int. J. Psychoanal.* 29:114–123, 1948.
5. Bowlby, J. Grief and mourning in infancy and early childhood. *Psychoanal. Study Child.* 15:9–52, 1960.
6. Bowlby, J. Childhood mourning and its implications for psychiatry. *Am. J. Psychiatry* 118:481–498, 1961.
7. Glueck, S.; Glueck, E. 500 delinquent boys. In *Unravelling juvenile delinquency.* New York: The Commonwealth Fund, 1950.
8. Johnson, A.M.; Szurek, S.A. Etiology of antisocial behavior in delinquency and psychopathology. *JAMA* 154:814–817, 1954.
9. Clarke, J. The precipitation of juvenile delinquency. *J. Ment. Sci.* 107:1033–1034, 1961.
10. Shoor, M; Speed, M.H. Delinquency as a manifestation of the mourning process. *Psychiatr. Q.* 37:540–558, 1963.
11. Brown, F. Childhood bereavement and subsequent crime. *Br. J. Psychiatry* 112:1043–1048, 1966.
12. Kirkpatrick, J. Bereavement and school adjustment. *J. School Psychology* 3:58–63, 1965.
13. Fulton, R.; Markusen, E. Childhood bereavement and behavior disorders: A critical review. *Omega* 2:107–117, 1971.
14. Norton, A. Incidence of neurosis related to maternal age and birth order. *Br. J. Social Medicine* 6:253–258, 1952.
15. Barry, H.; Lindemann, E. Critical ages for maternal bereavement in psychoneurosis. *Psychosom. Med.* 22:166–181, 1960.
16. Archibald, H.C. Bereavement in childhood and adult psychiatric disturbances. *Psychosom. Med.* 24:343–351, 1962.
17. Hilgard, J.R.; Newman, M.F. Parental loss by death in childhood as an etiological factor among schizophrenic and alcoholic patients compared with a non-patient community sample. *J. Nerv. Ment. Dis.* 137:14–28, 1963.
18. Birtchnell, J. Depression in relation to early and recent parent death. *Br. J. Psychiatry* 116:299–306, 1970.
19. Birtchnell, J. Early parent death and mental illness. *Br. J. Psychiatry* 116:281–288, 1970.

20. Birtchnell, J. Recent parent death and mental illness. *Br. J. Psychiatry* 116:307–313, 1970.
21. Cobb, S.; Bauer, W.; Whiting, I. Environment factors in rheumatoid arthritis. *JAMA* 113:668–670, 1939.
22. Lindemann, E. Psychological aspects of mourning. *The Director* 31:14–17, 1961.
23. Brewster, H.H. Separation reaction in psychosomatic disease and neurosis. *Psychosom. Med.* 14:154–160, 1952.
24. McDermott, M.; Cobb, S. Psychogenic factors in asthma. *Psychosom. Med.* 1:204–234, 1939.
25. Lidz, R. Emotional factors in hyperthyroidism. *Psychosom. Med.* 11:2, 1949.
26. Parkes, C.M. Effects of bereavement on physical and mental health—A study of the medical records of widows. *Br. Med. J.* 2:274–279, 1964.
27. Peller, S. *Cancer in Man.* New York: International Universities Press, 1952.
28. Rees, W.D.; Lutkins, S.G. Mortality of bereavement. *Br. Med. J.* 4:13–16, 1967.
29. Parkes, C.M.; Benjamin, B.; Fitzgerald R.G. Broken heart: A statistical study of increased mortality among widowers. *Br. J. Med.* 1:740–743, 1969.
30. Parkes, C.M.; *Bereavement: Studies of Grief in Adult Life.* New York: International Universities Press, 1972.
31. Maddison, D. The relevance of conjugal bereavement for preventive psychiatry. *Br. J. Med. Psychol.* 41:223–233, 1968.
32. Parkes, C.M.; Brown, R.J. Health after bereavement: A controlled study of young Boston widows and widowers. *Psychosom. Med.* 34:449–461, 1972.
33. Pugh, T.F.; MacMahon, B. *Epidemiologic Findings in U.S. Mental Hospital Data.* Boston: Little, Brown, 1962.
34. Stein Z.; Susser, M. Widowhood and mental illness. *Br. J. Prev. Soc. Med.* 23:106–110, 1969.
35. Hollingshead, A.B.; Redlich, F.C. *Social Class and Mental Health, A Community Study.* New York: John Wiley & Sons, 1958.
36. Clayton, P.J. The clinical morbidity of the first year of bereavement: A review. *Compr. Psychiatry.* 14:151–157, 1973.
37. Clayton, P.J.; Halikes, J.A.; Maurice, W.L. The bereavement of the widowed. *Dis. Nerv. Syst.* 32:597–604, 1971.
38. Clayton, P.J.; Desmarais, L.; Winokur, G. A study of normal bereavement. *Am. J. Psychiatry* 125:169–178, 1968.
39. Kraus, A.S.; Lilienfeld, A.M. Some epidemiologic aspects of the high mortality rate in the young widowed group. *J. Chron. Dis.* 10:207–217, 1959.
40. Young, M.; Benjamin, B.; Wallis, C. The mortality of widowers. *Lancet* 2:454–456, 1963.
41. Cox, P.R.; Ford, J.R. The mortality of widows shortly after widowhood. *Lancet* 1:163–164, 1964.
42. Kutscher, A.H.; Kutscher, I.O. (eds). *For the Bereaved.* New York: Frederick Fell, 1971.
43. Ciocco, A. On mortality in husbands and wives. *Hum. Biol.* 12:508, 1940.
44. Maddison, D. The factors affecting the outcome of conjugal bereavement. *Br. J. Psychiatry* 113:1057–1067, 1967.
45. Richter, C.P. On the phenomenon of sudden death in animals and man. *Psychosom. Med.* 19:191–198, 1957.
46. Weiss, J.M. Somatic effects of predictable and unpredictable shock. *Psychosom. Med.* 32:397–408, 1970.
47. Weiss, J.M. Effects of coping behavior in different warning signal conditions on stress pathology in rats. *J. Comp. Physiol. Psychol.* 77:1–35, 1971.
48. Weiss, J.M. Psychological factors in stress and disease. *Sci. Am.* 226:104–113, 1972.
49. Ader, R. Experimentally induced gastric lesions, results and implications of studies in animals. *Adv. Psychosom. Med.* 6:1–39, 1971.
50. Fredrick, J.F. Physiological reactions induced by grief. *Omega* 2:71–75, 1971.
51. Schildkraut, J.J.; Kety, S.S. Biogenic amines and emotion. *Science* 156:21–30, 1967.
52. Coppen, H.J. Depressed states and indolealkylamines. *Adv. Pharmacol.* 65:283–291, 1968.
53. Rushing, W.A. Individual behavior and suicide, in Gibbs, J.P. (ed.): *Suicide.* New York: Harper & Row, 1968.
54. Bunch, J. Recent bereavement in relation to suicide. *J. Psychosom. Res.* 16:361–366, 1972.

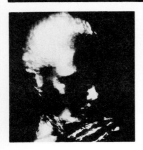

6

Research

Are you afraid of dying? Perhaps that question is too direct! Do you have some concerns about dying? Are these concerns more related to yourself (e.g., experiencing pain) or more related to how others will cope without you? Have you ever wondered how we can reliably and validly measure these concerns? Does knowing that I have a high death concern help me plan my life differently? This chapter by Richard Schulz explores these questions and may be appropriately followed by these Appendix exercises.

E.   Confronting the Realization of Death

I.   Life and Death Attitudes: Dyadic Encounter

K.   Planning for Living

Death Anxiety: Intuitive and Empirical Perspectives

Richard Schulz

An Intuitive Perspective

"Of all things that move man, one of the principle ones is his terror of death" (Becker 1973, 11). This statement is the premise of Ernest Becker's provocative book *The Denial of Death*. Becker argues that "the idea of death, the fear of it, haunts the human animal like nothing else; it is a mainspring of human activity—activity designed largely to avoid the fatality of death, to overcome it by denying in some way that it is the final destiny for man" (Becker 1973). While Becker argues his case better than most, he would be the first to admit that his basic premise is not a particularly new slant on the significance of death to man's existence. How to deal with the end of life has been a major focus of all contemporary and ancient religions and the central problem of philosophers from Epicurus of ancient Greece to Heidegger and the modern existentialists.

It would be impossible to review here the innumerable views of death proposed in man's recorded history. Most writers would agree on one point, however: death is a paradox. It is both a destructive and creative force. The basic premise of the paradox is that man fears or is anxious about death, and it is this fear or anxiety that directly and indirectly motivates much of his behavior. On one hand, man's fear of death has been identified as the genesis of neurosis (Meyer 1975) and psychosis (Becker 1973); on the other hand, man's pleasure of existence and many of his good works have been attributed to his fear of death.

One might ask, does man really fear death and, if so, what exactly does man fear about death? With the exception perhaps of Gary Gilmore, the convicted murderer who asked to be executed, it is reasonable to assume

This material was first published in *The Psychology of Death, Dying, and Bereavement*, pp. 18–39. Copyright 1978 Addison-Wesley Publishing Company. It is printed here in slightly modified form by permission.

that most persons in Western society consider death, at best, a mediocre experience. Although the supporting data are not available, it is likely that death is not on our minds much of the time, and for most persons it looms far enough in the future that we experience little anxiety over the prospect of dying and being dead. On the other hand, death is an experience that few people seek out. We are, in fact, willing to spend fortunes to avoid it. The question to be answered, then, is, what is it about death that makes it such an undesirable prospect? Anyone can easily generate at least a partial list to answer this question. The reader may be surprised to find how long this list (presented below) can actually get.

Physical and Psychological Components
In brief, the negative aspects of death and dying can be classified under two general and interactive categories: physical and psychological suffering. They are interactive because each can intensify the other and neither exists in isolation.

Fear of physical suffering. As the causes of death change in our society, so does the probability of experiencing physical discomfort. Slow degenerative processes, such as cancer, are more often the cause of death today than fifty years ago. While it is possible to control the pain often associated with cancer, the best methods available are not always used. We have all heard stories of persons with terminal cancer who experienced months and sometimes years of excruciating pain before death. A related concern that has elements of both physical and psychological suffering is the deterioration of the body that is sometimes a consequence of a degenerative disease such as cancer. Breasts or limbs are removed, lesions develop that don't heal, and body systems cease to function normally. An individual who has lived an active and vital life can be devastated easily by such events, and for those of us who are presently healthy and vigorous, the thought of such deterioration can be frightening indeed.

Fear of humiliation. This is a more purely psychological fear but it is often born out of physical suffering. It is the fear of becoming a coward in the face of death either because of the physical suffering (e.g., pain) we might experience or because we dread the thought of not existing, of being dead.

Interruption of goals. For some individuals, the thought of death is anxiety-arousing because death will interfere with the achievement of their goals. Length of life is often measured in terms of accomplishments rather than in time. This is particularly true for academics. When asked how long he wants to live, a university professor might reply, long enough to write two more books. More mundane examples can be found in our own personal experiences and the interview protocols reported by Kübler-Ross (1969). Persons who are old or severely ill often talk about living long enough to experience a particular event such as a birthday, wedding, anniversary, and so on. Thus, an individual might become fearful or anxious if he feels that death might deny him the opportunity to achieve certain goals or experience particular events.

Impact on survivors. Another source of death anxiety might be the psychological and economic impact of one's death on emotionally involved survivors. The parent with a large family depending on him or her for economic and emotional support may worry about the impact of his or her death on the children. It could be argued that purchasing life insurance is one way of buying off some of this death anxiety.

Fear of punishment. Religious persons who have a strong belief in an afterlife in which one atones for deeds committed while living may fear the prospect of being punished for misdeeds. As our society continues to become more secularized, however, this source of death anxiety should decline.

Fear of not being. "Man is the only creature who must live with the constant awareness of the possibility and inevitability of nonbeing" (Coleman 1972, p. 71). Unless the individual chooses suicide, he must live with the fact that death will come at some unknown time and place. According to existentialist thinkers, it is this awareness of inevitable death that leads man to existential anxiety—a deep concern over the meaning of life. This concern manifests itself through questions about whether one is leading a fulfilling and authentic life. Viewed from the existential perspective, the idea of nothingness can arouse anxiety so general that it influences our entire lives.

Fear of the death of others. All of the possible sources of fear and anxiety described up to now are reasons why we might fear our own death. However, we may also fear the death of those around us. We may become anxious at the thought of having to experience vicariously the psychological and physical suffering of those close to us. In addition, we might fear the loss of an important relationship. To the extent that we perceive an individual as a source of many of our positive outcomes we should dread that person's death.

Fear and Anxiety

The terms *fear* and *anxiety* have been used here interchangeably. A distinction often made by psychoanalysts is that *fear* is experienced in reference to specific environmental events or objects while *anxiety* is a negative emotional state that lacks a specific object. The apprehension evoked by thoughts of death and dying has properties of both fear and anxiety. There are specific things one can fear, such as the pain and associated psychological suffering. In addition, thinking about death may arouse amorphous and unspecified anxieties about the many unknowns associated

> **. . . thinking about death may arouse amorphous and unspecified anxieties. . . .**

The idea of not being is for some persons incomprehensible and unsettling.

with death: we do not know when, where, or how we will die, or if there is an afterlife. The idea of not being is for some persons incomprehensible and unsettling.

Since specific fears are grounded in the environment, they are amenable to treatment. For example, a person's fear of the pain of dying may be eliminated if he can be assured that appropriate drug therapies will be made available to him should he become terminal. Similarly, the knowledge that dying persons are treated with respect and compassion may reduce the fear of an undignified death. The fact that these fears still exist lends credence to the argument that these are problems in our culture.

Death anxiety is a much stickier problem. Clearly, it is ethically impossible to specify the time, place, and manner of death for most persons. Nor is it possible to convincingly demonstrate what it is like to be dead, although some persons claim to have knowledge of this (see Moody 1976). Most likely we will never be able to do anything about these causes of anxiety. While this anxiety may be a burden, it may also be a great boon to mankind. According to the psychoanalyst Zilboorg (1943), the behaviors and psychological energies invested in self-preservation are products of death anxiety. Most of the time these anxieties are repressed and must remain repressed if we are to function normally, but they exist and, like boiling water in a teakettle, exert their pressures on man's behavior. When the pressures become too great and the kettle boils over, the anxieties manifest themselves in neurotic and psychotic behaviors (Becker 1973; Meyer 1975). Taking this perspective to the extreme, one might argue that many of man's great individual achievements may be attributable to death anxiety. Becker (1973) argues fervently that many of man's heroic achievements represent an attempt to master this anxiety and conquer death. Most of us know persons who are motivated to transcend their physical mortality through their products—the artist who hopes his work will live forever or the politician who wants his accomplishments recorded in history books.

While this view of death anxiety may have some intuitive appeal, little research is available to either refute or support it. Indeed, it may be impossible to test many of these notions using empirical methods. And it can perhaps be argued that some of these ideas were never meant to be tested empirically. Nevertheless, while literature abounds with speculation about the nature and meaning of death, we also have available large quantities of research on death anxiety.

An Empirical Perspective: Death Anxiety Research

Death anxiety has been measured in a variety of populations and settings with a wide assortment of assessment devices ranging from projective techniques (such as the Rorschach and Thematic Apperception Test) to the measurement of galvanic skin response, a physiological correlate of anxiety. It is the aim of this review to bring order to the existing death anxiety literature and direction to the field by critically evaluating the various methods used to assess death anxiety, deriving conclusions warranted by the available data, and suggesting the direction that future research should follow. Before this literature is examined, one qualifier is in order. The distinction between death fear and death anxiety described earlier has not been made by empirical researchers. As a result, the two terms are used interchangeably in the discussion that follows.

Methodological Issues

Both direct and indirect techniques have been used to assess death anxiety. Direct techniques include questionnaires, check lists, and rating scales, while indirect techniques include projective tests, the measurement of galvanic skin response, and reaction times during death-related word association tasks. Direct techniques are by far the more frequently used, and at present there are six widely used death anxiety questionnaires (Boyar 1964; Collett and Lester 1969; Lester 1967a; Sarnoff and Corwin 1959; Templer 1970; and Tolor and Reznikoff 1967). An example of one death anxiety scale is presented in Table 1. After reading each statement, the respondent decides whether a particular statement is true or false for himself. These responses are then coded according to a key, and a death anxiety score is derived.

Only Boyar's (1964) Fear of Death Scale (FODS) and Templer's (1970) Death Anxiety Scale (DAS) have been validated. Validation is a procedure for determining whether a scale measures what it was designed to measure—in this case death anxiety. Exactly how this should be done varies with the type of scale used. Boyar attempted to validate his scale by administering it

Table 1 Templer's Death Anxiety Scale

Content
I am very much afraid to die.
The thought of death seldom enters my mind.
It doesn't make me nervous when people talk about death.
I dread to think about having to have an operation.
I am not at all afraid to die.
I am not particularly afraid of getting cancer.
The thought of death never bothers me.
I am often distressed by the way time flies so very rapidly.
I fear dying a painful death.
The subject of life after death troubles me greatly.
I am really scared of having a heart attack.
I often think about how short life really is.
I shudder when I hear people talking about a World War III.
The sight of a dead body is horrifying to me.
I feel that the future holds nothing for me to fear.

From: D. Templer, The construction and validation of a death anxiety scale, *Journal of General Psychology* 82 (1970): 167.

to subjects before and after viewing a highway accident movie intended to increase their death anxiety. Fear of death scores rose significantly more in the experimental group than in the control group, which saw an innocuous movie. Templer validated his scale both with psychiatric patients in a state mental hospital and with college students. High death anxiety psychiatric patients independently assessed by a clinician were found to have significantly higher DAS scores than control patients. The remaining four scales (Collett and Lester 1969; Lester 1967a; Sarnoff and Corwin 1959; Tolor and Reznikoff 1967) have not been independently validated, although intercorrelations among the scales are high enough to lend each a degree of concurrent validity. Durlak (1972a) found positive intercorrelations ranging from .41 to .65 among five of the scales. He inexplicably omitted Templer's DAS from his study, although Templer (1970) reported a positive .74 correlation between his scale and Boyar's (1964) FODS.

Two remaining scales (Dickstein 1972, 1975; Krieger, Epsting, and Leitner 1974) have neither been validated nor compared to the six scales discussed above. Krieger, Epsting, and Leitner's (1974) "Threat Index" has the interesting feature of being theoretically based but has poor test-retest reliability ($r = .49$ with one of 13 subjects dropped). Test-retest reliability is a measure of the reliability of the scale over time. That is, if an individual completes the same scale at different times, his scores should be very similar even though several months may have passed between the first and second time the scale was administered. This is based on the assumption that the scale measures permanent dispositional characteristics of the individual, which should not vary greatly over time.

Most death anxiety scales treat death anxiety as a unitary concept. This is based on the probably erroneous assumption that death anxiety is a single type of fear or anxiety. The one exception is the Collett and Lester (1969) scale, which is divided into four subscales measuring anxiety over death of self, death of others, dying of self, and dying of others. These subscales are roughly equivalent to the fear of nonbeing and the fear of the process (the pain and suffering) of dying as they apply to oneself and those close to us. Collett and Lester found low intercorrelations among their subscales, especially between the two subscales dealing with self and the two dealing with others, suggesting that death anxiety is a multidimensional concept. An individual may, for example, fear the process of his own dying and not be fearful about the dying process of those close to him. Durlak's (1972a) intercorrelation study showed that other scales correlate best with the death-of-self subscale of Collett and Lester. Many of the inconsistencies in the death anxiety data will probably be clarified once researchers begin paying closer attention to the components of death anxiety instead of treating it as a unitary concept. One such attempt is made below in the section on sex differences, where it is argued that inconsistencies in the literature are resolved when the cognitive and affective components of death anxiety are isolated. The accurate assessment of death anxiety is further complicated by recent findings that the method of administering a death anxiety scale affects reported death anxiety. Schulz, Aderman, and Manko (1976) found significantly lower reported death anxiety among college students on the Templer (1970) and Sarnoff and Corwin (1959) scales when administered individually rather than in group sessions. Death anxiety as measured by a group-administered questionnaire was not significantly different from death anxiety as assessed by the "bogus pipeline method" (Jones and Sigall 1971), in which a fake "emotion monitoring device" is attached to subjects to keep them honest. The rationale underlying the bogus pipeline is that subjects do not want to be second-guessed by a machine, and when asked to predict what the machine says about their attitudes, they respond without many of the social biases that obscure straight paper and pencil measures on sensitive topics. The findings of Schulz, Aderman, and Manko (1976) suggest that there may be a private and public component to death anxiety and that the private attitudes are more likely to be expressed when the respondent is anonymous.

In addition to the problems of the "unitary concept" assumption, death anxiety scales have been criticized by some researchers for their inability to discriminate between private and "unconscious" death anxiety. For example, Fulton (1961) has argued that even with a valid and reliable measuring instrument, a researcher can still only tap the "epiphenomenal" or surface-level attitudes of subjects, while Rheingold (1967) has stated that even the most elegant instrument can measure only public attitudes "passively acquired from culture or religion" (p. 33) and completely miss those attitudes and feelings existing at the unconscious level. In order to delve into the unconscious, according to Rheingold, it is necessary to turn to projective techniques and the intuitive insights of the psychotherapist. It is difficult to argue against such an approach except by pointing out its subjective nature. More objective measurements of unconscious death anxiety are possible by comparing reaction time, recall reaction time, galvanic skin response for death-related and neutral word associations, or through use of the Color-Word Interference Test (Stroop, 1938). Presumably, these indirect techniques assess death anxiety on a level beneath that accessible by questionnaires, although results from such studies must be interpreted with care.

Researchers have assumed that high galvanic skin response or slow reaction time during death-related word association tasks indicate "perceptual defense" and hence death anxiety (Alexander and Adlerstein 1958; Feifel and Branscomb 1973). Using a different indirect technique, Lester and Lester (1970) found that recognition of blurred death-related words was faster than recognition of blurred neutral words. They explained that "perceptual facilitation" makes evolutionary sense since survival requires hasty recognition of threatening stimuli. Since most investigators of unconscious death anxiety use word association rather than recognition tasks, the focus of this research has been on processes of perceptual defense rather than perceptual facilitation.

Another indirect technique is analysis of dream content. Handal and Rychlak (1971) had several judges (inter-rater reliability = .89) classify dreams reported in subjects' morning-after journals as positive, negative, or

> . . . indirect techniques assess death anxiety on a level beneath that accessible by questionnaires. . . .

. . . death anxiety can be tapped at any one of three levels: public, private, and unconscious.

neutral and as death-related or non-death-related. They considered a high frequency of negative and/or death-related dreams to be evidence of unconscious death anxiety.

Taken together, these studies indicate that the measurement of death anxiety is indeed a more complex task than early researchers had anticipated. At present, it appears that death anxiety is not a unitary concept and may be comprised of four or more subcomponents. To complicate matters even further, it appears that death anxiety can be tapped at any one of three levels: public, private, and unconscious. Table 2 shows the three levels crossed by possible subcomponents. Although it is unlikely that each of fifty-seven possible cells can be clearly differentiated operationally, death anxiety researchers should nevertheless be sensitive to the complexity of their task, if confusion is to be avoided in the future.

Demographic and Personality Correlates of Death Anxiety
Though many variables have been found to relate to death anxiety, few clear and consistent patterns have emerged. The search for such patterns in the data is reviewed below.

Sex. Although several early studies yielded no systematic sex-related differences in death anxiety (Christ 1961; Rhudick and Dibner 1961; Swenson 1961; Jeffers, Nichols, and Eisdorfer 1961), it now appears fairly certain that, on the level assessed by questionnaires, females fear death more than males. Templer's (1970) DAS has been administered to samples of apartment residents, hospital aides, psychiatric patients, ninth graders, and high school students and their parents (Templer, Ruff, and Franks 1971; Iammarino 1975), and in all cases females scored higher than males. This finding was replicated by several other researchers.

Table 2 Specific death fears by different assessment methods

Specific Fears Relating to Death of Self*	Level of Assessment		
	Public	Private	Unconscious
Pain			
Body misfunction			
Humiliation			
Rejection			
Nonbeing			
Punishment			
Interruption of goals			
Negative impact on survivors			
a. psychological suffering of survivors			
b. economic hardship			

*All these fears can be experienced vicariously in relation to the death of someone close to us. In addition, the fear of abandonment can be experienced directly.

Only when death anxiety is broken up into its components do researchers find any evidence of a greater fear of death among males. According to Thematic Apperception Test (TAT) responses, males have more fear of the effects of their death on dependents (Diggory and Rothman 1961) and more fear of the violence of death (Lowry 1965). In contrast, women show more fear of the dissolution of the body and the physical pain associated with death (Diggory and Rothman 1961).

Degner (1974) identified two clusters of responses to the concept of death by having subjects fill out 36 semantic differential scales. Among males she found an "evaluative" dimension to be strongest and an "emotional" dimension to be weakest. In an earlier study, Folta (in Degner 1974) found the reverse to be true for women. These studies suggest that there may be a cognitive and emotional component to death anxiety, with women viewing death in more emotional terms and men viewing death in more cognitive terms.

Consistent with these findings is the preliminary work of Krieger, Epsting, and Leitner (1974) with their Threat Index, a scale that measures death anxiety by measuring the "cognitive distance" subjects place between the concepts "death" and "self." Males tend to have higher death anxiety scores than females—a finding directly contrary to that obtained when Lester's Death Anxiety Scale is used. Since the Threat Index is a cognitive measure and Lester's Death Anxiety Scale is a more affective one, these results, and those of Degner and Folta, can be understood if it is accepted that male death anxiety tends to be cognitive and female death anxiety more emotional. Further support for the existence of these two components of death anxiety is the lack of correlation between Lester's affective Death Anxiety Scale and the more cognitive Threat Index (Krieger, Epsting, and Leitner 1974) and also the lack of correlation between Lester's Death Anxiety Scale and Boyar's FODS, which is also supposedly a more "cognitive" scale (Krieger, Epsting, and Leitner 1974; Berman & Hays 1973). Finally, Krieger et al. reported a very high positive ($+.73$) correlation ($p < .01$) between the two cognitive scales: the Threat Index and Boyar's FODS. In summary, these findings suggest that researchers who use affectively oriented death anxiety scales will find higher death anxiety among females than males while the reverse is likely to be true when cognitively oriented death anxiety scales are used.

Age. Although most of the death anxiety data have been collected from college students and the aged, there is some pertinent data available for every age group, from infants to the very old. Hall and Scott (in Hall 1922) attempted to assess death concern in children by asking adults to recall their earliest experiences with death. Using this retrospective technique, they concluded that the young child's view of death is characterized by specific objects and feelings associated with a specific death. A more informative study on children's views of death was conducted by Nagy (1959), who directly interviewed 378 boys and girls three to ten years old. Nagy's results yielded three relatively discrete developmental phases: for ages three to five, death

> . . . for ages three to five, death is seen as a temporary departure or sleep. . . .

is seen as a temporary departure or sleep; for ages five to nine, death is seen as final and is personified as either a separate person or the dead person himself; beyond nine years of age, children recognize death as not only final, but also inevitable. Nagy's data suggest that the association between death and anxiety is established as early as three years of age, when death is viewed as separation.

According to Rothstein (in Kastenbaum and Aisenberg 1972), death anxiety is relatively low throughout young adulthood until the middle adult years. Relying on extensive interview data, he found that death anxiety peaks in the middle years. This is especially true for men, perhaps because this is the first time men become aware of their own vulnerability as a result of deaths among friends and acquaintances their age. Contrary to Rothstein's findings, Feifel and Branscomb (1973) found that subjects over the age of fifty tended to answer "no" to the question, "Are you afraid of your own death?" more frequently than younger subjects. On the other hand, a study by Templer, Ruff, and Franks (1971) yielded results contrary to both Rothstein and Feifel and Branscomb. Testing over 2,000 subjects of various ages, they found no significant correlation between age and death anxiety scores.

This discrepancy in findings remains unresolved and is further complicated by a study of death anxiety at the unconscious level. Feifel and Branscomb (1973) found that the same elderly subjects who reported below-average overt death anxiety exhibited unconscious death anxiety that was just as high as that of younger subjects. Corey (1961) similarly found that older adults tend to show avoidance of death in projective tests. While no explanation can account for all these data, they can perhaps in part be understood if it is assumed that people are more likely to deny their fears as death becomes a more immediate threat. Researchers frequently invoke the concept of denial to explain low death anxiety scores in populations such as the aged, who because of their nearness to death are expected to have high death anxiety. Unless other corroborating data are available, such interpretations of low scores are unjustified. Individuals who score low in death anxiety just may not be very concerned with death, regardless of their temporal nearness to death. The study by Feifel and Branscomb (1973) is one example of a study where a denial interpretation can be entertained. The relative discrepancy between overt death anxiety and unconscious death anxiety in the same population of elderly subjects could be the result of denial influencing the expression of overt death fears.

Physical health. Evidence on the relationship between health and death anxiety follows a pattern similar to that of death anxiety and age. There is conflicting evidence on overt death anxiety and a possibility of denial among subjects most threatened by impending death. Lucas (1974) studied 60 hemodialysis and surgery patients and did not find their DAS scores to be significantly different from the normal mean scores reported by Templer (1970). Templer, however, found a significant negative correlation between scores on the DAS and a measure of physical health, indicating that the higher an individual's death anxiety, the lower his physical health status. Swenson (1961) suggested that people who are unhealthy might look forward to ending it all and so fear death less than the healthy. His finding that individuals in poor health tended to look forward to death more than fear it supports this view, although his sample included only aged individuals. Feifel and his colleagues (Feifel 1974; Feifel, Freilich, and Hermann 1973) found that terminally ill patients reported fearing death no more frequently than other subjects but demonstrated higher death anxiety on an unconscious level. Kübler-Ross (1969) reports some impressionistic data based on interviews with 200 terminal patients. She found that although patients experience a great deal of shock and anxiety when first informed of their terminality, most patients eventually came to accept their impending deaths. In a review of the literature on the feelings and attitudes of dying patients, Schulz and Aderman (1974) concluded that the predominant response of most terminal patients is depression rather than anxiety shortly before death. In sum, there is little evidence that persons closer to death, because of their health status, exhibit greater overt death anxiety than their healthy counterparts, and there is no evidence to suggest that extraordinary denial processes are operating in these populations.

In general, the link between belief in afterlife and religiosity has been amply demonstrated.

Religiosity.   While Lester's review (1967a) reported considerable confusion on the relationship between religious beliefs and death anxiety, recent findings have been refreshingly clear. It is possible that the disparate results from earlier studies (e.g., Faunce & Fulton 1958; Kalish 1963) are attributable to different conceptualizations of religiosity. Indicators of extrinsic religiosity (frequency of church attendance) might result in a positive relationship between religiosity and death anxiety, but religiosity measured in terms of fundamental values might produce the reverse relationship. Recent studies show that degree of religiosity (measured by self-report of beliefs and churchgoing) is unrelated to death anxiety for the general population (Feifel 1974; Kalish 1963; Templer 1970) but is negatively related when subjects are religiously involved (Templer 1972a; Shearer 1973). That is, for Templer's sample, which included many ministers, religiosity was correlated with low levels of death anxiety.

Belief in afterlife has been suggested as an intervening variable reducing death anxiety for highly religious people. Jeffers, Nichols, and Eisdorfer (1961) found that individuals with strong religious commitments were more likely to believe in afterlife and also showed less fear of death than less religiously committed persons. Osarchuck and Tatz (1973) found that for subjects scoring high in a Belief in Afterlife Scale, a death-threatening slide show induced still greater belief in an afterlife. In general, the link between belief in afterlife and religiosity has been amply demonstrated. Osarchuck and Tatz (1973) and Kalish (1963) reported that active Protestants and Catholics had higher belief in afterlife when compared to religiously inactive persons of any faith. The other link—the relationship between belief in afterlife and death anxiety, independent of degree of religiosity—is in need of further study.

. . . suicidal individuals have lower death anxiety than comparable nonsuicidal populations.

Emotional disorders. Research on the death anxiety of psychiatric patients is inconsistent. Brodman, Erdman, and Wolff (1956) and Templer (1971a) found psychiatric illness positively associated with high death anxiety. Similarly, Templer and Ruff (1971) reported above average DAS means for samples of psychiatric patients. However, contradictory findings are reported by Feifel and Hermann (1973). Using a wide range of death anxiety measurement devices, they found no differences between the death anxiety of mentally ill and normal subjects. They also found degree of mental illness to be unrelated to death anxiety.

Working with samples of "normals" from the general public, Templer (1970, 1972a) reported small positive correlations between Templer's DAS and the neuroticism scales of the Eysenck Personality Inventory and the Welsh Anxiety scale, respectively. Other scales of general anxiety correlate similarly with the DAS (Templer 1970; Lucas 1974), as does the Minnesota Multiphasic Personality Inventory (MMPI) depression scale (Templer 1971a). Using projective measures, Rhudick and Dibner (1961) found significant positive correlations between death concern and four MMPI scales of neurotic preoccupation. These findings indicate that death anxiety shares features with more general forms of anxiety, neurosis, and depression. While it is important not to ignore this aspect of death anxiety, it is also important to note that Templer (1970) reports data suggesting that death anxiety is a concept distinct from general anxiety. The intercorrelations among various death anxiety scales are consistently and significantly higher than their correlations with general anxiety.

It might be expected that people who attempt suicide would fear death less than the general population. Lester (1967a) found this to be the case when he administered his and Boyar's (1964) FODS to attempters and threateners of suicide and compared their scores to those of subjects who never considered suicide. Similarly, Tarter, Templer, and Perley (1974) found a significant correlation between the DAS and the judged "potential for rescue" following the act of attempted suicide. One possible interpretation of these data is that those who fear death less are more serious about acting on their suicidal desires. The only evidence contrary to these findings comes from an unpublished study carried out by Lester and reported in his review (1967a). He found that suicide-threateners fear death more than suicide-contemplators, who in turn fear death more than those who have never considered taking their lives; Lester admits this evidence is weak because of the small sample studied. The best conclusion is that suicidal individuals have lower death anxiety than comparable nonsuicidal populations.

Need for achievement, sense of competence, and purpose. At least three hypotheses have been generated relating need for achievement, sense of competence, and sense of purpose in life to death anxiety: (1) individuals with high need for achievement (nAch) will fear death more because it ends their chance for further achievement (Diggory and Rothman 1961); (2) individuals with a high sense of competence will fear death less because they are satisfied with their lives (Goodman 1975); and (3) persons with low fear of death will have a greater purpose in life because a crucial step in developing the latter is confronting death without fear (Frankl 1965).

Two studies (Nogas, Schweitzer, and Grumet 1974; Ray and Najman 1974) investigated the first hypothesis and failed to find a relationship between nAch and death anxiety, although Ray and Najman pointed out that the undergraduate samples used were too high in need for achievement to provide a sufficiently wide range of scores. The second hypothesis was partially supported by Nogas, Schweitzer, and Grumet (1974), who found a significant negative correlation between death anxiety and sense of competence. The data may indicate, however, that sense of competence includes competence in confronting death. The third hypothesis is supported by convincingly high negative correlations (ranging from $-.54$ to $-.82$) between overt death anxiety and Crumbaugh and Maholick's (1964) Purpose in Life Test (Blazer 1973; Durlak 1972b, 1973). Ignoring the fact that correlations say little about causality or about direction of causality, Blazer and Durlak suggest that children taught to accept death will become adults with more meaning in their lives.

Cognitive style. A provocative study by Mishara, Baker, and Kostin (1972) indicated that college students differing in cognitive style hold different attitudes toward death. Cognitive style was determined by the Kinesthetic Figural After-effects task, which classifies subjects as "augmenters" if they overestimate the width of a wooden block held between their fingers after holding a wider "intervening stimulus" block. Subjects who underestimate the block's width after the intervening stimulus are classified as "reducers." Augmenters tend to magnify stimulus intensity; they tend to be more comfortable with stimulus deprivation and less comfortable with aversive stimuli. When asked to imagine the final year of their lives, augmenters avoided mentioning death (presumably an aversive stimulus) significantly more than reducers. While no death anxiety scale was administered in this study, these data suggest that augmenters have higher death anxiety than reducers.

This attempt to link death anxiety to cognitive functioning is a refreshing change from the usual pattern of relating death anxiety to other questionnaire measures.

Other variables. A host of other variables have been researched as possible correlates of death anxiety. No significant correlations were found for the following variables: projective measures of fear of failure (Cohen & Parker 1974); a dependency scale (Selvey 1973); guilt about hostility (Selvey 1973); race (Pandey 1974; Pandey and Templer 1972); and Eysenck's Extraversion Scale (Templer 1972b). Three of four studies relating death anx-

> . . . college students differing in cognitive style hold different attitudes toward death.

. . . the concept of denial has been invoked to explain the lack of increased death anxiety scores among dying subjects.

iety to Rotter's I–E locus of control scale reported no relationship (Selvey 1973; Dickstein 1972; Berman 1973); only Tolor and Reznikoff (1967) found a significant relationship between Rotter's I–E scale and death anxiety. Externally oriented subjects had significantly greater death anxiety than subjects with internal orientations.

Denial of Death Anxiety

The idea that death anxiety can exist at both the conscious and unconscious level has been a theme throughout this chapter. While researchers have occasionally found consistencies between self-reported and unconscious death anxiety, more often than not the two are discrepant. When such discrepancies occur, researchers typically invoke the concept of repression, or denial, of death anxiety to explain these findings.

Handal and Rychlak (1971) found a much higher proportion of negative and death-related dreams among subjects scoring high or low on self-report death anxiety scales than among those with moderate scores. They concluded that many of those with low conscious death anxiety were denying their deeper fears. Feifel and his colleagues (Feifel and Branscomb 1973; Feifel and Hermann 1973) concluded that death anxiety is greater at unconscious than at conscious levels, especially for aged and unhealthy subjects. For this reason, the concept of denial has been invoked to explain the lack of increased death anxiety scores among dying subjects. Similarly, the failure to find a relationship between death anxiety and contact with death may be attributed to the exclusive use of conscious death anxiety measures in these studies.

Other evidence of denial of death anxiety makes use of Byrne's (1964) Repression-Sensitization scale. Subjects who tend to repress threats (according to the Repression-Sensitization scale) also tend to be low in conscious death anxiety as measured by the DAS (Templer 1971b). Templer found no evidence for the relationship between Repression-Sensitization score and unconscious death anxiety. Apparently repressors, while low in conscious death anxiety, are not high in unconscious death anxiety either.

Templer (1971b) also found a .30 correlation between DAS and unconscious death anxiety as measured by a galvanic skin response to death-related stimulus material. This moderately positive correlation suggests that the two levels of death anxiety are not totally independent.

Donaldson (1972) argues that operational and theoretical definitions of denial must be determined before conclusions are drawn about its existence. The discrepancies between conscious and unconscious death anxiety found in the research reviewed above represent a step in this direction. Research employing discrepancy between conscious and unconscious death anxiety as a variable and searching for its correlates appears promising. The internal dynamics resulting from disharmony between different levels of a person's attitudes toward death may prove to be more important than death anxiety itself.

Environmental Influences on Death Anxiety

Three classes of environmental variables are found in the literature. Researchers have examined the effects of educational intervention, contact with death, and the impact of the family on death anxiety. Lucas (1974) and Templer, Ruff, and Franks (1971) reported high correlations ($r = .59$) between spouses' DAS scores; child-parent correlations were less ($r = .40$) but tended to be somewhat higher when the two are of the same sex. Although these data say nothing about the relative importance of environment and genetics as determinants of death anxiety, they do support the notion that the environment, through parents' influence, affects death anxiety (Templer, Ruff, and Franks 1971).

Lester and Templer (1972) found a striking developmental trend in child-parent correlations. During adolescence, daughter-parent DAS correlations decreased steadily and were statistically insignificant by age eighteen or nineteen. No explanation is offered for the apparent tendency for adolescent boys to continue to be influenced by their parents while their sisters are cutting the death anxiety apron strings. Another finding of family influence was reported by Iammarino (1975). Ninth-graders living with only one parent feared death more than their two-parent peers. This could be interpreted as evidence that separation anxiety can be an antecedent of death anxiety. More generally, this serves to demonstrate the effect of family environment on death anxiety.

Since death anxiety has been shown to be a socially influenced phenomenon, one might expect it to respond to direct intervention. However, attempts to verify the success of intervention, in the form of nursing curricula and college courses, have met with mixed success. Nurses nearing graduation accept death more than students earlier in their training (Yeaworth, Kapp, and Winget 1974). Their death anxiety is lower (Lester, Getty, and Kneisl 1974), and thoughts of death are less frequent (Snyder, Gertler, and Ferneau 1973). With the exception of Lester and his colleagues, most researchers attribute the changes in death anxiety to the nursing curriculum, ignoring alternative explanations such as contact with patients. All that can be concluded with certainty is that something in a nursing student's experience reduces death anxiety.

Several specific "death education" programs have been evaluated, but only one caused a significant reduction in death anxiety. Murray (1974) found nurses' DAS scores significantly reduced after a six-week course. It is possible that the practical work of the students interacted with the program to lessen death anxiety, since courses for college students have not been found to change death anxiety significantly (Bell 1975; Leviton 1973; Wittmaier 1975).

While death education courses will certainly continue in colleges and nursing schools, an indirect approach to lessening death anxiety was shown to be effective by Templer, Ruff, and Simpson (1974). They evaluated the death anxiety of subjects before and after therapy dealing exclusively with

> **. . . adolescent boys . . . continue to be influenced by their parents while their sisters are cutting the death anxiety apron strings.**

reduction of depression. DAS scores declined significantly along with depression, demonstrating that depression and death anxiety covary to some extent.

In spite of many attempts, no study has shown that contact with death or with high-risk situations influences death anxiety. Self-report of previous death-threatening experiences is unrelated to death anxiety (Durlak 1973; Berman 1974). Nurses' death anxiety is not related to the patient death rate on their unit (Shusterman and Sechrest 1973) or within their area of specialization (Lester, Getty, and Kneisl 1974). Parachute jumpers (Alexander and Lester 1972) and widows (Kalish and Reynolds 1974; Rhudick and Dibner 1961) score no higher than controls on death scales, although Swenson (1961) found that widows tend to deny their death anxiety when direct methods are used. The mixed pattern of results obtained on environmental determinants of death anxiety is most likely attributable to the lack of conceptual and methodological rigor in designing and executing research in this area. Researchers should know at what level death anxiety is being assessed and should be sensitive to possible confounding variables when carrying out their research.

Future Research

This review of the death anxiety literature suggests that future research should move in three directions. First, researchers should be sensitive to the multidimensionality of death anxiety. Much of the confusion of past research may be avoided by recognizing that death anxiety is comprised of several independent components, each of which can be tapped at a public, private, and unconscious level. An immediate goal should be the investigation of the various subcomponents of death anxiety. Some components— such as anxiety over nonexistence and the anxiety over the process of dying (that is, the humiliation, pain, and suffering) in relation to self and others— have been identified. Other components might include anxiety about the impact of one's death on survivors and about having one's plans interrupted.

A second endeavor should be the untangling of discrepancies between conscious and unconscious death anxiety. The consequences of this discrepancy may eventually prove more interesting and important than simple death anxiety per se. One perspective on this problem is presented in a recent excellent review of the psychological death literature by Kastenbaum and Costa (1977). These authors suggest that fear of death and death anxiety are two different and independent phenomenon. Thus, an individual may be high on specific fears associated with death and yet exhibit little death anxiety. Viewed from this perspective, there is no reason to expect a consistent relationship between conscious and unconscious death anxiety. At any rate, further attempts at enlarging the list of paper-and-pencil correlates of death anxiety appear to be of little use in understanding or demonstrating its relevance to human behavior.

Third, an effort should be made to demonstrate the functional or behavioral consequences of death anxiety. One such example is Templer's (1972b) study of death anxiety in smokers. Templer found that while nonsmokers and smokers did not differ in death anxiety, smokers with high death anxiety tended to smoke less. Another example is Kastenbaum and Briscoe's (1975) study of street-crossing behavior. The authors demonstrated the feasibility of relating naturalistically observed behavior to unobserved psychosocial variables: they found strong relationships between risk-taking in street-crossing and suicidal tendencies, marital status, and desired and expected life span.

Schulz and Aderman (1977) investigated the relationship between physicians' death anxiety and the length of their patients' survival in the hospital. It was hypothesized that a physician high in death anxiety would be less willing to admit that his patients were terminal and therefore more likely to use heroic measures to keep them alive. Thus, these patients should survive longer once admitted to the hospital than the terminal patients of physicians with low death anxiety.

To test this hypothesis, 27 physicians at a community hospital were told that the researcher was calling a variety of professional people as part of an attitude survey that dealt with attitudes toward death. After explaining that they were to indicate their agreement or disagreement using a scale from -3 to $+3$, the following five statements (Sarnoff and Corwin 1959) were read to each physician:

1. I tend to worry about the death toll when I travel on highways.
2. I find it difficult to face up to the ultimate fact of death.
3. Many people become disturbed at the sight of a new grave, but it does not bother me.
4. I find the preoccupation with death at funerals upsetting.
5. I am disturbed when I think of the shortness of life.

The 27 physicians interviewed were divided into three groups reflecting degree of death anxiety: high ($n = 8$), medium ($n = 7$), and low ($n = 9$). Their hospital records were examined to determine the number of patients each physician treated, the number that died, and the average length of stay in the hospital of dying patients and nondying patients. The relevant data are presented in Table 3.

The length of stay for dying patients varied directly as a function of the physicians' death anxiety. Patients of physicians with high death anxiety were in the hospital an average of 14.49 days before dying while patients treated by physicians of medium and low death anxiety were in the hospital 9.98 and 8.45 days, respectively. One possible interpretation of these data is that physicians with high death anxiety admit terminal patients earlier and/or are more likely to use heroic measures to keep them alive. Table 3 also shows that the nondying patients do not differ as to length of stay in the hospital as a function of their physicians' death anxiety. The percent of deaths per group of physicians also does not vary as a function of level of death anxiety. Taken together these data suggest that death anxiety may

Table 3 Average stay in hospital of dying and nondying patients and percent of total patients who died (by level of death anxiety of attending physicians)

	Level of Death Anxiety of Attending Physicians		
	High (n = 8)	Medium (n = 7)	Low (n = 9)
Average stay of dying patients (in days)*	14.49	9.98	8.45
Average stay of nondying patients (in days)	11.20	9.76	10.46
Percent of total patients treated who died	3.25	5.32	3.32

*$F(2,22) = 3.52, p < .05$

affect a physician's policy regarding the treatment of terminal patients. These data are only correlational, and much additional information would be necessary to substantiate this hypothesis.

This experiment represents one way of relating death anxiety to some specific behavioral outcomes. To the extent that death anxiety can be related to and influence an individual's functioning, the pursuit of this concept should become a useful and important endeavor.

Conclusion

Thinking about death has been one of man's major preoccupations. Many early speculations were based on intuition and individual case studies and yielded a rich and complex perspective on what it is that man fears about death and how these fears affect his functioning. Some researchers (Becker 1973; Meyer 1975; Zilboorg 1943) have used this perspective to argue that death anxiety has been the inspiration for many great individual achievements. Turning to the empirical studies of the relationship between death anxiety and a multitude of other variables, we found the existing empirical approach to be somewhat simplistic. Death anxiety does not appear to be a unidimensional concept. Instead, it appears to have many components, each of which can be assessed at different levels. However, recent research shows signs of tapping into the richness of this topic.

References

Alexander, I. E., and A. M. Adlerstein. 1958. Affective responses to the concept of death in a population of children and early adolescents. *Journal of Genetic Psychology* 93:167–77.

Alexander, M., and D. Lester. 1972. Fear of death in parachute jumpers. *Perceptual and Motor Skills* 34:338.

Becker, E. 1973. *The Denial of Death.* New York: Free Press.

Bell, W. 1975. The experimental manipulation of death attitudes: A preliminary investigation. *Omega: Journal of Death and Dying* 6:199–205.

Berman, A. 1974. Belief in afterlife, religion, religiosity, and life-threatening experiences. *Omega: Journal of Death and Dying* 5:127.

————. 1973. Smoking behavior: How is it related to locus of control, death anxiety, and belief in afterlife. *Omega: Journal of Death and Dying* 4:149-55.

Berman, A., and J. E. Hays. 1973. Relationship between death anxiety, belief in afterlife and locus of control. *Journal of Consulting and Clinical Psychology* 41:318.

Blazer, J. 1973. The relationship between meaning in life and fear of death. *Psychology* 10:33-4.

Boyar, J. I. 1964. "The construction and partial validation of a scale for the measurement of fear of death." Unpublished doctoral dissertation, University of Rochester, Rochester, New York.

Brodman, K., A. Erdman, and H. Wolff, 1956. *Manual for the Cornell Medical Index*. Ithaca, New York: Cornell University Medical College.

Byrne, D. 1964. Repression-sensitization as a dimension of personality. In B. A. Maher (ed.), *Progress in Experimental Personality Research, vol. 1*. New York: Academic Press.

Caldwell, D., and B. L. Mishara. 1972. Research on attitudes of medical doctors toward the dying patient: A methodological problem. *Omega: Journal of Death and Dying* 3:341-46.

Christ, P. E. I. 1961. Attitudes toward death among a group of acute geriatric psychiatric patients. *Journal of Gerontology* 16:56-59.

Cohen, R., and O. Parker. 1974. Fear of failure and death. *Psychological Reports* 34:54.

Coleman, J. C. 1972. *Abnormal Psychology and Modern Life*. Glenview, Illinois: Scott Foresman and Co.

Collett, L. and D. Lester. 1969. Fear of death and fear of dying. *Journal of Psychology* 72:179-81.

Corey, L. G. 1961. An analogue of resistance to death awareness. *Journal of Gerontology* 16:59-60.

Crumbaugh, J. C., and L. T. Maholick. 1964. An experimental study in existentialism: The psychometric approach to Frankl's concept of noogenic neurosis. *Journal of Clinical Psychology* 20:200-207.

Degner, L. 1974. The relationship between some beliefs held by physicians and their life-prolonging decisions. *Omega: Journal of Death and Dying* 5:223.

Dickstein, L. 1972. Death concern: Measurement and correlates. *Psychological Reports* 30:563-71.

————. 1975. Self-report and fantasy correlates of death concern. *Psychological Reports* 32:147-58.

Diggory, J. C., and D. Z. Rothman. 1961. Values destroyed by death. *Journal of Abnormal and Social Psychology* 63:205-10.

Donaldson, P. J. 1972. Denying death: A note regarding some ambiguities in the current discussion. *Omega: Journal of Death and Dying* 3:285-90.

Durlak, J. 1972a. Measurement of the fear of death: An examination of some existing scales. *Journal of Clinical Psychology* 28:545-47.

————. 1972b. Relationship between individual attitudes toward life and death. *Journal of Consulting and Clinical Psychology* 38:463.

————. 1973. Relationship between various measures of death concern and fear of death. *Journal of Consulting and Clinical Psychology* 41:162.

Faunce, W. A., and R. L. Fulton. 1958. The sociology of death: A neglected area of research. *Social Forces* 36:205-9.

Feifel, H. 1974. Religious conviction and fear of death among the healthy and the terminally ill. *Journal for the Scientific Study of Religion* 13:353-60.

Feifel, H., and A. Branscomb. 1973. Who's afraid of death? *Journal of Abnormal Psychology* 81:282-88.

Feifel, H., and L. Hermann. 1973. Fear of death in the mentally ill. *Psychological Reports* 33:931-38.

Feifel, H., J. Freilich, and L. Hermann. 1973. Death fear in dying heart and cancer patients. *Journal of Psychosomatic Research* 17:161-66.

Frankl, V. E. 1965. *The Doctor and the Soul*. New York: Knopf.

Fulton, R. 1961. Discussion of a symposium on attitudes toward death in older persons. *Journal of Gerontology* 16:44-66.

Goodman, L. 1975. Winning the race with death, fear of death and creativity. Symposium, American Psychological Association Convention, Chicago, Illinois.

Hall, G. S. 1922. *Senescence*. New York: Appleton.

Handal, P. J., and J. F. Rychlak. 1971. Curvilinearity between dream content and death anxiety and the relationship of death anxiety to repression-sensitization. *Journal of Abnormal Psychology* 77:11-16.

Iammarino, N. K. 1975. Relationship between death anxiety and demographic variables. *Psychological Reports* 17:262.

Jeffers, F. C., C. R. Nichols, and C. Eisdorfer. 1961. Attitudes of older persons to death. *Journal of Gerontology* 16:53–56.

Jones, E. E., and H. Sigall. 1971. The bogus pipeline: A new paradigm for measuring affect and attitude. *Psychological Bulletin* 76:349–64.

Kalish, R.A. 1963. Some variables in death attitudes. *Journal of Social Psychology* 59:137–45.

Kalish, R., and D. Reynolds. 1974. Widows view death. *Omega: Journal of Death and Dying* 5:187.

Kastenbaum, R., and R. Aisenberg. 1972. *The Psychology of Death.* New York: Springer.

Kastenbaum, R., and L. Briscoe. 1975. The street corner: A laboratory for the study of life-threatening behavior. *Omega: Journal of Death and Dying* 6:33.

Kastenbaum, R., and P.T. Costa. 1977. Psychological perspectives on death. In M. R. Rosenzweig and L. W. Porter (eds.). *Annual Review of Psychology* 8:225–49.

Krieger, S., F. Epsting, and L. M. Leitner. 1974. Personal constructs, threat, and attitudes toward death. *Omega: Journal of Death and Dying* 5:299.

Kübler-Ross, E. 1969. *On Death and Dying.* New York: Macmillan.

Lester, D. 1967a. Experimental and correlational studies of the fear of death. *Psychological Bulletin* 67:27–36.

———. 1967b. Fear of death of suicide persons. *Psychological Reports* 20:1077–78.

———. 1971. Sex differences in attitudes toward death: A replication. *Psychological Reports* 28:754.

———. 1972. Studies in death attitudes. *Psychological Reports* 30:440.

Lester, D., C. Getty, and C. Kneisl. 1974. Attitudes of nursing students and nursing faculty toward death. *Nursing Research* 23:50–53.

Lester, D., and G. Lester. 1970. Fear of death, fear of dying, and threshold differences for death words and neutral words. *Omega: Journal of Death and Dying* 1:175–79.

Lester, D., and D. Templer. 1972. Resemblance of parent-child death anxiety as a function of age and sex of child. *Psychological Reports* 31:750.

Leviton, D. 1973. Death education and change in students' attitudes. *Final Research Report,* National Institute of Mental Health Research Grant MH 21974–01. Washington, D.C.

Lowry, R. 1965. Male-female differences in attitudes toward death. Doctoral dissertation, Brandeis University.

Lucas, R. 1974. A comparative study of measures of general anxiety and death anxiety among three medical groups including patient and wife. *Omega: Journal of Death and Dying* 5:233.

Meyer, J. E. 1975. *Death and Neurosis.* New York: International Universities Press.

Mishara, B., H. Baker, and I. Kostin. 1972. Do people who seek less environmental stimulation avoid thinking about the future and their death? Proceedings of the Annual Convention of the American Psychological Association 7:667–68.

Moody, R. A. 1975. *Life after Life.* Atlanta: Mockingbird Books.

Murray, P. 1974. Death education and its effect on the death anxiety level of nurses. *Psychological Reports* 35:1250.

Nagy, M. 1959. The child's view of death. In H. Feifel (ed.), *The Meaning of Death.* New York: McGraw-Hill.

Nogas, C., K. Schweitzer, and J. Grumet. 1974. An investigation of death anxiety, sense of competence, and need for achievement. *Omega: Journal of Death and Dying* 5:245.

Osarchuck, M., and S. Tatz. 1973. Effect of induced fear of death on belief in afterlife. *Journal of Personality and Social Psychology* 27:256–60.

Pandey, R. E. 1974–75. Factor analytic study of attitudes toward death among college students. *International Journal of Social Psychiatry* 21:7–11.

Pandey, R. E., and D. Templer. 1972. Use of the death anxiety scale in an inter-racial setting. *Omega: Journal of Death and Dying* 3:127–30.

Ray, J. J., and J. Najman. 1974. Death anxiety and death acceptance: A preliminary approach. *Omega: Journal of Death and Dying* 5:311.

Rheingold, J. C. 1967. *The Mother, Anxiety, and Death.* Boston: Little Brown.

Rhudick, P. J., and A. S. Dibner. 1961. Age, personality and health correlates of death concern in normal aged individuals. *Journal of Gerontology* 16:44–49.

Sarnoff, I., and S. M. Corwin. 1959. Castration anxiety and the fear of death. *Journal of Personality* 27:374–85.

Schulz, R., and D. Aderman. 1974. Clinical research and the stages of dying. *Omega: Journal of Death and Dying* 5:137–43.

———. 1977. Physicians' death anxiety and survival of patients. Unpublished manuscript.

Schulz, R., D. Aderman, and G. Manko. 1976. Attitudes toward death: The effects of different methods of questionnaire administration. Paper presented at the meeting of the Eastern Psychological Association, New York, April.

Selvey, C. 1973. Concerns about death in relation to sex, dependency, guilt about hostility, and feelings of powerlessness. *Omega: Journal of Death and Dying* 4:209–19.

Shearer, R. E. 1973. Religious belief and attitudes toward death. *Dissertation Abstracts International* 33:3292–93.

Shusterman, L., and L. Sechrest. 1973. Attitudes of RNs toward death in a general hospital. *Psychiatry in Medicine* 4:411–26.

Snyder, M., R. Gertler, and E. Ferneau. 1973. Changes in nursing students' attitudes toward death and dying: A measurement of curriculum integration effectiveness. *International Journal of Social Psychiatry* 19:294–98.

Stroop, J. R. 1938. Factors affecting speed in serial verbal reactions. *Psychological Monographs* 50:38–48.

Swenson, W. M. 1961. Attitudes toward death in an aged population. *Journal of Gerontology* 16:49–52.

Tarter, R., D. Templer, and R. Perley. 1974. Death anxiety in suicide attempters. *Psychological Reports* 34:895–97.

Templer, D. 1970. The construction and validation of a death anxiety scale. *Journal of General Psychology* 82:165–77.

———. 1971a. The relationship between verbalized and nonverbalized death anxiety. *Journal of Genetic Psychology* 119:211–14.

———. 1971b. Death anxiety as related to depression and health of retired persons. *Journal of Gerontology* 26:521–23.

———. 1972a. Death anxiety in religiously very involved persons. *Psychological Reports* 31:361–62.

———. 1972b. Death anxiety: Extraversion, neuroticism, and cigarette smoking. *Omega: Journal of Death and Dying* 3:53–56.

Templer, D., and C. Ruff. 1971. Death anxiety scale means, standard deviations, and embedding. *Psychological Reports* 29:173–74.

Templer, D., C. Ruff, and C. Franks. 1971. Death anxiety: Age, sex and parental resemblance in diverse populations. *Developmental Psychology* 4:108.

Templer, D., C. Ruff, and K. Simpson. 1974. Alleviation of high death anxiety with symptomatic treatment of depression. *Psychological Reports* 35:216.

Tolor, A., and M. Reznikoff. 1967. Relationship between insight, repression-sensitization, internal-external control, and death anxiety. *Journal of Abnormal Psychology* 72:426–30.

Wittmaier, B. 1975. The impact of a death course. Unpublished manuscript, Kirkland College, New York.

Yeaworth, R., F. Kapp, and C. Winget. 1974. Attitudes of nursing students toward the dying patient. *Nursing Research* 23:20–24.

Zilboorg, G. 1943. Fear of death. *Psychoanalytic Quarterly* 12:465–75.

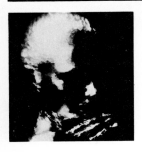

7

Research

What would you say to a child whose pet dog has just died? Or perhaps a parent? How do you think children would respond to the following questions? What makes things die? How do you make dead things come back to life? When will you die? What will happen then? Gerald Koocher has explored these questions with children and reports his findings below. The following Appendix exercises may be appropriate at the completion of your reading:

      E.   Confronting the Realization of Death

      I.   Life and Death Attitudes

Talking with Children about Death

Gerald P. Koocher

Many volumes have been written on the meaning of death, and its psychological concomitants. Many authors have attempted to describe the ways in which man learns about death and tries to cope with this universal phenomenon. Most of the recent literature on death and dying tends to focus on those confronting their own death, or those attempting to cope with the loss of people close to them. These works focus on adults for the most part, and are thus subject to a common fallacy that goes something like this: "Children look like grown-up people only smaller; therefore they probably think like grown-ups about most things." In point of fact, the opposite is the case. Children are far from being miniature adults when it comes to the quality of their thought processes. The adult literature on death and dying is simply not relevant to the child, in most cases.

Physicians, theologians, educators, and psychologists are often called upon for advice about how best to explain death to children, and many have taken up the challenge through books and magazine articles. For all of the writing that has been done in this area, however, there is embarrassingly little in the way of empirical research. That is to say, few of these authors have taken the time to talk extensively with children about death, and to report the children's answers. Whatever the reason for this state of affairs, the lack of empirical data in this area leaves a significant void. Virtually all professionals who work with children are aware of the need for accurate information on how their ideas about death develop. The purpose of this paper is to begin to fill the void caused by our ignorance of this area.

In her book on children's attitudes toward death, Mitchell[4] points out that very little research has been done on the development of these attitudes, although well before age six most children have discovered death in fact or

This material was first published in the *American Journal of Orthopsychiatry,* vol. 44, no. 3, pp. 404-411, April 1974. Copyright 1974 by the American Orthopsychiatric Association. Reprinted by permission.

conversation and are very interested in finding out more about it. Mitchell also notes that most of the research in this field is of the "opinion poll" variety, and there has been little effort to refine or improve on this. In the now classic studies by Anthony[1] and Nagy,[5] data is interpreted in ways that credit the child with superordinate levels of abstractive ability; Anthony's subjects were chiefly her own siblings.

In the present study, children were to be asked four questions, the answers to which were to be analyzed in developmental terms. The questions were: "What makes things die?" "How do you make dead things come back to life?" "When will you die?" and "What will happen then?" Answers were grouped according to the child's level of cognitive development, in order to best understand the reasoning that went into the answers. It was anticipated that answers to these four questions would vary predictably according to the developmental stage of the child.

Subjects

The subjects were 75 children ranging in age from six to fifteen years. They were drawn from among participants in various summer recreation and school enrichment programs in a midwestern university community. The sexes were approximately equally represented, and roughly 20 percent of the sample was nonwhite. The median socioeconomic status of the sample was three on a five-point scale devised by Hollingshead and Redlich,[2] and might be described as "middle class."

Measures

To obtain an estimate of intellectual level of each subject, the Similarities Subtest of the Wechsler Intelligence Scale for Children was used. It is comparatively simple to use, and yields good estimates of a child's verbal concept formation, abstract reasoning, and general intellectual level. Children who did not obtain at least average scores on this subtest (scaled score of 10) were not included in the study.

Criteria suggested by Phillips[6] formed the basis for classifying the children according to their level of cognitive functioning. Each child was tested with three conservation tasks (*i.e.,* mass, number, and volume) and one task in hypothesis formation. If the child failed one or more conservation tasks, he was placed in the "preoperational" group. If he passed all three of those but failed the hypothesis formation task, the child was classified as "concrete-operational." If the child dealt with all four tasks successfully, he was classified as "formal-operational."

Procedure

The examiner introduced himself to prospective subjects as a person who is interested in finding out what children think about different things, and in seeing how well they can solve certain puzzles. Each child was told in advance that he would be rewarded with a candy bar "for spending the time to tell us what you think about these things." Each child was then tested to determine his cognitive development and estimated intellectual level. During the same session the questions on death were asked verbatim, with no elaboration aside from the probes, "Anything else?" or, "Can you tell me any more about it?" When in doubt, the children were encouraged to guess or, "Just give the best answer you can think of."

Although this procedure involved three separate parts—the similarities subtest, the cognitive development tasks, and the death questions—no distinction as such was made to the child. In this way the whole procedure took on a unity as a questioning and problem-solving activity. Thus, any potential stress associated with the impact of bringing up the discussion of death was minimized. It was one way of communicating to the child the message that, "All of these questions are important, and all should be approached as puzzles to solve or phenomena to explain."

The examiners were prepared to follow up with psychological assistance any children who appeared anxious or upset following the questioning; however, this proved to be unnecessary. One child did not want to estimate when he might die, and was not pressed further once he declined to answer; this child was willing to answer the other questions asked. Most of the other children seemed very interested in making their ideas about death known, and were quite willing to elaborate on them in great detail. A frequent response when the children were allowed to choose their candy bars following the procedure was, "Is that all you wanted to know?" This finding was in marked contrast to the feelings of a few parents and teachers who expressed reservations about allowing their children to participate in the study. Often these adults would refer incidentally to their own experiences with death, and recall their own anxiety. Contact with parents following the interviews confirmed the initial observation that the children showed little or no adverse reaction to being interviewed on this topic. Some of the parents volunteered that they were pleased someone had talked with their children about this.

The examiners who administered and scored the tests were all graduate students in clinical psychology. All were unaware of the major hypotheses of the study. All had completed one full year of graduate study, including practicum courses in the administration of objective and projective psychological instruments.

> Most of the . . . children seemed very interested in making their ideas about death known. . . .

Results

From the outset it should be noted that no statistically significant differences attributable to the race or sex of the subjects were found.

What Makes Things Die?
The answers to this question were found to be of three different varieties, ranging on a continuum from the very concrete to the very abstract. While not mutually exclusive, the categories are appropriately descriptive of children's thinking on the subject. The categories, with actual examples, are listed below.

Category 1. This group includes fantasy reasoning, magical thinking, and realistic causes of death that are marked by egocentric reasoning as demonstrated in one or more special cases. This sort of response is characteristic of the "preoperational" child. Often these explanations are closely tied to the child's individual experiences. In the examples listed, the examiner's comments are bracketed.

Carol (age 7.3): They eat poison and stuff; pills. You'd better wait till your mom gives them to you. [Anything else?] Drinking poison water and stuff like going swimming alone.

Naomi (age 6.5): When they eat bad things, like if you went with a stranger and they gave you a candy bar with poison on it. [Anything else?] Yes, you can die if you swallow a dirty bug.

David (age 7.8): A bird might get real sick and die if you catch it. [Anything else?] They could eat the wrong foods, like aluminum foil. That's all I can think of.

Brian (age 8.2): Poison, marijuana, not heroin, because that's the same as marijuana. [Anything else?] You could die from styrofoam cups and wood [How?] If you swallow a whole bunch and get sick.

These responses are fairly typical of the children under age eight. It should be remembered, however, that the categories described here are not mutually exclusive and span many ages. That is to say, a primitive response, such as those listed above, might well be given as a partial answer by an older child. In addition, the answers of some children will include items from one or more categories.

Category 2. This group includes specific means of inflicting death, with or without intention. Naming specific weapons, poison, or other means including assaultive acts are all included here. This category of response is most typical of the child at the "concrete-operational" stage of development.

Jeff (age 10.3): The fact that they stop living. Diseases can kill you or you can get stabbed or use a gun; there are millions of ways. Do I have to tell you all of them? [As many as you want to tell.] You could crash their brains out or shoot them, there are millions of ways.

Debra (age 12.0): Accidents, cars, guns, or a knife. Old age, sickness, taking dope, or drowning. [Anything else?] Nope.

Todd (age 7.5): Knife, arrows, guns, lots of stuff. Do you want me to tell you all of them? [As many as you want.] Hatchets and animals, and fire and explosions too.

Kenny (age 9.5): Cancer, heart attacks, old age, poison, guns, a bullet, or if someone drops a boulder on you. [Anything else?] That's all.

This type of response was the most common and spanned the broadest age range, from about seven to twelve. Children in this group generally addressed the question, "What makes things die?," in terms of specific causes of death rather than general processes. Older children would also list specific causes of death, but often paired these with the more abstract responses typical of *Category 3.*

Category 3. This group includes relatively abstract clusters of more specific possibilities. The idea of physical deterioration, naming classes of potential causes, or the recognition of death as a natural process are all included in this group. The responses in this category are typical of those offered by the "formal-operational" children.

Ed (age 15.7): Death in a physical sense? [Yes.] Destruction of a vital organ or life force within us.

George (age 13.5): They get old and things, and their body gets all worn out, and their organs don't work as well as they used to.

Dean (age 10.2): When someone gets too old. You could also die of a sickness, or if you couldn't have enough to eat. [Anything else?] Well, when you get old you can just wear out eventually.

Paula (age 12.2): When the heart stops, blood stops circulating, you stop breathing and that's it. [Anything else?] Well, there's lots of ways it can get started, but that's what really happens.

Most of the children interviewed who were over age twelve gave this sort of response, but so did some children as young as nine or ten. One exceptionally bright example was Tina, age 8.5, who noted:

Sometimes they just die when they don't have the things they need to live, like food and water or clean air.

How Do You Make Dead Things Come Back to Life?
According to Piaget,[7] children at the "preoperational" stage of cognitive development, generally age seven and below, might be expected to describe one or more means to accomplish this feat. Kübler-Ross[3] agrees somewhat, stating that the child does not develop a realistic conception of death as a permanent biological process until age nine or ten. At the "preoperational" stage, the child is unable to share the experiences of others to a significant degree, and is not fully able to distinguish animate from inanimate objects. Since he has had no personal experience with death (i.e., he himself has

> . . . the child does not develop a realistic conception of death as a permanent biological process until age nine or ten.

never died), the child at this level might not be expected to regard death as permanent.

Eight children in the present study did tell ways in which they thought the dead might be revived. These eight children ranged in age from 6.0 to 7.1 years, and all were found to be "preoperational" in terms of Piaget's[7] description. These eight also gave Category 1 answers to the question, "What makes things die?" Although no children under age six were included in this study, it seems reasonable to conclude that they would also tend to view death as reversible. Typical responses included:

You can't revive them unless you take them to the emergency room and get them doctored up. Then they'll be okay.

Help them, give them hot food, and keep them healthy so it won't happen again.

No one ever taught me about that, but maybe you could give them some medicine and take them to the hospital to get better.

If you know a lot of science, and give them some pills, you can do it.

Older children considered the question seriously, but recognized death as a permanent condition. Some representative responses included:

If it was a tree you could water it. If it's a person you could rush them to the emergency room, but it would do no good if they were really dead already.

By thinking about them; then they can live in our mind, but you can't really make them come alive again.

Maybe some day we'll be able to do it, but not now. Scientists are working on that problem.

When Will You Die?
In answer to this question, all but one of the 75 subjects were willing to make an estimate. These ranged from a low of seven by a six year old, to a high of 300 years by a nine year old. When the subjects are grouped by age and cognitive development, however, some interesting variations can be observed. Once again it must be remembered that the "preoperational" child, as described by Piaget,[7] is unable to make use of the experiences of others to his advantage. Thus, such children (i.e., approximately age seven and below) would be expected to base their estimates more on fantasy than on reality and the observation of others.

Table 1   Children's estimates of when they will die (age)

Age Group	Number of Subjects	Mean Estimates	Standard Deviation	F
6-8 [preoperational]	20	86.6	66.01	
9-11 [concrete-operational]	35	81.3	12.68	27.10[a]
12-15 [formal-operational]	20	81.4	9.54	478.85[a]

[a] Indicates that *F* is significantly different from the 6-8 age group beyond the $p < .001$ level. The 9-11 and 12-15 group did not differ significantly, producing an *F* of only 9.54.

The children's responses to this question are summarized in Table 1. Although the average estimates of all three age groups fell quite close together, the variability of these estimates was quite diverse. As indicated in Table 1, variance of these estimates decreases significantly ($p < .001$) as the subjects' ages move beyond eight. That is to say, there was a very wide range or variance of estimates in this youngest group of children that was significantly greater than the range of variance of estimates by the two older groups. The older groups did not differ from each other on this measure to a significant degree. This change occurs, rather predictably, at the point when the child first becomes capable of using the observed experience of others in his own mental problem solving.

> **I think I'm going to be reincarnated as a plant or animal; whatever they need at that particular time.**

What Will Happen When You Die?
A wide variety of responses to this question was obtained. Answers were grouped in nonexclusive categories, with response rates as follows: references to being buried were given by 52 percent of the children; references to being judged, going to heaven or hell, or other hints at any sort of afterlife by 21 percent; references to having a funeral by 19 percent; specific predictions of how death would occur by 10 percent; references to some aspect of sleep by 7 percent; references to being remembered by others by 5 percent; references to reincarnation by 4 percent, and references to cremation by 3 percent. A sampling of responses follows:

Larry (age 9.5): They'll help me come back alive. [Who?] My mother, father, and grandfather. They'll keep me in bed, and feed me, and keep me away from rat poison and stuff.

Willie (age 8.1): You go to heaven, and all that will be left of you will be a skeleton. My friend has some fossils of people. A fossil's just a skeleton.

Debbie (age 13.3): It will be an accident, and I'll be rushed to the hospital, and I'll die of a piece of bone in my blood stream. They'll perform an autopsy, and then cremate me.

Boyd (age 11.3): I'll feel dizzy and tired and pass out. They they'll bury me and I'll rot away. You just disintegrate, and only your bones will be left.

Mark (age 12.0): I'll have a nice funeral, and be buried, and leave all my money to my son.

Meta (age 10.8): If I tell you then you'll laugh. [No, I won't, I want to know what you really think.] I think I'm going to be reincarnated as a plant or animal; whatever they need at that particular time.

George (age 14.9): I'll rot. You just decay and then turn back into material like the earth. That's it.

Discussion

Kübler-Ross[3] provides an eloquent context for discussing the findings of this study. She writes:

> . . . far better . . . to respond to the child's ideas than to allow magical or unspoken fears. . . .

The most meaningful help that we can give any relative, child, or adult, is to share his feelings before the event of death and allow him to work through his feelings, whether they are rational or irrational. [p. 180]

It is apparent that children's ideas about death are quite different at different age levels. These differences assume dramatic proportions when the death of a relative, or even a pet, forces an adult into the awkward and uncomfortable position of explaining to a child what has happened. Yet, it seems imperative that we help the child to understand what has happened and share his feelings of loss in a way that will help him to adapt and grow appropriately.

The present data lead to some suggestions for discussing death with the child who has suffered a loss. First, the reactions of the children to the questioning procedure suggests that there should be no "unspoken barriers" to this topic of conversation. Children are capable of talking about death, and seem to want to do this. They are pleased by the attention of understanding adults. Silence teaches them only that the topic is taboo; it cannot help them to cope with their feelings of loss. Second, the data in the present study suggest that the best explanations for children, especially those under age seven or eight, will be those that are simple, direct, and draw as much as possible from the child's own experiences. In this way the relative concreteness of the younger child will produce the least possible distortion.

Still another suggestion follows from an examination of the more magical answers given by younger children to the questions, "What makes things die?," and "How can you make dead things come back to life?" Those adults who would undertake explaining death to a young child would also be wise to ask the child to explain back again what he has been told. This would offer the opportunity to detect and correct any gross distortions or misperceptions on the part of the child. From the variety of causes of death that children are apt to think about, one can conclude that it is far better to explore and attempt to respond to the child's ideas than to allow magical or unspoken fears to play upon a child's imagination.

Keeping in mind the fantasies that childhood reasoning might lead to regarding the permanence of death is also important. For some children in this study there were ways in which ". . . you can make dead things come back to life." By implication, death need not be permanent if someone will only look after the corpse properly. This view could easily give rise to guilt and anxiety when the child learns that the body has been buried rather than nurtured back to health.

While no data were gathered on church affiliation or parental theism, it seems a bit surprising that little in the way of detailed religious concepts of death and its concomitants was elicited. In fact, only seven percent of the children in the study used the word "god" in answering the questions. Another 21 percent referred to this somewhat indirectly, mentioning heaven, hell, judgment, or some unearthly afterlife, but still this may seem rather low. There are many possible explanations, not the least influential of which might be media portrayals of death, including cartoons, comic books, television westerns, televised accounts of war news, etc. The weight of religious content in all of these is minimal. One might also think in terms of the growing disillusionment with religion as a mode of coping with death. This might be particularly reflected in the population for this study, because of the prevalence of this point of view in the university community.

Along these same lines it is worth comparing the present findings with those of Nagy.[5] She noted that Hungarian children between five and nine years old generally personify death. That is to say, they speak of death as if it were a person, and in this way keep it at a safe distance since, "Only those die whom the death-man carries off." Kübler-Ross[3] also notes that children of this age group tend to ". . . regard death as a bogey-man who comes to take people away" (p. 179). Not a single child in the present study gave a personification type response when discussing what might happen at the time of death. This finding probably reflects cultural differences, but certainly suggests a different sort of coping mechanism than Nagy found in her sample. Kübler-Ross cites Nagy as a reference and reports no new data. This might lead one to suspect that she has not looked for any cultural differences, but is simply repeating Nagy's assertions.

In the present study, answers to the question, "What will happen when you die?" are more difficult to interpret than are the others. While most children mentioned the idea of being buried, some giving graphic details of the interment process, there was a wide range of responses. It is particularly interesting to note that only five percent discussed their death in terms of how others might react. Rather, most of the subjects focused on concrete or stereotyped accounts of what would happen, such as detailed accounts of their funerals or of "rotting away" in the grave.

Perhaps the "coping mechanism" used instead of personification is hinted at in these findings. In the present sample, even children who were capable of above average levels of verbal abstraction were consistently specific and concrete in their replies. Perhaps American children are more inclined to use specificity of detail as a means to mastery and hence "control" over death rather than personification. That is to say, "If I know what is going to happen to me when I die, then I won't have to worry about it now." If this is indeed the case, then seeing that death is talked about with children becomes especially important.

> "If I know what is going to happen to me when I die, then I won't have to worry about it now."

References
1. Anthony, S. 1940. *The Child's Discovery of Death.* Harcourt, Brace, New York.
2. Hollingshead, A. and Redlich, F. 1958. *Social Class and Mental Illness.* John Wiley, New York.
3. Kübler-Ross., E. 1969. *On Death and Dying.* Macmillan, New York.
4. Mitchell, M. 1967. *The Child's Attitude to Death.* Schocken Books, New York.
5. Nagy, M. 1948. The child's theories concerning death. *J. Genet. Psychol.* 73:3–27.
6. Phillips, J. 1969. *The Origins of Intellect: Piaget's Theory.* Freeman, San Francisco.
7. Piaget, J. 1960. *The Child's Conception of the World.* Littlefield, Adams & Co., Paterson, N.J.

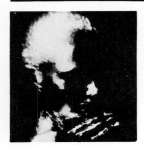

8

Practice

Take a moment and imagine someone you know who has experienced a death in the family. What physiological, psychological, and behavioral indication did this person present which let you know they were in pain? How did they cope? Did they rely on themselves or perhaps other resources available to them? Who would you turn to if you experienced a death? How would you help someone else who has had a loved one die? Attempt the following exercises in the Appendix when you have read the chapter.

C. Awareness of Grief Process

H. Fantasizing Grief Reaction of Significant Others

Fundamentals of Bereavement Intervention

Larry A. Bugen

When you think of dying and bereavement, what sorts of images come to mind? Perhaps a wife walking up and down a hospital corridor. Perhaps a husband crying during a funeral service. Or you might see a cancer patient crying out in pain or a child kneeling at a tombstone. Certainly none of these scenes are very pleasant and as I write them, I hesitate to dwell on them for any length of time. Leave these events to the specialists in death: the doctors, funeral directors, religious leaders, etc. Helplessness and avoidance underscore human bereavement as well as other human losses. To be terminally ill or bereaved is to face the threat of being out of control and in emotional and psychological pain. Who desires to face such hardships?

Ernest Becker (1973) has declared that the human being is the only animal to our knowledge who must face each day with the knowledge that he or she will eventually die. The heaviness of this diurnal plight leaves us with only one alternative—denial. Becker suggests that we must deny death in order to cope from day to day. Certainly some truth exists here. In order to cope effectively and lead relatively healthy lives, we need to involve ourselves with issues and events other than death. Baking an apple pie, playing basketball, gardening, reading a book, or going to a movie all qualify. This chapter, however, is not concerned with these more pleasant aspects of living.

The purpose of this chapter is to help each of us face death, the process of dying, and the process of helping more effectively. Efforts will be directed toward combating the helplessness and avoidance so many of us feel in these circumstances. This chapter will provide a basis for understanding human grief and managing it more effectively while appreciating the full spectrum of the helping role. All of us, sooner or later, will face death. A

. . . "death of
spouse" was . . .
the most intense
and highest rated
life event out of a
list of forty-three.

friend may die. Or a friend of a friend may die. A neighbor, pet, relative, colleague, or even we ourselves may soon face a death experience. Learning to face death and dying as a crisis of living is a courageous task but one that all of us can learn to cope with.

Death as a Life Crisis

Our lives are certainly filled with a great deal of change. Many changes we masterfully create, plan, and carry out ourselves. In a sense, we deliberately choose them. This kind of change may include marriage, childbirth, or a mortgage. Other changes seem to sweep over us with awesome power, leaving us helpless in their wake. Mandatory retirement, illness, menopause, and certainly death are this kind of change. The former changes may be termed *incremental life crises*. They are any new bond (a) deliberately chosen (b) which requires an emotional or behavioral time commitment (c) in order to further embellish our lives. The latter changes may be called *decremental life crises*. They are (a) any unexpected or unavoidable loss (b) which threatens our preferred way of living (c) in relation to others, ourselves, or the environment. The essential distinction is that incremental changes reflect the deliberate increase in commitment to others, self, and environment that we make, while decremental changes reflect the nondeliberate decrease we make in our commitment to others, self, or environment.

Death is one of the most profound decremental life crises. Holmes and Rahe (1967) found that "death of spouse" was considered to be the most intense and highest rated life event out of a list of forty-three. Each item in their scale was weighted in terms of the amount of readjustment necessary to cope with the event. The subjects in their study also rated "death of a relative" in the "top five." These results objectively tell us what we already know. Death is a very upsetting process in our lives.

In order to understand death as a life crisis, we must grasp (a) the components of a crisis and (b) the components of managing a crisis. As figure 1 portrays, the components of any crisis may be understood in terms of (a) perception of the crisis, (b) characteristics of the crisis, and (c) reaction to the crisis. The components of crisis management may be in turn understood in terms of (a) situational supports and resources and (b) coping mechanisms.

Components of Death as a Crisis

Perception of Death as a Crisis
No situation, however bizarre or unusual, can be considered a crisis unless individuals perceive it to be. It is important to clarify that death as a process or event is a stressor. Stressors are the myriad of moments and events in our

	Components of crisis			Components of crisis management	
	Perception of crisis	Characteristics of crisis	Reactions to crisis	External resources	Internal (coping) resources
Incremental crisis					
Decremental crisis					

Figure 1 Model depicting the relationships of incremental and decremental crisis to components of crisis and crisis management.

> . . . perception of stress as a crisis is subject to wide variation. . . .

lives which evoke, or have the potential to evoke, a stress reaction. Getting a speeding ticket, a failing grade, a raise, a divorce, or a kiss all qualify as stressors. "Stressors" refer to the stimulus situation, while "stress" refers to our response. Death, at first glance, must be considered a stressor until we understand an individual's response to it.

The perception of stress as a crisis is subject to wide variation among individuals. Imagine two students receiving a letter grade of C in a college algebra course. One student may joyously grab three friends and dart to the nearest bar to rejoice. A second student may instead grab a gun and shoot the professor. The final grade was certainly a stressor for both students; however, it was a crisis for only one. This actual event at a university exemplifies the wide range of potential behaviors that may be elicited in response to perceived events.

In a similar fashion, two individuals diagnosed with acute leukemia may perceive their illnesses differently and consequently respond in quite different ways. One person may become politically active regarding legislative issues such as "laetrile" or the "right-to-die" movement and thereby find a new purpose in living in response to the threat of cancer. A second person may quit a job, withdraw from people, and manifest an intense and prolonged depression.

A number of variables may contribute to the differences—genetic predisposition, age, sex, hormonal level, drugs, dietary factors, belief in preventability, and certainly pain. And the differences may depend largely

It is important to identify how an individual perceives a threatening stressor such as death.

upon the presence or absence of symptoms. Someone losing hair because of chemotherapy, and in a great deal of pain, will probably perceive his or her situation differently from someone else free from these manifestations.

An additional factor affecting anyone's perception of stressors is his or her conditioning history. Crises may occur as a result of stressful life events interacting with previous experiences. The more susceptible someone is to crises, the more that person is likely to distort our perception of stressful events. Cantankerous Aunt Minerva may have led her entire life reacting to daily events with a fit of rage followed by a yet more intense outburst. Events ranging from fender benders to sticky door locks were all capable of eliciting this omnipresent rage. Uncle Leroy, in comparison, was capable of riding out the most threatening storms with unexpected ease. Uncle Leroy would cope well with hurricane destruction or parking violation. When these two individuals face death—their own or that of someone close—each may display his or her characteristic response to this new stressor. This somewhat predictable interaction of prior conditioning with novel stressors is at variance with the prescribed stage model offered by Kübler-Ross (1969). Her model hypothesizes that individuals progress through five stages in response to death as a stressor: (a) denial, (b) anger, (c) bargaining, (d) depression, and (e) acceptance. This model has been criticized by Bugen (1977) because of the prescriptive flavor of the preordained sequencing. The human organism attempts to maintain a homeostatic balance with the surrounding environment. That means that when this fragile balance is threatened by physiological or psychological forces, the human organism engages in problem-solving activity designed to reestablish this delicate balance. A crisis such as death, however, confronts us with a problem that appears to have no immediate solution. We will usually try behaviors that have worked in the past. We may quickly discover that when confronting death the old strategies aren't working. At this point we must explore new and more effective methods of dealing with the crisis.

It is important to identify how an individual perceives a threatening stressor such as death. Someone experiencing a grief reaction may be just beginning to explore his or her array of problem-solving skills and may view the situation as potentially manageable. Someone else may feel at the end of the line and need active professional intervention.

Characteristics of Death as a Crisis

A second component of crisis is concerned with the nature of the crisis itself. Once death as a stressor is perceived as a crisis, what characteristics seem to underlie the event? From the number of characteristics to be presented, one appears to be most vital to our understanding. Every crisis involves the notion of *loss.*

Death involves innumerable losses. A terminally ill person faces the loss of bodily functions, mobility, friends, and potentiality. Bereaved friends and relatives face many losses also. A family may need to give up a home and a preferred life-style should a breadwinner die. A grief-stricken father may need to adjust to losing his nurturant role upon the death of his child. This notion of losing a part of oneself when someone dies is a central concept in understanding the prolongation of grief.

As long as a bereaved person feels as though his or her own life has been irreparably changed by the death of a loved one, the grief will inhibit establishing new roles in the world. Every loss we experience involves a *shift of roles*. Therefore, part of the problem-solving process faced by the bereaved entails this kind of adjustment.

Every loss we experience involves a *shift of roles*.

Two characteristics of death as a crisis have been mentioned: loss and role shift. A third characteristic is *suddenness* or *unexpectancy*. A death experience can move through a family network, or a country, as in the case of President John F. Kennedy, like a destructive freight train out of control. A sudden death leaves families and friends in shock and disbelief. A sudden loss of this kind is particularly distressing since the bereaved seldom get an opportunity to say good-bye to their loved one. It has been suggested that sudden death results in more prolonged and intense grief periods because a prior period of anticipatory grief was not possible. It is generally believed that having time prior to an expected loss actually helps us cope more effectively.

A fourth characteristic of death as a life crisis is that it shrouds *an important event*. This may seem a simplistic notion on the surface, however, death as a stressor will not be perceived as a crisis unless a bereaved individual considers it to be an important event. The death of one's mailman will certainly not cause as much grief as the death of a parent.

A fifth characteristic relevant to death as a life crisis concerns *externality*. Recall the distinction made earlier between incremental and decremental crises. It was suggested that incremental crises were deliberately chosen and therefore may be viewed as internally determined. Marriage would be an example in this culture. Death is a decremental crisis, however, and is usually viewed as an external force which invades all of us at one time or another. This view is most literally represented among the children who conceive the death-man or -woman coming to get them. The entire belief in externality is being seriously questioned by researchers who believe that in many ways we unwittingly will our own cancer and time of death. Certainly suicide represents yet another example of internality as a locus for death.

A sixth characteristic of death as a life crisis relates to the *potential for change*. Every crisis may be viewed as either a threat or a challenge. Crises are turning points in our lives. A good deal of grief work is usually required before a bereaved individual can appreciate this dynamic. A husband who had been financially dependent upon his wife may, after she dies, eventually recognize that he has potential for change and develop a new career for himself. Any death may cause survivors to feel as though they have been "done in" or may be experienced as an opportunity to develop new strategies, interests, or resources.

. . . grief
involves
physiological,
psychological,
and behavioral
components.

A seventh characteristic is that crises usually represent an *insoluble problem* in the immediate future. For the awesomeness and strangeness of something new like death is felt to be an experience impossible to absorb. An individual must ask, "What do I do now?" "How do I handle it?" "My previous ways of coping don't seem to be working very well."

A final characteristic of death as a life crisis relates to duration. Crises are *acute* situations rather than chronic. There is an implication that crises as acute events will be of relatively short duration. Unfortunately, there seems to be little agreement on how protracted is normal grief over a death. Lindemann (1944) and Caplan (1964) are of the opinion that most grief can be worked through in six to eight weeks. Other theorists and researchers, such as Parkes (1964), Clayton (1973), and Bugen (1977), suggest longer periods. Some of the disagreement is due to an oversimplification of grief or reaction to crisis. As we shall see, grief involves physiological, psychological, and behavioral components. Some components may be resolved in a six-week period while others are not.

Reaction to Crises

Much of our understanding of crisis reactions can be traced to Erich Lindemann's work. In his early investigation of psychoneurotic patients, relatives of patients who died in the hospital, bereaved disaster victims, and relatives of members of the armed forces, Lindemann concluded that most people experiencing the crisis of acute grief or bereavement usually have five related reactions: (1) somatic distress; (2) preoccupation with the image of the deceased; (3) guilt; (4) hostile reactions; and (5) loss of patterns of conduct. Lindemann's observations can be conveniently catalogued as physiological, behavioral, and psychological.

Physiological. Lindemann discovered the following symptoms: sensations of somatic distress which assumed a repetitive wave pattern lasting from twenty minutes to an hour at a time; light feelings in the throat region; shortness of breath accompanied by choking; a need for sighing; an empty feeling in the abdomen; lack of energy and muscular power; and dizziness.

Selye's (1974) contribution of the General Adaptation Syndrome offers a further guide to our understanding of the physiological response to grief. Selye reports that a common biochemical response underlies all stress reactions. Objective indices of prolonged stress include adrenal enlargement, thymus atrophy, and gastrointestinal ulcers. Of interest is Lindemann's observation that peptic ulcers and ulcerative colitis are found in severe cases of stress. The high level of adrenocorticoids in the blood during stress seems to account for their presence. Further data substantiating the role of the pituitary-adrenocortical axis in response to acutely stressful situations is provided by Hofer, Wolff, Friedman, and Mason (1972). These investigators found that mourning parents of leukemic children could still be differentiated from nongrieving parents by excretion of adrenocorticoids two years after their child's death.

Behavioral.   The behavioral response to grief is perhaps the most ignored of all reactions of life crises. This is surprising because behavior is more readily observed than either physiological or psychological response. Essentially, behavior in response to death may be viewed as alteration in our patterns of living. A terminally ill or bereaved person may withdraw from social interaction, dress haphazardly, avoid washing, cleaning the house, or going to work, and may spend much time staring at mementos.

Repetitive behavior may often seem bizarre or strange. A parent whose baby dies of the Sudden Infant Death Syndrome may continue to peep into the baby's bedroom throughout the day and look at the empty crib, to buy baby food, or to get up at night to check on the baby. This repetitive behavior is in effect therapeutic because each sequence helps the parent face the harsh reality of the infant's death and come closer to accepting and managing the death.

Patterns of sleep and sexuality may also become disturbed in response to loss. At bedtime a griever may not be able to slow down his or her thoughts to allow sleep or may be too filled with anxiety to allow the relaxation necessary for sleep. Similarly, obsessive thoughts and anxieties may inhibit the sex drive and place a strain on sexual relations during the grief process. Anticipatory counseling in this area is particularly helpful.

A concept which may have some utility in our understanding of abnormal grief patterns is "helplessness proliferation." Occasionally a griever will allow one behavior to feed into another so that withdrawal from people, places, and oneself becomes the rule. First, an individual may choose not to prepare food, then not to eat, and eventually not to leave the house. A helper who observes this pattern must be careful not to confuse normal grief with an escalation of helplessness.

Psychological.   Perhaps the most widespread psychological reaction to grief is the belief that "I am the only person who has ever felt this way." "There's no one around who can understand what I am going through." We will shortly see that much comfort can be afforded by the presence of similar others. A mastectomy patient, for example, usually believes adjustment is impossible until other mastectomy patients share their progress.

Death will undoubtedly be perceived as a threat to present roles and goals. Assuming the new roles of bereaved widow, widower, or parent brings new responsibilities along with the unwanted vacuum of spent hopes and dreams. A parent may have had a large emotional investment in vocational, educational, and recreational plans for his or her child. The child's death causes a role shift that is difficult to manage.

Helplessness and loss of control may also be experienced during a death crisis. When the pleasures and meaningful moments of life seem independent of our efforts, we feel helpless. Watching a loved one die slowly produces an overwhelming sense of helplessness and loss of control.

When we experience a loss, we may be obsessed or preoccupied with thoughts and images. A bereaved person may have repetitive pictures of the

> . . . behavioral response to grief is perhaps the most ignored of all reactions. . . .

death scene, hospital scene, or perhaps a policeman's statements. Such thoughts and images are healthy and suggest a process of gradual coping. Our minds typically "let in" just about what we can handle. Over time, the reality of a situational crisis such as death becomes less harsh and more easily managed. This process of ego mastery will extend throughout a grief process. Three common examples of repetitive thoughts are: "What caused the death?" "Why did she have to die?" "He will never be a part of the life I wanted him to be a part of."

Emotional responses to loss include anxiety, depression, anger, or even relief. Individuals may maintain an emotional state for some time during a death experience. Three different conceptual approaches seem to exist in regard to understanding emotional reactions to loss.

Some theorists suggest that persons move through crises in roughly predictable stages. Most of these stage-theorists, such as Kübler-Ross (1969) and Kavanaugh (1972), qualify their sequencing by noting that stages invariably intertwine and overlap. Kavanaugh outlines the following: (a) shock and denial; (b) disorganization; (c) volatile emotions; (d) guilt; (e) loss and loneliness; (f) relief; and (g) reestablishment. A second approach visualizes an array of emotions which may characterize an individual from moment to moment or day to day depending upon external events, mind sets, etc. The third approach to understanding emotional concomitants to grief suggests that each individual is unique and will manifest his or her own pattern of emotional response. A truly objective analysis of our pattern of grief would probably reflect an interaction of all three models. The important point is that a full spectrum of emotions and patterns of expression seem to surround our reactions to crises. We shall see shortly that openness to this normal diversity is required in order to be an effective helper.

Numerous other psychological patterns are responses to death as a crisis. Some are inability to concentrate, sudden loss of capacity to memorize or reason, inadequate decision-making, guilt, and a belief in preventability. Poor concentration is the result of the large amount of energy consumed by the emotions of grief. As Bugen (1977) has pointed out, preventability essentially echoes the concern that something more could have been done to divert the eventuality. More than any other variable, a belief in preventability may contribute to prolonged grief.

Components of Crisis Management

Now that a global picture of death as a crisis has been presented, one essential question remains: How do we handle death as a crisis in our lives? In order for anyone to successfully navigate the choppy waters of bereavement, it is necessary to have both *internal* and *external* resources. By internal resources, we mean our resourcefulness and ability and desire to cope. External resources are the people, agencies, customs, and other situational supports that facilitate movement through crisis.

Situational Supports and Resources

Individuals who are threatened by a terminal illness or have experienced a bereavement are in a vulnerable position. Morley (1970) has described four approaches that helping persons and agencies might take to reckon with this increased vulnerability. It is imperative that helpers understand the full spectrum of intervention strategies appropriate to death as a life crisis.

The kind of help we can call *environmental manipulation* requires someone who knows the resources of a community. This may be a friend next door who knows "who does what" in the community and refers a bereaved person to the appropriate setting, depending upon the need. This "environmental manipulation" may refer a leukemic father to a local chapter of an organization such as Make Today Count. A bereaved parent may be referred to a local chapter of the Sudden Infant Death Syndrome organization. A grieving widow may eventually be made aware of Parents Without Partners or a local grief group at a neighborhood church. A mastectomy patient may be put in touch with other mastectomy patients who have successfully dealt with their own life-threatening illness. All of these examples of environmental resources are important in combating many aspects of grief.

Such resources encourage a bereaved or terminally ill person to minimize the belief that he or she is psychologically unique. They may also see that the many repetitive thoughts and images they experience are quite expected. A person unable to sleep or who is manifesting other somatic signs of distress may be physiologically helped by judicious use of medication or an exercise/movement program. By participating in a variety of group activities, usually held in places other than homes, a griever will be helped behaviorally to forestall the tendency to escalate helplessness.

Crisis resolution is promoted by having a variety of well integrated resources available to members of a community. They may include agency counseling, pastoral care, neighborhood crisis clinics, or friends next door, and they should know about one another. If agencies or individuals have not heard of one another or are reluctant to utilize one another's strengths, the handling of crises may be hampered. A funeral director may be the first to observe an intense grief response. If grief counselors are not available through that setting, it behooves the funeral director to make an appropriate referral. In a similar fashion, a doctor unable or unwilling to meet minimal psychosocial needs of a patient and his or her family should find an available ombudsman in the hospital or community setting.

One last point about environmental manipulation resources is that they must be more than available, they must be actually used. It does not matter how varied or well integrated the helping resources of a community are if persons in need are reluctant to use them. Barriers to utilization may need to be explored. If, for instance, a locally sponsored bereavement group is poorly attended, publicity, setting, or transportation may be a problem.

A second kind of help outlined by Morley involves *general support* of the person in crisis. Most of us can qualify as helpers in this way. The

It is imperative that the helpers understand the full spectrum of intervention strategies. . . .

One misconception is that it is somehow better for us helpers to be talking rather than listening.

primary behavior for a good helper will be interested listening without deep probing or confrontation. The importance and effectiveness of good listening by anyone *cannot* be overstated. Both family and friends may be particularly helpful here. Letting seven-year-old Mary talk about how sad she is that her turtle died may mollify her grief significantly.

Before we elaborate on what constitutes good listening and other basic helping skills, we will list some minimal helping skills as summarized by Butcher and Maudal (1976).

We must possess sufficient empathic ability in order to understand a problem being presented.

We must be capable of listening attentively.

We must be capable of eliciting appropriate material which relates to the problem.

We must listen objectively without imposing personal values and preferences.

We must assess appropriately the individual's problems, conflicts, assets, and resources within the context of the immediate crisis situation. Decisions regarding crisis intervention or crisis therapy depend on this.

We must have current knowledge regarding community resources for purposes of referral.

We may have some added effectiveness if we are a member of the same subculture as the people who might utilize the resource.

Butcher and Maudal's outline, you will note, refers to both personal and social resources, and repeatedly emphasizes the role of effective listening. One of the most difficult notions for many of us to understand and accept is that one human being can help another merely by listening. Different levels of listening can, according to Gordon (1974): (a) invite a troubled person to discuss his or her concerns; (b) facilitate catharsis and release of emotions; (c) keep the responsibility on the person who owns a problem; (d) foster exploration into deeper and more basic feelings; (e) communicate one's willingness to be a helper; and (f) communicate one's acceptance of the person, troubles and all.

A truly silent conspiracy awaits the terminally ill and bereaved. Death and dying so intimidates both professional and lay members of the community that most of us hesitate to try to be good listeners because of basic fears and misconceptions. One misconception is that it is somehow better for us helpers to be talking rather than listening. We therefore feel a pressure to have answers where few exist. A second misconception is that, as helpers, we should not experience any discomfort, anxiety, or confusion while working with the bereaved and terminally ill. In fact, however, such feelings are our normal response to a highly threatening topic and can become a valued part of our empathic responses to others.

Four levels of listening response have been outlined by Gordon: (a) passive listening (silence); (b) acknowledgment responses; (c) door openers; and (d) active listening. Our passive listening actually communicates acceptance and concern even though we may say nothing. In addition to the many moments when saying nothing is quite appropriate, we may find some additional situations where just our physical presence would be a help. Imagine the following phone conversation:

Helper: Hello, Bob. I was just calling to see how you are and ask if I can do anything to help.

Bereaved: Thanks anyway, Jim. I think I just want to be alone tonight.

Helper: I don't want to be pushy, Bob, but I'm not doing anything tonight either. If it is all right with you, I would feel good just coming over to sit for awhile.

Bereaved: Well, I guess that would be O.K.

In order to communicate that you really are paying attention, it is usually helpful to use an acknowledgment response from time to time. It helps to use both nonverbal and verbal cues to indicate that you are tuned in. Examples would include nodding, leaning forward, smiling, frowning, and numerous other body gestures. Holding a hand or hugging someone can be an incredibly powerful, facilitative gesture in releasing pent-up emotions. Verbal grunting such as "Uh huh" or "Oh" or "Yes" are also important cues in maintaining rapport.

Occasionally a griever will need additional encouragement or urging to talk about the loss or share some feelings. Door openers can serve this need: "Can you tell me what happened next?" "How did your husband deal with the suddenness of it all?" "I wonder how you are feeling now, as we talk about Joe's death." Door openers are intended to be open-ended statements or questions which attempt to lead the person to more self-disclosure.

Silence, acknowledgment responses, and door openers are relatively passive listening skills and do have a number of shortcomings. The griever has no way of being certain that he or she is being understood. In addition, these responses often fail to encourage explorations of underlying feelings and thoughts.

If we as helpers want to facilitate deeper explorations, we can use *active listening.* Active listening combines two separate skills: empathy and reflection. Empathy is the capacity to reach deep inside ourselves to our prior emotional experiences in order to understand how another person feels. It is not necessary to have experienced a death in order to understand someone else's bereavement. Each of us many times over has experienced some kind of loss with its concomitant grief. It may have been a divorce, mandatory retirement, rejection from a school or job of our choice, or the loss of friends through a job transfer. Reflection is our attempt to express our understanding of another's emotional pain. We go beyond the words they are using. The following dialogue may serve as an example.

Rhonda: I am going to Houston for more blood work tomorrow. Since I lost my remission last month, the doctors want me to get ready for another damn new drug.

Helper: The whole routine of starting a new procedure must be frustrating for you.

> **It is not necessary to have experienced a death in order to understand someone else's bereavement.**

Rhonda: All that nausea and losing my hair, too! I don't want to make any more decisions. I want to just ride it out my way. I'm tired of everybody having the right answer for me.

Helper: Sounds frustrating as hell! You must feel like throwing in the towel sometimes.

Rhonda: I do get awfully tired of trying to be brave. Sometimes I just feel like a worn-out tire.

Helper: Just like a deflated, worn-out tire needing support.

Rhonda: Yes (sobs).

Most reflection is not intended to operate at deep emotional levels. When our efforts are merely to encourage another person to continue speaking we may choose to paraphrase what they have just said and reflect this back to them.

Bob: The things that nurse and doctor said to me were absurd.

Helper: Some of the things you just heard from the staff sounded incredible to you?

It is important to underscore that being a good helper means building a trusting relationship. All of the listening skills briefly outlined here are intended to help build the trust necessary to bridge the gap which alienates the bereaved from the nonbereaved. An array of skills which require years of training and experience are not necessary for our basic humanness is usually enough—if we reach out and let it flow!

A third kind of help described by Morley is termed *generic*. This approach requires the helper to have a knowledge of crisis in general and death in particular. It is regrettable that special expertise in the field of death and dying is conspicuously absent. There are financial counselors, employment counselors, marriage counselors, retirement counselors—but where are our grief counselors? Funeral homes are beginning to offer grief counseling, but the adequacy of training and the cost of these services raise serious questions about the spread of such a movement. Hospital chaplains and various paraprofessional groups are attempting to meet the need. However, generic experts in the field of death and grief management are long overdue and are not on the horizon.

The final kind of help described by Morley is called *individually tailored*. The crisis worker at this level is usually a psychologist, psychiatrist, or social worker. This professional, with knowledge of personality theory and abnormal psychology, can intervene at the deepest psychodynamic level.

But when is the crisis serious enough to require professional psychological or medical help? If the bereaved person is showing morbid grief reactions, as described by Lindemann, they would include: (a) delay of reaction, (b) distorted reactions, (c) medical diseases being manifested, (d) alterations in relationships to friends, (e) furious hostility against specific persons, (f) acquiring symptoms belonging to the deceased, and (g) prolonged loss of social interaction patterns. These criteria are ambiguous at best. In certain instances, for example, furious hostility may be considered quite therapeutic. Distinctions between normal and abnormal grief are difficult to make for several reasons. (a) There are no agreed-upon criteria for acceptable "working through." (b) The time factors for acceptable crisis transitions are poorly defined. (c) There is confusion about physiological, behavioral, and psychological distress levels. And (d) there are cultural biases. Whatever the criteria for their intervention might be, to have professionals who could offer individually tailored counseling in a community would greatly enhance the network of death-concerned resources.

> . . . we probably maintain . . . coping resources and call them forth when needed.

Coping Resources

The terminally ill and bereaved face a difficult problem. They must each learn to say good-bye to previous patterns of living as they face the end of their transitional period. Throughout the course of our lives we each learn a variety of techniques to help us with difficult moments or periods of time. These techniques are problem-solving approaches which, we hope, facilitate our movement through a crisis. If they are successful at doing what they are intended to do we probably maintain them in our repertoire as coping resources and call them forth when needed. It is important to note that a crisis usually develops at a time when our previously learned methods of coping prove inadequate in our present circumstance.

No transition period in our lives can tax the efficacy of our coping resources to such as extent as death and dying. In order to understand the problem facing the bereaved it is convenient to portray the task as a two-step problem. First, each bereaved person must learn to grieve the termination of relationships which no longer can be maintained. Second, each person must eventually begin to construct new relationships and rewarding patterns of interaction with the world about them.

All of the helping skills and situational resources discussed earlier can help these processes. In addition, early work by Erich Lindemann is particularly pertinent to our understanding of the first task. In order to extricate oneself from the bondage to the deceased, Lindemann suggests that the griever must (a) accept the pain of the bereavement; (b) review his or her relationship with the deceased; (c) become aware of changing patterns of one's emotional reaction; (d) accept the varied fears of losing control and going insane; (e) express the accompanying sorrow and sense of loss; (f) find an acceptable formulation for a future relationship with the deceased; and (g) verbalize guilt feelings.

The above processes are both demanding and draining. We can understand why shock, denial, and avoidance are ready alternatives to dealing with grief work. Much of the process of saying goodbye occurs in the privacy of our hearts and minds. The loneliness and emotional pain that accompany grief work truly test the rational problem-solving strategies we generally like to rely on. A time does come eventually when the second task of re-establishment can begin.

. . . crisis is a time to learn new behavior, to grow, and to change.

As pointed out earlier, crisis is a time to learn new behavior, to grow, and to change. The success of our attempts to cope will in part depend upon the creative problem-solving needed at that time. The process of constructing new relationships and establishing new patterns of rewarding interaction may proceed according to the following steps: (a) a difficulty is felt; (b) the source of the difficulty is found; (c) possible solutions are suggested; (d) consequences are considered; and (e) a solution is accepted.

The process is seldom this smooth and may well have to be reassessed along the way. Accepted solutions may not work because the problem was inaccurately perceived, because the solution may be inappropriate, or perhaps because the solution was poorly implemented. Both tension and discomfort will probably be on the rise throughout this process. Even though someone may be struggling to find an answer, the problem may reach crisis proportions. New childrearing patterns, new dating and social skills, and new vocational interests may all confront a recent widow or widower. The solution to these dilemmas of reestablishment will depend partly on the creative coping resources of the individual as well as the situational resources available. Barriers to successful coping may also need to be uncovered. Sex role stereotypes inhibiting some men from emotional release or role shifts may need to be explored.

Coping is an active process. It is more than merely adjustment to a way "things used to be!" Death and dying are powerful, dynamic experiences in our lives. In order to cope effectively with such momentous transitions, we must learn to make equally momentous changes. Through the use of our own inherent resources, as well as those around us, we can continue to grow and flourish.

References

Becker, E. 1973. *The denial of death.* New York: The Free Press.
Bugen, L. 1977. Human grief: A model for prediction and intervention. *American Journal of Orthopsychiatry* 47: 2, 196–206.
Butcher, J. N., and G. R. Maudal. 1976. Crisis intervention. In I. B. Weiner (ed.), *Clinical methods in psychology.* New York: John Wiley.
Caplan, G. 1964. *Principles of preventive psychiatry.* New York: Basic Books.
Clayton, P., J. Halikas, W. Maurice, and E. Robins. 1973. Anticipatory grief and widowhood. *British Journal of Psychiatry* 122: 47–51.
Gordon, T. 1974. *Teacher effectiveness training.* New York: Wyden.
Hofer, M., C. Wolff, S. Friedman, and A. Mason. 1972. A psycho-endocrine study of bereavement: Part 1. 17-Hydroxycorticosteroid excretion rates of parents following death of their children from leukemia. *Psychosomatic Medicine* 34: 481–91.
Holmes, T., and R. Rahe. 1967. The social readjustment rating scale. *Journal of Psychosomatic Research* 11: 219–25.
Kavanaugh, R. 1972. *Facing death.* Baltimore: Penguin.
Kübler-Ross, E. 1969. *On death and dying.* New York: Macmillan.
Lindemann, E. 1944. Symptomatology and management of acute grief. *American Journal of Psychiatry* 101: 141–48.
Morley, W. E. 1970. Theory of crisis intervention. *Pastoral Psychology* 21: 14–20.
Parkes, C. M. 1964. Effects of bereavement on physical and mental health—A study of the medical records of widows. *British Medical Journal* 2: 274–79.
Selye, H. 1974. *Stress without distress.* New York: Lippincott.

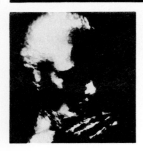

9
Practice

Most of us cherish pictures and other tokens belonging to a loved one who has died. The extent to which we "cling" to these objects can sometimes differentiate appropriate from inappropriate coping. In this chapter Vamik Volkan describes how such objects can facilitate working through the grief process. The following exercises in the Appendix would be helpful at the completion of your reading:

      M.   Saying Good-bye to a Loved One

      N.   The Final Rite of Passage: A Technological Update

A Study of a Patient's "Re-Grief Work"

Vamik Volkan

Uncomplicated grieving may be seen as nature's exercise in loss and restitution. Persons who suffer from pathological grief reactions are, however, either caught in the struggle of loss and restitution without coming to a resolution or bolstered by a restitution which is symptomatic.

In order to define more precisely the nature of pathological grief and to gain an understanding of its psychodynamics, more than 50 patients were studied at the University of Virginia between 1966 and 1971; each had lost by death a close relative, and each displayed a diversity of clinical symptoms dating from this known loss. Re-grief work as a method of brief psychotherapy evolved during this investigation.[1] Initial findings typical of these cases of pathological grief have been presented in previous papers;[2,3] another paper describes the methodology and theoretical considerations of re-grief work.[4]

Sixteen patients have been treated by re-grief work therapy, and five of these were included in a pilot project designed to measure the effectiveness of this process. Results of the pilot project will be discussed in future publications.

This paper describes the problem of a patient with pathological grief reaction and reports in detail techniques used in his treatment. Some time has passed since Showalter and the present writer disclosed the technique of re-grief work,[4] and it is felt that providing further detail will be useful to other therapists responsible for patients whose problems arise from unfinished grieving.

This material was first published in the *Psychiatric Quarterly,* vol. 45, no. 2, pp. 255–273, 1971. Copyright 1971 by the New York State Department of Mental Hygiene. It is printed here in slightly modified form by permission.

Re-Grief Work

> . . . the pathological mourner is in a state of chronic hope and chronic effort to regain the one who died. . . .

The short-term psychotherapy of re-grief work helps the patient suffering from pathological grief to resolve the conflicts of separation—however distant in time this resolution may be from the death itself, or from the period within which normal grief would have spent itself. The author has attempted[2, 3, 5] to show that the clinical entity of pathological grief, with its predictable symptomatology and characteristic findings, lies between uncomplicated grief and those reactions to death which turn into depression or other identifiable neurotic, psychosomatic or psychotic conditions. Only those patients who occupy middle ground are suitable for re-griefing; and re-griefing may in some cases be a key by which some disturbed patients who labor under a diagnosis of severe and even chronic mental disorder can be restored to their previous level of functioning.

In the first report of our re-grief work[4] we indicated that it could be divided into three phases, each of which requires different maneuvers. In actual practice these phases overlap, and appear in no fixed order, but the therapist can nevertheless use the concepts involved. They are: *demarcation, externalization,* and *reorganization,* the latter referring to the achievement of a state in which psychic energies can be directed toward new objects. The process typically takes two months, the patient being seen four times a week.

Since the pathological mourner is in a state of chronic hope and chronic effort to regain the one who died—or, as Bowlby[6] describes his situation, is engaged in "the persistent seeking of reunion" with the dead—he is helped during the first phase to make rational distinctions between what actually belongs to himself and what actually belongs to the lost one. The taking of a detailed history promotes this end. We shy away from questioning the patient, however, and conduct our history-taking in nondirective exchange. These patients, especially those suffering from the chronic type of grief reaction, inevitably arrive at the subject of the death and the deceased, and the hours are filled with memories of events in which he played a part. During this phase we ask the patient to bring a picture of the dead person, and ask him to look at it and describe the appearance of its subject.

The *externalization phase*—actually a continuation of *demarcation*—follows. In this the patient is encouraged to repeat his accounts of the past and to recall circumstances of the fatal illness (or accident), the conditions in which he learned of the death, his reaction to beholding the body, the events of the funeral, etc. Anger usually appears at this point if the therapy is going well—anger diffused and directed first toward others and then toward the dead. Abreactions—what Bibring[7] describes as "emotional reliving"—may then occur, demonstrating to the patient the actuality of his repressed impulses. The therapist, using his understanding of the psychodynamics involved in his patient's need to keep the lost one alive, explains and interprets the relationship to the lost one. When the patient begins to re-grieve we assume that certain impulses such as death-wishes are surfacing, and that the patient is ready to have them interpreted, experiencing relief at being able to talk about taboo impulses, and becoming able to handle guilt at his anger.

The pathological mourner typically uses the mechanism of splitting, which we bombard by asking at an appropriate time how he became aware that the dead person was in fact no longer alive. The question will obtain good results if it is put at an emotionally suitable time and not posed as an intellectual exercise. The patient may show genuine surprise, and blurt out something like: "I thought he was not breathing any more. But gee! I didn't really look!" The therapist has helped him to revisit the point where the splitting took place, and to reevaluate reality.

It is characteristic of our patients' experience that the funeral rites did not go well. The patient often did not see the coffin lowered into the ground. Asked at an appropriate time, "How do you know he is buried?" the patient will surprise himself by realizing that one part of his awareness never did believe that burial had been accomplished. He is then likely to feel anger at those who stood in the way of his participation in the funeral ceremony. It has been pointed out to him that one part of himself felt and indeed knew that death had occurred, but that another part of himself had continued to behave as though nothing had happened. Disorganization occurs in the patient during this phase, and he may be flooded with primary process thinking. If necessary, he may be hospitalized. Most of the patients we studied came from an in-patient psychiatric unit, but we have also been successful with re-grief work conducted on an out-patient basis.

The patient grieves and feels sadness in the final phase of treatment. He has been enabled to feel, experience, and verbalize his taboo impulses. He now sees that he wanted something from the dead, or that the dead represented part of himself. Suggestions and interpretations for his continued life in the face of his loss are provided. Since most of these patients have not visited the grave, they are asked to do so as part of the treatment, and then to examine their feelings about the visit. When possible, the therapist may actually have an hour with the patient at the graveside. Few have provided a tombstone since they have denied the reality of the grave, and the therapist helps them to take this step. He also provides help as the patient seeks to direct his energies toward new objects.

Our procedures for re-griefing, although retaining the original plan described earlier, have undergone a few changes in concept and techniques since the institution of this therapeutic modality. Experience has led to stronger emphasis on the explanations and interpretations made by the therapist, and to the meanings which the patient has condensed into the known loss. Rado[8] uses the term *interceptive interpretation* which we have modified to our purpose in describing our interception of the development of transference neurosis as it occurs in long-term insight therapies. We in-

> . . . one part of his awareness never did believe that burial had been accomplished.

tercept the transference phenomenon prematurely in order to abort its ripening into a transference neurosis.

Since the studies of Abraham[9] and Freud,[10] *internalization processes* like the introjection and identification in mourning have been investigated extensively. I indicated in previous reports that in pathological mourning the process of establishing and maintaining the introject of the dead is not completed, so that total identification does not occur—as Pollock[11] also found—but the temporary identification of "merging"[12] may appear. I have reported elsewhere[5] my view of the *externalization processes* used by pathological mourners, and the theoretical considerations to which they give rise. These processes become possible through the adoption and use of inanimate objects which I have named *linking objects,* refining the former[3] terminology of *symbolized objects.*

There are four occasionally overlapping categories of linking object. They are: (1) articles worn by the dead—e.g., a dress, a watch; (2) objects seen as an extension of the dead owner's body, as a camera represents vision; (3) articles recalling the appearance of the dead, either realistically (a photograph) or symbolically; and (4) articles at hand when the death news was received or when the funeral took place, and which are part of the last moment in which the dead person was considered to be living. Linking objects have no intrinsic characteristics in common, but their use is highly consistent. They are not put to appropriate use, but are jealously hoarded. It is always possible to keep them at a distance and to avoid them altogether. They hold an eerie fascination, and are not to be confused with the inherited article which is simply a keepsake. I have elsewhere[5] made the distinction between the linking objects and the fetish, and between linking and transitional objects.

As soon as we recognized the importance of these linking objects, we focused on them in the second phase of re-grief work, feeling that they mark in an externalized way the locking in of the process of mourning, and hold the keys to it. They are not hard to identify; after the treatment is under way and the therapist has obtained information and made a formulation as to the reason for pathological mourning, he may ask: "What sort of token from the dead person do you keep?" The reply usually points to a highly symbolized object.

The process of re-griefing has, like that of uncomplicated grief, a recognizable beginning and end; its course is more predictable—especially in respect to its resolution—than that of most interpretive therapies.

Re-Grief Work Applied

The course and outcome of a patient's treatment will be examined under three headings: (1) an account of the treatment process; (2) analysis of dreams occurring during treatment; and (3) psychoanalytic observation of the patient after re-griefing has been completed.

Identification.   A 23-year-old married Jewish man, exhibiting the classic symptoms of pathological grief, was hospitalized on the first anniversary of his father's death. Mike was the oldest child of a surgeon; his mother was a manic-depressive who had been hospitalized several times during his childhood, leaving him sensitized to separation. During his childhood and pubertal years, she had been seductive toward him when she was manic, and this had frightened him. Her instability made it necessary for him to seem to be extremely self-reliant although his unacknowledged basic dependence persisted.

The father, who had been dominated by his father, the clan leader, and over-shadowed by an elder brother, seemed bewildered by his wife's behavior. It was only after the elder's death "liberated" him toward the end of his life that he presented a model for his son, in whom he then began to take an active interest, preparing him for medical school and supporting his plans for marriage. The son responded with constructive attempts at identification with him.

At Mike's puberty his father checked his testicles to be sure that both had descended so that he would one day beget a child. This act made the boy anxious about his manhood, and in spite of his father's reassurances he felt that only by impregnating a woman would he prove himself. When Mike was 22 the father died suddenly in his sleep while on vacation, and Mike could not go through his mourning successfully. He made his girl friend pregnant at about this time.

Treatment.   After Mike had been told that he had not finished grieving for his father and that some of his symptoms arose from this fact, he made a contract for goal-limited therapy. He was told that hospitalization might prove necessary—although this turned out not to be the case—and that the treatment would be completed when he became able to grieve over and accept his father's death. During a two-month period from May 1, 1968 (one week after the first anniversary of the death) to July 1, 1968, I had 25 sessions with him.

During the first three hours he exhibited symptoms and preoccupations typical of those who suffer from pathological grief. He made jokes and unintentional remarks connected with his death wishes. He described introjective attempts at reunion with his father, speaking of the strange feelings that seized him when he handled things the dead man had handled. He treasured his father's electric razor, but when he used it he was obsessed with the idea that his whiskers would "merge" with those of his father in the instrument, which he could not bring himself to clean for six months.

He indicated that he had depended on his father for narcissistic supplies. "When he died, a rug was pulled out from under my feet. Where will I turn now?" He felt that he had contributed to his father's death. In describing a difference between them he spoke of his father as being *"mortally*

> ... strange feelings . . . seized him when he handled things the dead man had handled.

How could his father die and leave him alone? Who was going to look after him now?

hurt" by something he had said. He disclosed an unconscious fear that his father would come back and hurt him, joking, "I can't talk against the dead so much, because if you knock them down they come back." He felt that his father was both dead and not dead, and had repeated dreams of seeing him as a hospital patient. He recalled the aborting of his normal grief reaction. "Suddenly I was the head of the family. My uncle said I should take care of the women. No one thought of *my* shock!"

In the fourth hour I requested that he make a list of objects related to himself and his dead father which had peculiar meaning for him. The list began with a beefsteak which the father had bought and which Mike felt a compulsion to eat after he learned of the death, in an effort to internalize him. Then came the razor, a key case, the father's camera, a particular photograph of the father, and things the father had written. My understanding of linking objects had at that time not yet been formulated; it was work with this patient which pointed to their recognition.

The first item brought in was a letter written by the father in which he blamed Mike for buying a motorcycle. Free association elicited an account of its purchase, and subsequent sale at the insistence of parents who felt it to be dangerous. Mike had felt his manly pride injured by this episode. I asked him to copy the letter, and to consider the differences between himself and his father as he noted the manifest differences in handwriting.

In the third week he brought a picture of his father which the mother had sent him after the death. It had come in a folder which he had not opened to reveal the photograph except for an occasional glimpse. The folder was wrinkled; Mike had once put it under dripping water, demonstrating an unconscious wish to weep over the dead father, and an equally unconscious wish to drown him. Drowning related to the actual cause of death, since he had died in his sleep after a day of snorkeling during which he had taken in sea water.

After talking about the picture, the patient said he was afraid of weeping. I then made my first "id interpretation" by stating that he was in truth afraid of drowning. I suggested that he look at the photograph, and that if he wept and felt as though he were drowning, I would help him. He removed his glasses and indicated unwillingness to look. I told him not to look until he was ready, and after considerable delay he did open the folder. At first he felt shock and indicated that the picture did not entirely resemble the father in his dreams. He then reported the *Operation on the Leg Dream* (described under the heading which follows). He went on to compare his father's physical appearance with his own. Unable at first to touch the picture, he began, at my suggestion, to touch the frame; when his fingers brushed the face he was reminded of the razor, and had an abreaction. He cried aloud, the tears rolling down his cheeks for 15 minutes. Narcissistic outcry followed. How could his father die and leave him alone? Who was going to look after him now?

We used the photograph also at the next session, at which the weeping was chronic, the patient attributing it to "a cold." Demarcation exercise continued with a comparison of the appearance of father and son. Mike recalled the night when news of the death had reached him in a motel room he occupied with his future wife. He remembered a dream of that night which had oedipal significance, in which his father punished him for driving his car too fast. The recollection led to an angry outburst against his mother and uncle, who had treated him as a child while burdening him with adult responsibilities. On the night of the death the uncle had warned him over the telephone not to try driving home alone, but at the same time he gave him responsibility for the legal affairs arising out of his father's death. Toward the end of the first month of treatment Mike did demarcation exercises with both the razor and the key chain, using the former in my office, and clarifying the present ownership of the key chain. He reported the *Birthday Present Dream,* and was encouraged to talk about the funeral.

Once at home he yelled, "Get out! Get out!" to the dead father he felt within himself.

Mike's mother had found her husband dead in bed. She had initially supposed that the blue color of an uncovered leg came from varicose veins in need of attention. Trying to cover the leg, she felt its chill and screamed for help, realizing that death had taken place. From his mother's account of this Mike had developed the picture of his father as a dead body with a blue leg. Feeling that he had had a "spiritual merging" with his father, he declined to view the body of the man who, in his view, had only begun to live—i.e., get away from the grandfather's domination—at the time of his death.

Mike had left the cemetery before the interment, and I verbalized the doubts I suspected were springing from his unconscious, flooding him with id impulses. I asked if the father had really been inside the coffin and if, in fact, the coffin had been buried. He replied angrily. His splitting response to reality was being assailed by the direct interpretations of this phase of treatment. A flooding with primary process thinking was permitted to promote the subsequent reorganization of more practical reality testing and a new adaptation to his life circumstances. He took a second psychological test at this point (May 1) in treatment. He seemed bewildered, and uncertain whether his father were alive or dead. Once at home he yelled, "Get out! Get out!" to the dead father he felt within himself. His abreactions continued.

His wife had to take him to the hospital emergency room during this phase, and he returned again on the following night, having hurt his eyes through his failure to remove his contact lenses for sleep. With his permission I interviewed his wife to enlist her help. Within a week his emotional state had greatly improved. He said he "felt great," and his old symptoms—trance-like states, sleepiness, and laziness—disappeared in the first week of the second month.

The assassination of Senator Kennedy during this phase of Mike's treatment led to the same splitting in reality testing displayed at his father's death. Indicating that although he knew about the Kennedy death he did not fully realize what had happened, he said, "It is so absurd! It was so sudden!" He refused to watch the televised funeral until I asked him to do so.

**. . . he carried
out my suggestion
of visiting the
rabbi to go
through the
Jewish burial
ritual.**

He sighed, had an abortive crying spell, and explained that he felt empty, showing most of the symptoms described by Lindemann[13] as being characteristic of acute grief reaction. The sight of the Kennedy son acting as pallbearer had reminded him that he had been an "errand boy" at his father's services, and unable to participate in them fully or to express his feelings. He remembered being angry at those who wept. He had wanted to say, "Don't cry! *I* want to cry. After all, he was *my* father!" I asked him to name his emotion as he told me this with tears in his eyes. "Grief—O.K.," he replied, and I exposed his father's picture once more. This time his abreaction was different; it was more nearly silent, and genuinely sad.

The next step was to prepare him for a cemetery visit to include taking pictures of the grave and bringing them in for discussion. Typically, he had not visited the grave since the funeral. The pathological mourner can pretend that death has not occurred by acting as though the grave were nonexistent.[3] Mike was uncertain about being able to locate the grave, even doubted its existence. He commented disapprovingly on burial in sealed coffins of the kind selected for his father, and gave his view that immediate decomposition should be allowed to occur. I interpreted these thoughts as doubts about the reality of the death and fears that the dead man might rise. Since he had access to the medical school, he suggested that he make arrangements to see a cadaver because he had never had the experience of seeing a dead body. I did not interfere with his plan.

His preparation during the first part of June to visit the grave evoked two temporary symptoms—tube vision, which made him feel as though he were "sinking into a grave," and stomach trouble with loss of appetite, which is a symptom of acute grief. A psychoanalytical interpretation suggests that eating is sexualized[14] in a symptom typical of pathological mourners. His reluctance to make the visit was conscious. He postponed it for three days, first doing something to his car which delayed his departure so that he arrived at the family home after the cemetery closed for the night. He also "forgot" his camera, and was obliged to use his father's. On the second day at home he carried out my suggestion of visiting the rabbi to go through the Jewish burial ritual. That afternoon, instead of going to the graveyard, he went to an ophthalmologist for the treatment of a stye which had caused his eye to fill with "tears," and which he understood was caused by his emotion. He did go to the cemetery on the third day, and was virtually on top of his father's grave before he was aware of it. "For all practical purposes I was *in* it—I mean I was *on* it!" He knew that his father was buried six feet below, but at the graveside he felt him to be nearer; he was apparently not ready to "put" his father in the ground all the way. He reported that at the last minute he had taken the caretaker's dog with him to the grave, in spite of a determination to make this difficult pilgrimage alone. In telling about this he began to weep. At the next session he took back his father's picture, and reported the *Safeway Dream.*

He then returned on his own initiative to the cemetery, going alone this time. He reframed his father's picture, and put it on his desk. He brought in the pictures his father had taken on vacation, the film for which had remained undeveloped in the camera he had used at the cemetery. These snapshots, which had presented uncomfortable possibilities to him, had been developed, and he now was able to use them to test reality about his father's last days. His chief exhibit, however, was the series of 24 pictures taken at the cemetery, which he asked me to view in order. He had taken them according to his memories of the funeral, beginning with the approach to the cemetery and continuing with pictures of the gate and views from both sides of the road. He had managed to include his shadow in all of the pictures of the grave, and interpreted this maneuver himself as evidence of his wish to "go in." He laughed at the notion, and denied that it still made him nervous. During his second visit he walked on the grave and convinced himself that his father was indeed dead. This was toward the end of the second month of re-griefing, at about the time when he reported that he had gone to view a cadaver and had not been afraid of the reality. He reported the *Examination Dream* on June 24, and began to talk about his daughter instead of his father. The child's name began with the same initial as the father's, and the patient noted the "link" between the living and the dead.

At this point he took another psychological test and reported two dreams, the *Dead Father Dream* of June 26 and the *Minor Operation Dream* of June 30. We agreed that these dreams and the associations they evoked indicated the completion of the re-grief work, and the contract was accordingly terminated.

Summary of objects and events of the demarcation, externalization, and reorganizational phases of re-grief work. Re-grief work started: May 1, 1968. Re-grief work ended: July 1, 1968 (25 sessions altogether). (1) The father's letter; (2) the father's picture; (3) the razor; (4) the key chain; (5) the televised Kennedy funeral; (6) the father's camera; (7) the visit to the rabbi; (8) the undeveloped snapshots; (9) photographs of the cemetery; (10) the grave; (11) the view of a cadaver.

The Study of Dreams During Re-Grief Work

In our collection of dreams of patients undergoing re-grief work we found fairly predictable manifest content ranging from a life-and-death struggle in which the deceased, undisguised, was engaged, and the funeral, to situations reflecting an acknowledgment of separation and the anger it engendered. References to burial and a completed task appeared toward the end of the re-griefing. It is outside the scope of this paper to review the possible significance of manifest content. Spanjaard,[15] who did review manifest dreams from the psychoanalytic point of view, concluded that manifest content of dreams usually has a subjectively conflictual aspect, and that "this aspect offers us the opportunity to evaluate the most superficial layer of the conflict and thus to arrive at a construction of the poten-

> **During his second visit he walked on the grave and convinced himself that his father was indeed dead.**

tially most useful interpretation." He summarized by giving his opinion that "the role of the dreamer in the manifest dream is particularly important as a guide for the construction of one's interpretation, namely in relation to the current conflict." What I learned from my re-grief patients supports such a view. In a majority of these cases I could use the manifest content of dreams as "review dreams" like those suggested by Glover[16] and interpret them readily as an assessment of the patient's progress in overcoming his difficulties. The flow of change in the dreams reported here is typical of what is seen in the process of re-griefing.

The Content of the Dreams

Dream no. 1: Repeating dreams. A series of repeating dreams appeared between the father's death and the beginning of re-grief work. In these Mike saw his father undisguised, always alive, and usually engaged in some kind of life-and-death struggle. Mike knew that his father was alive but was at the same time convinced of his death. Whenever not engaged in a struggle, the father would be seen in a hospital, wearing a grim expression.

Dream no. 2: An operation on the leg. On May 23 Mike reported dreaming of being with his father in a shopping center. He was prepared to have an operation, perhaps a leg amputation. He looked at his father, who he knew was about to die.

Dream no. 3: The birthday present dream. On May 31 Mike reported dreaming of the receipt of a wrapped birthday gift. When it was unwrapped it appeared to be a telephone in pieces, to be put together. This was reported one month after re-grief work began, and just before the funeral memories were reviewed.

Dream no. 4: The Safeway dream. On the night after the visit to his father's grave (June 17) Mike reported:
"I was driving some type of vehicle on the sidewalk as I had done when I was a child. My dream took place in the downtown area of the university town. I was coming toward the university. I came near the Safeway Store, and after passing it I found myself at a place which looked like a slaughterhouse. [In reality, between the downtown area and the University Hospital there is a Safeway Store, next to which is a funeral home.] I saw a big dead cow and a newborn calf. Someone had slit open the cow's belly and had wrapped up the newborn calf and placed it in the belly of the cow."

Dream no. 5: An examination dream. The patient had this dream on the night of June 22, just after he had seen a cadaver. It was reported on June 24.
"I saw many of my classmates, and was getting ready to take an examination. I was anxious. Then the thought occurred to me that, after all, I

was not in school any more and there was no need for me to be anxious, I felt relieved."

Dream no. 6: The dead father dream.   This was reported on June 27.

"I had a dream about my father, but this one was different. In this dream my father was dead."

Dream no. 7: The minor operation dream.   This was reported on July 1.

"I felt that I had had a minor operation on my chest, performed recently. I also felt that I had the option of undergoing a major operation."

Analysis of the Dreams

These dreams permit many interpretations but will be examined here only in relation to re-grief work.

The first set of *Repeating Dreams* suggests that the father is not dead. Mike is having an internal struggle over whether not to kill him. This kind of dream is common to all patients suffering from pathological grief reactions.[2, 3]

The "operation on the leg dream" is a continuation of the series, showing Mike still engaged in the internal struggle about killing or not killing his father. His direct association concerns his father's help to him about going to medical school. Had the father invited his son to watch him perform an operation, this would have marked his initiation into manhood, but death had prevented.

There is an element of identification with the dead father. The patient's mother had emphasized the blue look of her husband's leg and her initial reaction that he needed an operation for varicose veins. In the dream Mike's identification led him to become the father who required a leg operation. Mike had said, "I looked at my father and knew he was dying." In reality, his mother had looked at her husband and become aware that he was dead.

The "birthday present dream" occurred at the end of demarcation exercises concerning what belonged to Mike and what had belonged to his father. In reality Mike at the time was engaged in assembling hi-fi equipment. After demarcation exercises he felt freed from his father—reborn. Communication (the telephone) with me had helped him—or gave promise of helping him—to accomplish this. Evidences of identification with the father can be seen in the use of the word "born" and "reborn"; Mike had spoken of his father's "rebirth" after the death of the grandfather. This dream preceded emotional outbursts at the internalized father in which he had called to his internalized father to "get out!" At the conclusion of this process he felt energetic, "like living again," and his symptoms abated.

The "Safeway dream," which followed the visit to the grave, represents the safety involved in examining the disturbing unconscious processes. He was on his way from a shopping center, the locale of the first dream reported in his re-grief work, to my office. In his direct association to this dream Mike himself suggested that he was the calf which was placed in and thus forced to merge with the dead cow. He felt that part of himself was buried with the dead father. Further association is disclosed when he said of his first visit to the grave . . . "for all practical purposes I was *in* it . . . I mean *on* it." Another association appears in his photographing his shadow "in" the father's grave.

The first part of his "examination dream" is typical of such dreams which, according to Freud,[17] occur only when someone has already passed an examination successfully. They convey to the dreamer the message, "Don't be afraid. Think how anxious you were before the examination, and yet nothing happened to you. You have already succeeded in what you had to tackle." In the second part of the dream, which followed his imperturbable viewing of a dead body, Mike rationalized that there was nothing to be anxious about. After this he enrolled in the university from which he had taken sick leave at the approach of the anniversary of his father's death.

Then in a dream he saw his father dead. In his association he reported that memories of his father were returning more freely, and that he could remember happy events in which they had both been involved, and could even laugh over some of them. He felt that "his energies were unbinding," and began to talk about terminating the contract with me. In the final dream of the "minor operation," the operation represented the re-grief work, now completed; the dream presented the option of undertaking a major operation (further treatment). . . .

The Investigation of Re-Grief Work Through the Psychoanalytic Microscope

Our pilot study followed the progress of its subjects after the completion of their re-griefing therapy to determine whether symptoms of pathological grief had returned. Mike's decision to go into psychoanalysis and the decision of another pilot-study patient to undertake psychoanalytic psychotherapy provided us with special access to this appraisal. Follow-up results of all the pilot-study patients will be given elsewhere.

Mike asked for psychoanalysis three months after the termination of our contract, showing no signs of pathological grief when he came to see me about it. He felt subjectively at this time that his problem concerning his father's death had been solved; he was no longer bothered by it. He had, however, become curious about himself and aware of certain personal characteristics which he wanted to do something about. His psychoanalytic contract gave me an opportunity to look through the psychoanalytic microscope at what had gone on in his re-grief work. He spent the first year of his analysis with me, but moved then to the city where his uncle lived. The move was made for financial reasons but also because of his wish to demonstrate to the uncle his capacity to follow in his father's footsteps and to prove his manhood to him. He continued his analysis with an analyst in the new location, and concluded it successfully.

I was closely in touch with the second analyst[18] in order to obtain his views of Mike, and his perceptions about re-grief work. Throughout his analysis Mike did not exhibit established symptoms referring to the core formulation of pathological grief reaction, the persistent attempt at reunion with the dead man. The father was dead, and father transference occurred in the usual fashion—the father was alive in the transference neurosis.

Mike was in analysis with me at the time of the second anniversary of the death. Anxiety and other incapacitating symptoms exhibited at the first anniversary were by then absent. Only one symptom appeared, the meaning of which was repressed and brought into his awareness only during analysis. On the anniversary night Mike quarreled with his wife and went to sleep in a motel, in the kind of environment in which he had received the news of his father's death. During the third anniversary no incapacitating symptoms appeared, and he told his new analyst about his night in the motel on the occasion of the second anniversary. The approach of the third anniversary prompted him to consider the possibility of taking a holiday at the vacation spot in which his father had died, but instead he devoted himself to securing an acceptance in medical school, and demonstrated successful assertive competence in beginning to get himself established.

The clinical findings, psychological test results, and dream analysis certainly indicated a change in his psychic state. As Showalter and I noted in an earlier paper,[4] "In the jungle of human behavior, events do not take place in isolated compartments as capsules but rather are intimately intertwined with many other memories and feelings representing different levels of development." It would be a mistake, however, to state that the technique of re-grief work was the *only* factor responsible for changing the patient's symptoms. Such an assumption would be as incorrect as the assumption of a behavior therapist who believes he is carefully refraining from making any interpretation to the female anorexia patient with whom he is lunching when he tells her, to encourage her to eat, that he has delivered a huge number of babies without harm to the mother!

As I have noted, Mike's father had conveyed to his 13-year-old son anxiety about the boy's ability to beget children when he was grown, and died before the son had an opportunity to prove his manhood to him, although at the time of the death Mike was having sexual relations with his wife-to-be. It became evident during his analysis that throughout his re-grief work Mike had thought of me as his oedipal father, and one of the determinants in his undertaking analysis was his desire to tell me about his child. The actual father was kept as the representative of the father of the oedipal age. Mike had been in acute involvement with him just before the death, had tried to identify with him, and saw this identification as a solution for the separation-individuation problems presented by the engulfing mother (who was represented in his dreams by the Gulf of Mexico). Since

"In the jungle of human behavior, events do not take place in isolated compartments . . . but rather are intimately intertwined with many . . . memories and feelings. . . ."

the death had been so ill-timed for the son, it was necessary for him to keep his father, and what he represented, alive. During the year following the death he had not only impregnated his future wife and married her, but he had purchased a flashy car and received word of his acceptance into medical school. In his analysis it became clear that these accomplishments and possessions intrapsychically represented an oedipal triumph by bypassing the necessary struggle for it, and produced guilt feelings. Guilt was manifested in his aimlessness, the loss of his car, the near-loss of his wife, and the loss of his opportunity to attend medical school, and pathological grief became his way of handling this guilt.

During re-grief work he saw me as a benign father who would teach him how to let go, how to learn to separate and to lose in order to achieve individuality. In an effort to identify with me he became a psychology major shortly after re-grief work terminated, and, later, after considerable analytic work, he re-enrolled in medical school.

He had no problem going into the analytical position, in spite of the fact that the techniques of re-grief work are quite different from those of psychoanalysis. His first dream after his analysis began was reported during the ninth hour:

"My brain was being operated on. My entire cerebral hemispheres were exposed and some squares of my brain were excised or modified or changed."

I felt this was a continuation of the "minor operation dream" of July 1, which represented the completion of re-grief work, but which offered an option to undergo a "major operation"—psychoanalysis. . . .

References

1. Volkan, V. Normal and pathological grief reactions—a guide for the family physician. *Va. Med. Monthly,* 93: 651-656, 1966.
2. ———. The University of Virginia study on pathological mourning. *Tip Dünyasi* (Istanbul) 42: 544-551, 1969.
3. ———. Typical findings in pathological grief. *Psychiat. Quart.,* 44: 231-250, 1970.
4. Volkan, V., and Showalter, C. R. Known object loss, disturbance in reality testing, and "re-grief" work as a method of brief psychotherapy. *Psychiat. Quart.,* 42: 358-374, 1968.
5. Volkan, V. The linking objects of pathological mourners. Paper read at the fall meeting of the American Psychoanalytic Association, New York City, December 19, 1970.
6. Bowlby, J. Process of mourning. *Int. J. Psycho-Anal.,* 42: 317-340, 1961.
7. Bibring, E. The mechanism of depression. In *Affective Disorders.* P. Greenacre (editor). International Universities Press. New York. 1953.
8. Rado, S. Adaptational development of psychoanalytic therapy. In *Changing Concepts of Psychoanalytic Medicine.* S. Rado and G. E. Daniels (editors). Grune and Stratton. New York. 1956.
9. Abraham, K. (1911). Note on the psychoanalytical investigation and treatment of manic depressive insanity and allied conditions. *Selected Papers.* Institute of Psychoanalysis and Hogarth Press. London. 1956.
10. Freud, S. (1917). Mourning and melancholia. *Collected Papers,* vol. 4. Institute of Psychoanalysis and Hogarth Press. London. 1956.
11. Pollock, G. H. Mourning and adaptation. *Int. J. Psycho-Anal.,* 42: 341-361, 1961.
12. Schafer, R. *Aspects of Internalization.* International Universities Press. New York. 1968.
13. Lindemann, E. Symptomatology and management of acute grief. *Am. J. Psychiat.,* 101: 141-148, 1944.

14. Fenichel, O. *The Psychoanalytic Theory of Neurosis.* Norton. New York. 1945.
15. Spanjaard, J. The manifest dream content and its significance for the interpretation of dreams. *Int. J. Psycho-An.,* 50: 221-235, 1969.
16. Glover, E. *Technique of Psychoanalysis.* International Universities Press. New York. 1955.
17. Freud, S. (1900). *The Interpretation of Dreams,* tr. by J. Strachey. Basic Books. New York. 1958.
18. Kirschner, G. I. Personal communication.

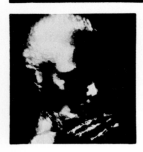

10

Practice

Do all people grieve in a similar fashion and require the same kinds of helping resources? Are cultural differences considered when techniques for treating the mentally ill are planned? A program that does pay attention to these differences is benefiting Spanish-speaking mental patients in a state hospital in Greater Los Angeles. The following exercises in the Appendix will be useful aids:

B.   Appropriate Death Fantasy

C.   Awareness of Grief Process

I.   Life and Death Attitudes: Dyadic Encounter

Therapy Through a Death Ritual

Ignacio Aguilar

Virginia N. Wood

Spanish-speaking people have always formed a significant proportion of the population in the Greater Los Angeles metropolitan area and have maintained their unique culture and their language. Although a goodly number of them had moved north from Mexico to settle the area before the English-speaking people came, they became a minority when the Anglo-Americans rushed to California in the mid-19th century. The subsequent history of prejudice, mistreatment, and violence has had profound effects—and the sense of being in a marginal group, apart from the mainstream of American life, has been accentuated by the fact that English was the only language taught in the elementary public schools, until perhaps the last two or three years.

A sense of marginality may be one factor that brings some Spanish-speaking adolescents and adults into state hospitals in this country. If such a feeling is a contributing cause of their illness, the prejudice and the lack of understanding they are likely to encounter in an American hospital aggravates rather than ameliorates it. Since the hospitals in most communities have few if any staff who speak Spanish, these patients are too often given their medicine and left alone until they are discharged. Psychiatric treatment for them is practically nonexistent.

In a state hospital, mental illness is usually viewed within the framework of particular methods or techniques, and whatever therapy the social worker prescribes is likely to be based primarily on the psycho-analytical school in which that worker has been trained. Often these techniques are not effective in treating culturally different patients unless they are modified to meet the patients' needs. As Slavson points out, "the individual cannot be understood apart from his family and social culture."[1]

This material was first published in *Social Work,* vol. 21, no. 1, pp. 49-54, January 1976. Copyright 1976 the National Association of Social Workers. Reprinted by permission.

The cultural values the patient brings with him . . . must be understood. . . .

Thus those who are providing therapy must not only understand the etiology of the illness, but should also have insight about the way the patient perceives his own illness within the context of his culture. If the overt symptoms can be classified within some classical framework of mental illness, this of course indicates the treatment in general, but consideration given to the patient's feelings and attitudes will help him get well too. The cultural values the patient brings with him to the hospital must be understood before the psychotherapeutic approach can be fully determined. Friedlander states it this way:

> In working toward the social adjustment of the individual and the group, social work needs to consider the cultural environment from which the individual clients or group come. These values may not be the same as those of the social worker himself or of a majority group that determines the policies of social work practice through its organization.[2]

This concept becomes even more important when one deals with patients whose cultural background is different from that of the social worker. Their values, their attitudes, and their perception of themselves in relation to their families, the society, and the institution itself must be taken into account. Not until then can one begin to tailor a therapeutic plan for the patient and to provide effective treatment that will return this individual to the community as a responsible person.

Metropolitan State Hospital in Norwalk, California has inaugurated a program for Spanish-speaking patients that is the first of its kind in California and in the United States. Many people in the area are of Mexican descent, although there is a substantial number of persons from Puerto Rico, Cuba, and other countries of Central and South America. This program is carried out in the Xipe-Totec Clinica de Salud Mental and has been in operation since November 1971.[3] It is still considered experimental, although the throes of initial organization are over and daily routines have become established. The program staff are all Spanish-speaking and, except for one person, are all of Mexican descent. However, they are still studying and learning about many aspects of mental and emotional disorders as they manifest themselves, particularly in Spanish-speaking people, and they are still devising techniques of treatment that meet the special needs of these people.

This article will focus on aspects of Mexican culture, rather than Latin American culture in general, and on techniques devised to meet the special needs of Mexican Americans, since a large proportion of the patients in the program are either Mexican or of Mexican descent. The clinic has between forty-five and fifty patients daily, and there are rarely more than ten of them who are of descent other than Mexican. Even though the techniques of treatment are based on the Mexican culture, all patients respond to them. Staff attribute this response to the unifying effects of the Catholic religion that Spain introduced throughout Latin America.

Death and Mourning

Death is among the many events that may lead to a psychotic break or nervous breakdown, especially when mourning and grief are not satisfactorily resolved. Death is a significant event in any culture, but the cultural ways of handling the highly stressful conditions related to it vary immensely. And as might be expected, a death in a Mexican family stimulates emotions and activities different from those seen in an Anglo-American family.

Weisman describes the Anglo-American situation:

> American culture, confronting death, has attempted to cope by disguising it, pretending that it is not a basic condition of life. . . . The unhappy result, all too often, is that the dying patient is left to die emotionally and spiritually alone. We do not even permit him to say goodbye. . . . Death is either an idolized extension of terrestrial life as we know it, or it is simply complete and unambiguous extinction.[4]

In contrast, the Mexican treats death and the dead with much respect, in the belief that the dead are always with us. The Mexican inherits a long tradition of belief that this life is merely an intermediate step on the way to another—perhaps not too much different from this one, perhaps better. There is an inevitability about this road from birth to death and an implicit feeling that one can do little but live one's days—working, raising children, praying, working. Always working. *La vida es trabajar y poco gozar* [Life is work, with little pleasure].

Perhaps the best expression of the fatalistic feeling toward life and death is expressed in an ancient Aztec poem:

> We only came to sleep,
> we only came to dream;
> it is not true, it is not true
> that we came to live on the earth.
> We became the green growth of spring;
> our hearts will again revive,
> they will again open their petals;
> but our body is like a rosebush;
> it gives a few flowers and withers.[5]

Most Mexicans are not familiar with this poem, but it expresses well the Mexican attitude toward death. This world is transient; life is merely a passage from one state of being to another; something of greater significance to us exists somewhere. Something of greater significance "somewhere" does not refer merely to the Christian concept of an everlasting life in some far-off heaven, but indicates that in this cosmos there must be a greater meaning and that death is merely a vehicle, a marker, on the road that must be traveled to achieve whatever awaits us. The Mexican handles the fear and uncertainty about death differently than the American or the European does. As Paz describes it:

Death is a significant event in any culture, but the cultural ways of handling the highly stressful conditions related to it vary immensely.

**. . . the Day
of the Dead,
November 2, is a
special day in
Mexico.**

For the resident of New York, Paris or London, death is a word that is never spoken because it burns the lips. In contrast, the Mexican frequents death, makes fun of it, caresses it, sleeps with it, fetes it; it is one of his favorite games and his deepest love. . . . Our songs, verses, fiestas and popular sayings demonstrate unequivocally that death does not frighten us because "life has cured us of fears."[6]

Customs in Mexico

Like those of most cultures, the Spanish-speaking people believe that one should not speak ill of the dead. There is a belief, often expressed, that they remain close enough to hear our words, and that they may revenge themselves upon the living. For this reason the Day of the Dead, November 2, is a special day in Mexico. It is a day of serious and meaningful ceremony, with implications of appeasement, forgiveness, and repentance. Altars are erected in homes, and food is set out to nourish the dead who may choose to return and visit their families. Paths to the house are strewn with marigolds to lead the dead back. The family may also decorate the tombs at the cemetery and take food to the graves where they sit, eat, pray, and commune with the dead. Failure to respect and care for the dead on this day that honors them brings fear, remorse, shame, and ultimately disgrace for the whole family.

Celebration of the Day of the Dead can perhaps best be described as a celebration of life-in-death. The figures associated with this day are death figures (skulls, bones, skeletons), but all are engaged in activities of life—dancing, singing, eating, and so on.[7]

When a person dies, a two-fold process is set in motion: there are the activities connected with burial and the honoring of the dead and the activities reaffirming the survivors' position in the world of the living. Indians in some parts of Mexico celebrate a death with a fiesta. If you ask them why they have music, dancing, and feasting, they always answer that they are celebrating the fact that this person has gone beyond and no longer has to be in this world of sorrow and unhappiness. People should be sad because they remain and glad because that person has gone—gone to something better than what there is here today.

In urban Mexico, when a person dies, the body is removed to a funeral home as soon as possible—or, if the family is poor, will be laid out in the largest room in the house. The family provides a constant watch over the body as it lies in state, and someone is always with the bereaved ones at home also. Friends, acquaintances, and neighbors continually visit the bereaved household, bringing food, drink, and other necessities and sitting with the family to offer condolences and to talk about the deceased. People may reminisce about the dead person in many ways—tell amusing but not irreverent stories, discuss personality traits, say anything that comes to mind, so long as they do not speak ill of the dead.

Family, friends, and acquaintances are all present at the burial, which is followed by a week or so of visiting to offer condolences. During this period, friends and neighbors sit with the family again, supply food and drink, and assist them in receiving the visitors. After this, life returns to the normal routine. Widows and widowers are expected to wear some sign of mourning and to refrain from social activities that may lead to courtship and marriage for six months to a year; sons and daughters, brothers and sisters, fathers and mothers, may return to their daily routine more rapidly.

The mourning process may be divided into eight stages: (1) the death of a significant person, (2) a state of depression in the bereaved, (3) initiation of the mourning process—consisting of *el velorio* [the wake] and *la tendida* [the lying in state], (4) initial acceptance of the loss of the loved one, (5) the burial, (6) a second state of depression, during which the bereaved becomes aware of unresolved feelings of hostility toward the dead and a sense of guilt for recognizing negative qualities of the dead person, (7) collective condolences during the week or so following the funeral, which provides a special way to resolve the sense of guilt, and (8) final acceptance of reality and the lifting of the depression. Remaining feelings of guilt and hostility are handled during the annual visit to the graveside on the Day of the Dead.

Remaining feelings of guilt and hostility are handled during the annual visit to the graveside on the Day of the Dead.

The Mexican American and the Mexican immigrant often miss part of this process in the United States. First, the circumstances preceding and surrounding the death itself may be more impersonal than in Mexico. In that country a family member who is ill is not bundled off to a hospital and seen rarely; Mexican hospitals provide rooms near the patient for the family to stay during the entire illness. Thus, when a family member dies, some or all of the family have been with the person during the final illness. In case of death by accident or death far away, part of the guilt and remorse lies in the fact that the person died alone, away from those close to him. A terminal illness in an American hospital with restricted visiting enhances this guilty feeling because it deprives family members of the opportunity to face the reality of approaching death and to make their own peace with the dying person.

Furthermore, the trend toward the breakdown of the extended family is likely to circumscribe the ritual surrounding death as it is performed in the United States. Because the family members may be separated—some still living in Mexico, others living in different communities in the United States—the support given to the bereaved after the death may not be as full and helpful as it would have been in Mexico.

The Mexican awareness of death goes beyond the death of a close relative or friend. A Mexican immigrant may mourn the loss of his native land in a way very like the mourning for a dead person. It is easy for a person of Mexican descent to imagine that the loss of a place of living or of something else important, or a shortcoming in coping with cultural norms is somewhat like death—the death of a part of him, which prevents his functioning in the prescribed way.

The Hospital Setting

. . . even though the problems of a Mexican and a non-Mexican may be the same, the signs and symptoms signaling that the person is not functioning may be different.

The problems that bring a person of Mexican descent to a mental hospital as a patient are fundamentally no different than those of non-Mexican patients. The differences lies in the cultural concepts of the patients: for instance, their attitudes toward male and female roles, the importance of family, the emphasis on work. That is to say, even though the problems of a Mexican and a non-Mexican may be the same, the signs and symptoms signaling that the person is not functioning may be different. Even more important, once the stress process is begun, cultural differences may act to aggravate the situation.[8] If these differences are not recognized and dealt with in the mental hospital, treatment may be seriously impeded.

Friedlander describes a stressful situation that seems particularly applicable to persons living in a place where their own culture is not that of the mainstream.

> A situation is potentially stressful when a reorganization of role relationships and a reallocation of social role functions must be made in an ongoing primary group. Accustomed and habitual modes of adaptation must, under such circumstances, be modified.[9]

The overall purpose when planning the Xipe-Totec Clinica de Salud Mental was first to place the patient within a familiar cultural setting. The aim was to relax the patient and remove additional stress caused through conflict with the Anglo-American culture by providing a place for treatment in which the Spanish language was spoken and familiar Latin music was heard, a place in which the decorations and furnishings, the recreational and other program activities, and the ways of work were adapted to Mexican customs and cultural styles.

Under such conditions, the patient is far more willing to trust the ward personnel and to discuss the problems that necessitated hospitalization. This trust in the personnel has to be established before the therapist can elicit the information that will make it possible to evoke appropriate responses in individual patients and in the group as a whole.

Catharsis is generally recognized as important in a psychotherapeutic relationship, but it is probably one of the most difficult responses to elicit freely in a patient. There are well-established techniques for triggering this process in Anglo-Americans, but it is not easy to apply them to persons of Latin extraction, since, in general, the character of the Latin is not so open as that of the Anglo-American. Thus it is likely to be especially difficult for the orthodox therapist to release an emotional outburst in the Latin patient.

The problem is compounded if the therapist is English-speaking and the persons under therapy are not, and it is further compounded if the therapist knows little or nothing about the patient's cultural background. In the experience at Metropolitan State Hospital, many culturally oriented techniques that elicit catharsis have been devised and used.

The therapist strives to produce emotional catharsis for bringing relief to the individual, but the main goal is to bring about a collective response in the group. As Yalom says:

> Catharsis—the expression of a strong emotion—is a valuable part of the curative process, but not a goal in itself. Strong expression of emotion enhances the development of cohesiveness.[10]

The development of group cohesiveness through catharsis is the most important element in the "funeral ceremonies" enacted at the Xipe-Totec Clinic to help patients resolve the mourning fixation.

The Ritual Drama

As already mentioned, collective mourning for the dead is essential if the technique is to be therapeutic for the patient. Whenever this technique is to be applied, the clinic team first discusses the indigenous cultural background and any other pertinent facts about the patient for whom an enactment of the ritual is being considered—that is, the target patient. When the time is ripe for the activity, the stage must be set; that is, the patient and the group must be prepared to participate and derive therapeutic benefit from the ritual drama.

What is presented is appropriately called a ritual drama, because it is a dramatic enactment of a solemn ritual. The technique must be treated with a great deal of respect and mysticism if it is to produce the desired results. First the mood—appropriately laden with cultural significance and ritualistic meaning—must be established in all patients by some means familiar to them. The reading of poetry about mother, child, or the dead has been found particularly effective. Gustavo Adolfo Becquer's "Dios mío, que sólo se quedan los muertos" [Dear God, how lonely are the dead] has always produced the desired reactions.

However, the procedure may start in a variety of ways. Occasionally the situation presents itself spontaneously. Perhaps the patient himself introduced the subject of death, or a gloomy day may have contributed to establishing the setting. Whatever the initiating conditions, the enactment never takes place abruptly; there are always preparatory statements that set the scene. Besides the reading of poetry, the therapist may encourage participation by such questions as "What would you say to your father if he were here now?" (Or your mother, husband, wife, sister—whoever the deceased may have been.) "What would you have said if you could have been with him when he died?" The preparatory period may be brief when the group is receptive, or it may be prolonged, but it rarely lasts longer than five minutes.

When a spontaneous enactment of the ritual seems fitting, the therapist determines during this exploratory or preparatory period whether the dead person is to be male or female. It is also decided during this period whether to have a *velorio* or a *tendida.* Both require that one of the patients take the role of the deceased. However, the *velorio* terminates with the closing of the coffin and the funeral procession; the *tendida* consists of having the target patient kneel by the body and say those things left unsaid during the actual event, after which all participants return to their seats. When the ritual has been planned beforehand, the exploratory stage tends to be shorter.

The exploratory period is followed by a rapid scene-setting. A blanket is quickly spread on the floor, the person selected as the deceased lies down on it, a second blanket is spread next to it that will later be used to cover the "corpse" when the "coffin" is closed. Candles are lit and placed at the head and foot of the bier; the lights are dimmed. The scene is set.

The therapist then says, "There is your father. Go to him. Say goodbye to him. Tell him all the things you never said when he died." This is the moment of catharsis. The patient approaches the bier and usually kneels beside it. As far as possible the scene should proceed spontaneously at this point. However, the therapist may have to encourage the patient to speak—even to the extent sometimes of standing behind him and speaking for him at first.

This is a delicate stage in the ritual. A *velorio* or a *tendida* has been recreated to evoke memories and feelings about the dead person. At a real *velorio* or *tendida,* revealing negative personal feelings about the deceased would not be sanctioned; it would be beyond the bounds of traditional appropriate behavior. Such feelings would not be expressed and resolved in real life until later—during the period after the funeral. Yet, if the catharsis that the therapist seeks is to be achieved through this dramatic enactment, the target patient must reveal whatever personal feelings of hostility, anger, or hate may be preventing a mature acceptance of the death.

This then is the paradox and the crucial problem for the therapist: how to make the patient feel that revealing negative feelings is appropriate at an enactment of the ritual long after death, although it would have been inappropriate at the actual ritual. If the situation is not handled carefully at this moment, the mood may be broken and the opportunity lost. The therapist must be sensitive to the mood of the group and of the target patient if the ritual drama is to be effective.

In the case of the *velorio,* after the patient has said everything he wants to, he closes the coffin by covering it with the second blanket. A funeral procession is formed, with a table representing the casket. Two pallbearers carry the casket, and the procession moves to the end of the hallway, where the "burial" takes place and flowers are put on the grave. While the burial is taking place, the *velorio* scene is cleaned up, lights are turned on again, the "corpse" returns to the group. The procession returns from the graveside to resume daily activities. Life must go on.

Clinic activities are resumed at this point, but in a way consistent with the events that have just occurred. This is usually the time for the coffee break, which gives everyone a chance to relax from the intense emotions released. Yet the setting also corresponds to a part of the mourning process outlined earlier—the period of collective condolences. The group is still considerate of the bereaved person and at the same time each person begins to resume his usual role. Group pressure thus acts to reinforce the acceptance of loss by the bereaved person and a return to his own life.

Reactions and Results

Reactions have sometimes been dramatic. One woman collapsed in a faint at the "bier" of her mother. A young man who had previously resisted treatment and been unresponsive cried bitterly over the "body" of his mother, who had died while he was in prison. A young girl became almost uncontrollably hysterical at the "burial" of a father. This last instance was entirely unexpected, as the girl was not the target patient and the clinic's knowledge of her case did not indicate the possibility of such a reaction.

The reaction of the group reinforces the emotional content of the ritual. There are always several women who spontaneously take on the role of mourners, kneeling around the "body" and reciting prayers. Men too seem to fall into appropriate roles. To an observer, a family almost seems to materialize for the patient; one can almost identify uncles, aunts, sisters, and brothers emerging from the group to comfort and support the grieving person.

The results of participation in this ritual have often been pronounced. A neurotic depression often becomes a healthy, normal depression, and after a day or so the patient's acceptance of the current situation becomes evident—in facial expression, and bodily attitudes as well as in verbal responses. The patient's response, when asked how he feels about the dead person, is a normal nonneurotic statement, "He's dead now."

One 14-year-old girl had been having hallucinations in which her father had appeared to her and told her she was "bad." This girl not only had unresolved feelings of grief and anger at the loss of her father, but also, after the father's death, had developed strong feelings against her mother. She resented the changes that had taken place, especially the family's move from Mexico to the United States, which resulted in her undergoing the physical and emotional changes of adolescence in strange surroundings. During the *velorio,* she slapped her "father's" face saying, "You were bad. You drank. You left us alone." Later she forgave him and asked his forgiveness, closed the coffin, and said, *"Descanse en paz* [Rest in peace]." She has had no further hallucinations of her father.

The ritual drama has been used at the clinic in even more symbolic ways, to bury undesirable things, such as one's past life. This also has been found effective. The effectiveness lies in the symbolism of the Mexicans' pervasive respect for death and their significant regard for the burial and the honoring of the dead—the mourning, the forgiveness, the interment, the final blessing—followed by the ultimate acceptance that one phase of life has ended and another is beginning.

Group pressure . . . acts to reinforce the acceptance of loss by the bereaved person and a return to his own life.

The clinic does not of course try to use this ritual drama to solve all problems, because many complex conditions cause a person to cease to function to the extent that he becomes a patient in a mental hospital. However, when there is reason to suspect that having unresolved feelings about the death of someone close is one of the precipitating conditions, it has been found that participation in this ritual drama frequently has a significant curative effect.

Conclusions

The effectiveness of the program for Spanish-speaking mental patients that is being carried out at the Xipe-Totec Clinica in the Metropolitan State Hospital, Norwalk, California, shows that cultural differences are a not-to-be-overlooked factor in considering techniques for treating the mentally ill. Experience at this clinic clearly indicates that it is important for a professional—whether social worker, psychologist, or other health service person—to incorporate this factor into his conception of his function, his relations, his psychic elements, and his self-image. Although the psychic elements are basically the same for all persons, the expression of these elements varies greatly according to the individual's cultural background.

The therapist who treats this type of patient must first endeavor to understand the patient's own world, the familial culture, and the national culture. Because the patient is expected to return to his own family and social setting, it is of utmost importance to learn about these aspects of his life and include them in the therapeutic plan. Hamilton sums it up this way:

> A person can be well-adjusted in a closed culture in which traditional and dogmatic influences perform the functions of a collective superego or conscience. Ideologies to which people completely submit or which they completely incorporate into their lives seem to create a condition of tranquility for the individual. Dislocation without reference to cultural roots and customs makes for tensions, insecurity, and anxiety. No treatment goal can be envisaged which does not involve a value judgment which is itself culturally determined.[11]

References

1. S. R. Slavson, *A Textbook in Analytic Group Psychotherapy* (New York: International Universities Press, 1964).
2. A. Walter Friedlander, *Concepts and Methods of Social Work* (Englewood Cliffs, N.J.: Prentice-Hall, 1958), p. 9.
3. *See* Ignacio Aguilar, "Clinica de Salud Mental—Xipe-Totec (Ward 210)," Norwalk, Calif.: Metropolitan State Hospital, 1971 (dittoed). *Xipe-Totec* is an Aztec mythological term meaning "Our Lord the Flayed One" and symbolically suggesting renewal and the god of spring.
4. Avery D. Weisman, *On Dying and Denying* (New York: Behavioral Publications, 1972), p. 101.
5. In Alfonso Caso, *El Pueblo del Sol* (Mexico, D.F.: El Fondo de Cultura Economica, 1953). p. 123. Translated into English by Virginia N. Wood.

6. Octavio Paz, *El Laberinto de la Soledad* (Mexico, D.F.: Fondo de la Cultura Economica, 1959); or Paz, *The Labyrinth of Solitude* (New York: Grove Press, 1961), p. 52.
7. Eduardo Matos Moctezuma, ed., *Miccaihuitl: El Culto a la Muerta* (Mexico, D.F.: Artes de Mexico, 1971); and Daniel Moreno, *El Humorismo Mexicano* (Mexico, D.F.: Artes de Mexico, 1971).
8. James P. Spradley and Mark Phillips, "Culture and Stress: A Quantitative Analysis," *American Anthropologist,* 74 (June 1972), pp. 518–529.
9. Friedlander, op. cit., p. 52.
10. Irwin D. Yalom, *Theory and Practice of Group Psychotherapy* (New York: Basic Books, 1970), p. 72.
11. Gordon Hamilton, *Theory and Practice of Social Case Work* (New York: Columbia University Press, 1951).

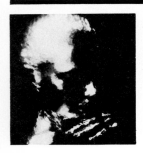

11

Practice

C an you imagine using your own mind to cure cancer? Carl and Stephanie Simonton suggest in this chapter that our belief systems not only contribute to our getting cancer, but also are instrumental in our combating it. Since fantasy and relaxation are important aspects in this process, the following Appendix exercises are recommended:

B.   Appropriate Death Fantasy

K.   Planning for Living

Belief Systems and Management of the Emotional Aspects of Malignancy

O. Carl Simonton

Stephanie S. Simonton

There are over 200 articles in the medical literature covering different aspects of the relationship between the emotions and stress to malignancy, as well as other very serious diseases. The interesting thing about the literature is that in all of these articles the conclusion is that there is a relationship between the two. None (to my knowledge) conclude that there is no relationship. The question is one of degree of importance and how to influence it, not whether or not emotions are a factor. So I'd like to begin with a quotation that has had a profound effect on my own thinking, and this is by a cancer specialist who was past president of the American Cancer Society in 1959, Dr. Eugene P. Pendergrass. I'm quoting from his presidential address, and these are his concluding remarks:

> Anyone who has had an extensive experience in the treatment of cancer is aware that there are great differences among patients. . . . I personally have observed cancer patients who have undergone successful treatment and were living and well for years. Then an emotional stress such as the death of a son in World War II, the infidelity of a daughter-in-law, or the burden of long unemployment seem to have been precipitating factors in the reactivation of their disease which resulted in death. . . . There is solid evidence that the course of disease in general is affected by emotional distress. . . . Thus, we as doctors may begin to emphasize *treatment of the patient as a whole* as well as the disease from which the patient is suffering. We may learn how to influence general body systems and through them modify the neoplasm which resides within the body.
>
> As we go forward . . . searching for new means of controlling growth both within the cell and through systemic influences it is my sincere hope that we can widen the quest to include the distinct possibility that within one's mind is a power capable of exerting forces which can either enhance or inhibit the progress of this disease.

This material was first published in the *Journal of Transpersonal Psychology,* vol. 7, no. 1, pp. 29–47, 1975. Copyright 1975. It is printed here in slightly modified form by permission.

To summarize what I consider the salient points from the literature and my own experience in working in these areas for four years now, the biggest single factor that I can find as a predisposing factor to the actual development of the disease is the loss of a serious love object, occurring six to eighteen months prior to the diagnosis. This is well documented in several long-term studies. Now the significant thing about this is that obviously not everyone who undergoes a serious loss, such as loss of a spouse or a child, develops a malignancy or any other serious disease. That's only one factor. The loss, whether real or imagined, has to be very significant; and even more important is the feeling that it engenders in the patient. The loss has to be such, and the response to the loss such, that it engenders the feeling of helplessness and hopelessness. Therefore, it's more than a loss—it's the culmination of the life history pattern of the patient. And this also is well-defined in the literature.

When we look at what constitutes the personality of the cancer patient, we find that there are many reputed authorities claiming there is no cancer personality. I can't see how one could be familiar with the literature and make this statement. I believe the work that has come out in *Type A Behavior and Your Heart* (Friedman & Rosenman, 1974) shows clearly that there is a life-history pattern in the development of heart diseases, and I believe that if we continue to look, we will find predisposing psychological factors in the development of all disease. Those predisposing factors most agreed upon as (negative) personality characteristics of the cancer patient are: (1) a great tendency to hold resentment and a marked inability to forgive, (2) a tendency towards self-pity, (3) a poor ability to develop and maintain meaningful, long-term relationships, (4) a very poor self-image.

I believe one of the big underlying factors behind all of the more superficial personality characteristics is basic rejection. The patient usually feels that he has been rejected by either one or both of his parents, and consequently develops the life-history pattern that we see so commonly in the cancer patient. All of us have a certain amount of this in our own personality. I probably have more than many. Of course, I developed cancer when I was 17, so I should have more than many. Just as Dr. Friedman, in *Type A Behavior and Your Heart,* points out the problems of personality in heart disease, he shows that they are very changeable. I strongly feel—and I certainly hope—that the cancer personality is changeable. Otherwise, I'm in a difficult spot. But if we don't bring it to the level of awareness, it is difficult to change. And just as Friedman and Rosenman point out in their book, the patient is very resistant to looking at the basic problem. That is, one very large factor contributing to heart disease is the person's response to stress. Supposing this same thing is true in cancer, which seems very strongly to be so, then as surely as the heart patient resists the fact that he has this type of personality, the cancer patient resists even more strongly. The heart disease personality is basically a much more socially acceptable personality than the cancer personality.

So how do we do anything about this? How do we go about changing this life history pattern? As I have stated before, this is a very difficult and responsible business in my experience. You're questioning things that so many people never consciously question. But let's look at some of the more pertinent factors that influence how patients present themselves and how they progress throughout the course of treatment. *I believe there are three extremely important factors that need to be recognized and brought to light. One is the belief system of the patient. The second is the belief system of the family and those people who surround the patient and are meaningful to him. The third is the belief system of the physician.* I'm going to elaborate on all of these and the role that I feel they play.

Let's begin with the belief system of the patient. I feel his beliefs about his disease, his treatment, and himself are very big factors, having a significant role in the course that his body takes during and after treatment. If we look at cancer as a disease, most patients see it as synonymous with death and something from without that there is almost no hope of controlling. Most patients have very negative feelings about treatment, whether it's radiation therapy, chemotherapy, or surgery. From the extensive psychological experimentation in expectancy, I can't see how any thinking person can help but see the relationship between what a person believes will happen as far as his treatment and disease are concerned and the eventual outcome. The psychological experimentation concerning expectancy points strongly toward this.

The last part, as far as the patient is concerned, is his set of beliefs about himself. Now I previously outlined the basic negative personality characteristics of the cancer patient. I said he had a very poor self-image. You see, he's got three strikes against him already! His belief about himself influences the course of his disease and his response to treatment. Therefore, this is an area where it is mandatory to modify early if you're going to modify the course of this disease significantly. Most patients see themselves as victims of the disease and not as having participated in the development of it. They also can see almost nothing that they personally can do to help themselves get well. Or at least this is the belief system that most of my patients present to me.

The belief system of the family is also vital, because we communicate what we believe to those around us. The patient is with the health-care personnel a small part of the time compared with how much of the time he is with his family. So you see, education of the family and changing their beliefs about the parameters of the disease are also vitally important in influencing the course of the patient.

The last area is the belief system of the physician. Most physicians are not aware of the fact that their thoughts about the treatment and the patient's own ability influence the outcome, but they most definitely do. . . . Expectancy of teachers influences children, and on down the line. You see, where the real problem comes in is when the physician's belief system parallels that of the initial belief system of the patient, namely, that the

His belief about himself influences the course of his disease and his response to treatment.

Too often in his visualization he sees the cancer as some big powerful thing, and the treatment as some little weak something that doesn't do much.

disease comes from without, that it's synonymous with death, that the treatment is bad, and the patient has little or nothing that he can do to fight the disease. This is all too common a belief among physicians. I know, because I have a large number of acquaintances who are cancer specialists, and I've heard them make statements like, "There is nothing that can be done." This, to me, indicates how they really feel about what a person can individually do to heal himself much more strongly than what they might intellectually tell me.

When we look at spontaneous remission or at unexpectedly good responses and try to figure out what happens in common, we find the same spontaneous occurrence of visualizing oneself being well. You analyze these people, you sit down with them and you find out what their thoughts are during that period of time, from the time they were given their diagnosis to the time that they were over their disease with no medical treatment: I have not found any patient that did not go through a similar visualizing process. It might be a spiritual process, God healing them, up and down the whole spectrum. But the important thing was what they pictured and the way they saw things. They were very positive, regardless of the source, and their picture was very positive. I find that the converse is true of my patients. Whenever I have a person visualizing, and I ask him to go through his visualization with me, how he pictures things tells me a tremendous amount about how he pictures his disease, his treatment, and his own ability to fight it. If I had nothing but one tool to use in looking at my patient's attitude, it would be how regularly he is relaxing and what his imagery is. This tells me so much more than he could tell me consciously, because he isn't even aware of what he's telling me. Too often in his visualization he sees the cancer as some big powerful thing, and the treatment as some little weak something that doesn't do much. He sees his white blood cells, his own immune mechanism, as really nonexistent, and he's trying to coax it into working. These are to me very unhealthy signs . . . because patients who verbalize these things are, in general, doing very poorly at the time they tell me this. Then we begin to take a different approach, not just using behavior modifications, but looking at the reasons behind why the person has these images of the disease, the treatment, and himself. We begin to work with him in a conscious way, to modify these images to the point that they will be more meaningful in his body's ability to fight the disease.

One of the things that I do early is to show the patient visually some of the best responses that I have ever seen, with some of the least side effects to the treatment. I do this so that he can have a very powerful image of what is possible. I show him a series of slides, not typical responses, but among the best I've ever seen. This is so he might see what the potential of the body is, both in getting rid of the disease and in the minimal reaction to treatment. When I arrived at Travis Air Force Base, I decided to duplicate two studies that had previously been done, correlating the patient's response with different personality characteristics and attitudes. I set up a study in which, at the completion of treatment, five staff members assessed each patient on their attitudes, from doubly positive to doubly negative, based on each one's clinical experience. I also had each staff member independently vote on what the clinical response had been, again based on their own experience, grading these responses from excellent to poor. Then when we averaged these together, giving one score for each patient, we found essentially a one-to-one correlation, which was similar to what Dr. Stavraky had found in her work in Canada. Those patients with positive attitudes had good responses, those with negative attitudes had poor responses, and out of 152 patients over an 18-month period, only two did not fall into the predicted categories (*see table below*).

These were 152 consecutive cases as they presented themselves in the department. Now out of the 20 patients who had excellent responses, 11 of them positive and 9 of them doubly positive, 14 had less than a 50 percent chance of a five-year cure, and only 6 of them had better than a 50 percent chance for a five-year cure. We found that the correlation was with attitudes and not with severity of their illness.

Now it should be strongly stressed that this was a very artificial environment, in a very protective atmosphere—that of a treatment center. These statistics did not last after they were out of that environment. Many patients who were very negative and had very poor responses changed after this study was over. In talking about it they said they didn't like the positivity, trying to see themselves getting well. After they got through treatment, there was a turn-around. They gained some degree of perspective, were much more pleasant to be with, and their health changed. Many of the patients with severe diseases had been very positive in this protective environment, but, when they got back to their home situation, they changed attitudinally, and we saw their diseases change correspondingly. So to try to extrapolate from this or draw any far-ranging conclusions is foolish, because the study was designed to look at patients under very controlled conditions. I did this study to see how our responses would correspond with the work done in Canada and UCLA, and found a very comparable correlation. I also learned many other things as a result of doing this study.

Clinical response	Attitude − −	−	+ −	+	+ +	Response totals
Excellent	0	0	0	11	9	20
Good	0	2	34	31	0	67
Fair	0	14	29	0	0	43
Poor	2	17	3	0	0	22
Attitude Totals	2	33	66	42	9	152

We have to assess the patients' belief structures. . . .

. . . Stephanie will discuss the specific aspects of this portion of the therapy, since she coordinates this in our office.

Stephanie Simonton: In order to explain the specifics of what our psychotherapy consists of, I think it would be best if I give you an overview of the type of practice we have and the type of patients we deal with. The treatment varies from patient to patient. We have to assess the patients' belief structures when we first see them and try to fit our treatment to their needs. We find that if we get into a conflict with their beliefs, they constantly fight us, and will almost get worse in spite of us, or *to* spite us.

We have a private practice with another radiation therapist in Fort Worth. The large majority of our patients come to us through normal referral channels from other physicians in our community, as most other cancer specialists receive their patients. These are about 80–90 percent of the patients we treat. We treat them with both medical treatment (radiation therapy or chemotherapy or whatever is appropriate) and psychotherapy. Most of them come to us not knowing that they are going to receive psychotherapy with their regular radiation therapy. It should be pointed out that of the patients that we receive through normal medical channels, who come to us with no preconceived ideas about what our treatment is, or any mental concept, over half of them will not participate in any form of psychotherapy. They will not attend group therapy. They will not use the relaxation and visualization techniques we prescribe. Many of them not only will not talk about, or allow us to talk to their families about, the psychological aspects of their disease, but they might even go back to their physician and ask to be referred to another doctor. That was a shock to me, yet as I continue to work with the patients, I am beginning to understand more of this. So let's begin with an understanding of where the consciousness of most of our patients is.

One of the other types of patients we are beginning to receive from our local community do not have active disease currently. They may be patients who have been free of disease for a year or two or three, but are coming to us for help in dealing with what we now know is one of the real residuals of cancer, and that is fear . . . the fear of recurrence, fear of reactivation—are they going to die? It is interesting to note that before a person has cancer, he may have a tennis elbow that aches occasionally. However, once he has had cancer, that aching tennis elbow suddenly represents the fear of metastases. Every time it hurts he thinks, "Is that a new cancer growing in there?" These patients need concrete techniques they can use to deal with aches and pains. Particularly after knowing that the mind participates in our becoming ill, it certainly doesn't help to worry and visualize cancer growing in new places.

The other type of patient that we have is generally referred from out-of-town and out-of-state. They are very few in number and we're extremely selective, but we are accepting some patients who come to us just for psychotherapy. They're usually receiving medical treatment from their local physician in their own community, or there may be no appropriate medical treatment for their case. They come to us believing there is a psychological component to their disease, and asking for help in understanding how to participate more positively in their future prognosis. These are extremely rewarding patients. They're probably the ones that we learn the most from, because they already have grasped so many concepts concerning their own disease process. Basically I think the biggest thing we do for these patients is give them reassurance and a greater awareness of themselves.

Now let me go over some of the concepts underlying our treatment, and then I'll get into the specifics of it. The first concept, and probably the hardest one for our patients to deal with, is our general concept of disease—the idea of personal responsibility. It's a difficult one. I think I can best refer to it as a double-edged sword. The idea that we have no participation in disease, that it's an outside agent acting on our body and we have nothing to do with its getting there, may be comforting in its denial. On the other hand, if you believe that concept, it doesn't make sense that you then can have any control in the progression of your disease. There's a double-edged sword there. In order to really grasp the concept that they can mentally influence their body's immune mechanism, they must eventually realize that their mind and emotions and body act as a unit and can't be separated. There is a mental and psychological participation, as well as a physical one, in the development of their disease. Once they can understand the psychological as well as physical reasons underlying their disease, they seem to get a better grasp on the future and how to deal with that. If you want to understand—and it took me a while to grasp it—how difficult psychotherapy is when you're ill, try an experiment. The next time you have the flu or a cold, ask yourself that very difficult question, "Why did I need this? What purpose does it serve?" It's a strange thing that happens to those of us, the staff, who work with the patients. If you're talking to a person who has cancer about his mentally participating in both the development and the progress of his disease, and suddenly you develop a cold, you have to get in touch with that. You can't continue to talk to them about influencing their cancer when you can't influence your own cold. So it causes all of us to do a great deal of self-discovery, which is not easy.

For some reason we have a conception of responsibility being the same as blame. This is one reason for our inability as a society to deal with the emotional aspects of our diseases. We feel that if we accept responsibility that we are to blame, should feel guilty, or have done something wrong. We try to convey the idea to the patient that it's just as if you were to deny your body food for too long: we know that you would eventually die. The same thing is true emotionally. A human being doesn't survive just by food, clothing and shelter. We have emotional needs that are very real and very concrete, and if these are denied, life loses its meaning. We will begin to seek the end of our life. We stress not that they should feel guilty, but that they have emotional needs that are not being met.

We do this in the beginning by trying to get patients to see what we call the "secondary gains of illness." One of the things we try to get them to do is to see how much different their life is now than before they developed the

> **The first concept, and probably the hardest one for our patients to deal with, is our general concept of disease—the idea of personal responsibility.**

. . . we were
trying to
accomplish in
. . . four to five
weeks . . . what
it takes years of
psychoanalysis to
do—if it's ever
accomplished.

disease. This is the clue to what we call the secondary gains. Let me give you an example of a woman who has breast cancer. Typically, a couple of years prior to the development of her disease, her children were suddenly growing up, graduating from school and beginning to enter their own lives. Her husband had become very preoccupied in his business and she had suddenly felt unneeded. Since the development of her disease, her husband is now showing her attention that he has not shown her in years. Now that's fine. It's good that he's giving her affection because she needs that. But what we try to get her to see is that if the disease is the only way she can get that, then the disease must continue in order for her to get that secondary gain, this affection. We don't try to get her to cut off that affection, but rather, we help her develop healthier ways of getting the support she needs emotionally. In essence the concept we use is not that one regains health first and then goes back to living a normal life, but that patients do better when they do both simultaneously.

I'm reminded of an unusual situation we had recently in one of our group therapy sessions, where we had two patients who had almost identical diseases. They were within a few years of age of each other, and both men had lung cancer that had spread to their brain. One man had had the disease for over a year, but had not missed work other than a few hours each time he had a treatment. Early in the development of his disease he had gotten in touch with a lot of things that were causing life to lose meaning for him. He started to spend more time with his family, taking his family with him on business trips. I remember him saying one day, "You know, I'd forgotten that I didn't look at the trees. I hadn't been looking at the trees and the grass and the flowers for a long time. And now I do that." It was interesting to watch him, every week he improved, getting stronger, healthier.

The other man who had lung cancer which had spread to his brain stopped working practically the day he received his diagnosis. He had gone home to sit in front of the television set all day. His wife said that what he did every day was to watch the clock to make sure she gave him his pain medication on time. He was in constant pain. He could not even bring himself to go fishing, which is something he liked to do. He died in a short period of time. The other man is still getting healthier day after day. This is the kind of thing that we try to show our patients. The treatment for both patients was the same medically, the diagnosis was the same, the patients' ages and physical conditions were almost identical. The difference was in attitude, the way the patients reacted once they knew the diagnosis.

When we began our psychotherapy, based on Dr. LeShan's findings that cancer patients have an emotional trauma 6–18 months prior to the development of the disease, we found ourselves trying to get patients in touch with the event, and to change certain things about their lives so that life could gain more meaning. In essence, we were trying to accomplish in a period of four to five weeks, in once-a-week group therapy sessions, what it takes years of psychoanalysis to do—if it's ever accomplished. As you can imagine, that became very frustrating. We then began to realize that not every woman who goes through a divorce develops cancer, not every man who retires from work develops cancer, not every person who experiences an unhappy marriage develops cancer as a result. And these are some of the common stresses we see. The difference, then, was not the stress: that was not the problem. The problem was the person's *reaction* to that stress. We try to get them to see that here is something they do have control over. They may not be able to control their husband when he makes them angry or their children when they frustrate them, but they can control how they choose to react to that situation. And I stress the word *choose.*

Now let me describe the actual tools we use. During the first week a patient comes to our office, he attends what we call an orientation session. He attends with as many family members and close friends as he would like to bring. We know that a person doesn't become sick in a vacuum nor does he get well in a vacuum. We do best when we mobilize all the forces within the person's environment. So early on, we try to educate the entire family. Many times the patient never brings his family back again after the first session. But we do generally get him to bring some of his family with him, at least his spouse. During the orientation session, we explain our concept of disease, how the mind interacts with the body, and how attitude plays a major role. We teach our patients a technique which we call relaxation and visualization. You might call it biofeedback without a machine, meditation, autogenic training. There are lots of names for it, but it is a basic relaxation technique in which the patients are told to visualize their disease, their treatment and their body's own immune mechanisms (we call them white blood cells to make it simple) acting on that disease. We tell them to do this three times a day, every day.

At that orientation, they are given a tape recording of the relaxation process that they can take home with them and listen to. All they have to do is put it on a cassette tape player and turn it on. We also give them the book, *The Will to Live,* a short paperback by Dr. Arnold Hutschnecker that more fully elaborates the principles of the mind-body concept. They are told at that session that they may attend what we call group classes or group therapy sessions once a week. Again, I estimate that over 50 percent of them will not come back at that point. Many of their families come to us and say they understand the psychological component in their relative's disease, but can't get him or her back to the group sessions.

In the group sessions, on a twice-a-week basis, we talk primarily about the relaxation and mental imagery process and how many times they are doing it. Again, we find that the majority of the patients, if they ever use the technique, use it rarely, once a day instead of three times a day, or maybe three times a week. We talk about why they are not using the technique. And very often the things that are preventing them from quieting themselves, from listening to themselves and mentally picturing their own disease process, are the very things that are causing life to lose its meaning. In the group we tend to discover those things that are preventing them from getting well.

We teach our patients a technique which we call relaxation and visualization.

. . . to hope that we will begin to look at disease in a new way. . . .

Let me give you an example of the kinds of things we talk about in groups. Remember the man I described to you who had lung cancer that had spread to his brain, the one who was doing poorly? He kept insisting that he was using the meditation or the relaxation technique three times a day. His wife said she did turn on the tape recorder and he was listening to it. So one day we had him describe to us what he visualized. We asked him what his cancer looked like to him and he said, "It looks like a big black rat." When we asked what his treatment looked like (he was receiving chemotherapy in the form of little yellow pills), he replied, "They look like little yellow pills and they go into my bloodstream and they look like tiny pills." We also asked what happened between the pills and the rat. He said, "Once in a while the rat eats one of the pills." We asked what happened when he did and he said, "Well, he's sick for awhile, but he always gets better and he bites me all the harder." When we asked about his white blood cells, he replied, "They look like an incubator. You know how eggs sit under the warm light? Well, they're incubating in there and one day they're going to hatch." That was his visualization, three times a day, which gives you a good idea of the way he visualized his disease.

I'll conclude by describing some of the studies we presently are engaged in. We instigated a control study with another radiation therapist in Fort Worth five months ago. Between his office and ours we treat approximately three-fourths of the patients given radiation therapy in the city. Both offices administer standard doses of radiation therapy, and our patients are treated on the same equipment, by the same technicians. The difference between the two is the psychotherapy administered to our patients. This study should show some interesting statistics, as to whether we can change both the quality and quantity of the patient's survival time by influencing his attitude. In addition to this, we are cooperating in a study with the Carl Jung Institute of Los Angeles, using Jungian analytical techniques to more fully study the psychological aspects of our patients.

A good deal of research has been done on the personality of the cancer patient. One of the most intriguing aspects of this work is the suggestion that the behavior pattern of the patient can even be correlated to the exact location of the malignancy. For instance, the breast cancer patient has a behavior pattern different from the lung cancer patient, etc. We are currently quantitating this in our patients.

I recently finished reading the book *Type A Behavior and Your Heart* and was very excited by the possible implications it could have on medicine in the future. The similarities between their work and ours has led me to hope that we will begin to look at disease in a new way, that instead of being entirely concerned with the disease process itself, we will also take into account the patient and his environment as a whole and see disease as a symptom of the general and total well-being of the patient.

References

Abse, D. W.; Wilkin, M. M.; Kirschner, G.; Weston, D. L.; Brown, R. S.; and Buxton, W. D. Self-frustration, nighttime smoking and lung cancer. *Psychosom. Med.* 1972, *34*, 395.

Andervont, H. B. Influence of environment on mammary cancer in mice. *National Cancer Institute,* 1944, *4*, 579–81.

Bacon, C. L.; Rennecker, R.; and Cutler, M. A psychosomatic survey of cancer of the breast. *Psychosom. Med.,* 1952, *14*, 453–60.

Bahnson, C. B. Psychophysiological complementarity in malignancies. *Annals N. Y. Acad. Sci.,* 1969, *164*, 319.

———. Second conference on psychophysiological aspects of cancer. *Annals N. Y. Acad. Sci.,* 1969, *164*.

———. The psychological aspects of cancer. Paper presented at the American Cancer Society's 13th Science Writer's Seminar, 1971.

Bahnson, C. B., and Kissen, D. M. Psychophysiological aspects of cancer. *Annals N. Y. Acad. Sci.,* 1966, *125*.

Bahnson, C. B., and Bahnson, M. B. Ego defenses in cancer patients. *Annals N. Y. Acad. Sci.,* 1969, *164*, 546.

Barrios, A. A. Hypnosis as a possible means of curing cancer. Unpublished manuscript, 1961.

———. Hypnotherapy: A reappraisal. *Psychotherapy: Theory, Research, and Practice,* 1970, *7*.

Beary, J. F., and Benson, H. A simple psychophysiologic technique which elicits the hypometabolic changes of the relaxation response. *Psychom. Med.,* March–April 1974, 115.

Bennett, G. Psychic and cellular aspects of isolation and identity impairment in cancer: A dialectic of alienation. *Annals N. Y. Acad. Sci.,* 1969, *164*, 352.

Benson, H. Your innate asset for combating stress. *Harvard Business Review,* July–August 1974, No. 74402.

Benson, H.; Beary, J. F.; and Carol, M. P. The relaxation response. *Psychiatry,* February 1974, 37.

Benson, H.; Marzetta, B. R.; and Rosner, B. A. Decreased blood pressure associated with the regular elicitation of the relaxation response: A study of hypertensive subjects. *Contemporary Problems in Cardiology, 1.*

Benson, H.; Rosner, B. A.; Marzetta, B. A.; and Klemchuk, H. Decreased blood pressure in pharmacologically treated hypertensive patients who regularly elicited the relaxation response. *The Lancet,* February 23, 1974, 289.

Booth, G. General and organic specific object relationships in cancer. *Annals N. Y. Acad. Sci.,* 1969, *164*, 568.

Butler, B. The use of hypnosis in the case of cancer patients. *Cancer,* 1954, *7*, 1.

Cutler, M. The nature of the cancer process in relation to a possible psychosomatic influence. *The Psychological Variables in Human Cancer.* Berkeley: Univ. Calif., 1954, 1–16.

Dorn, H. F. Cancer and the marital status. *Human Biology,* 1943, *15*, 73–79.

Dunbar, F. Emotions and bodily changes. *A survey of literature—Psychosomatic interrelationships 1910–1953.* (4th ed.) New York: Columbia Univ., 1954.

Dunham, L. J., and Bailar, J. C. World maps of cancer mortality rates and frequency ratios. *J. Nat. Cancer Instit.,* 1968, *41*, 155.

Editorial: The nervous factor in the production of cancer. *British Med. Jour.,* 1925, *20*, 113.

Eliasberg, W. G. Psychotherapy in cancer patients. *J. Amer. Med. Assoc.,* 1951, *147*, 525.

Evans, E. *A Psychological Study of Cancer.* New York: Dodd, Mead, 1926.

Everson, T. C., and Cole, W. H. Spontaneous Regression of Cancer. *Philadelphia,* 1966, *7*.

Ferracuti, F., and Rizzo, G. Psychological patterns in terdella psicologia del canceroso terminale. *Bollettino di Oncologia,* 1953, *27*, 3–53.

———. Psychological patterns in terminal cancer cases. Education & Psychology. *Delhi,* 1955, *2*, 26–36.

Fisher, S., and Cleveland, S. E. Relationship of body image to site of cancer. *Psychosom. Med.,* 1956, *8*, 304–09.

Friedman, M., and Rosenman, R. H. *Type A Behavior and Your Heart.* New York: Knopf, 1974.

Friedman, S. B.; Glasgow, L. A.; and Ader, R. Psychosocial factors modifying host resistance to experimental infections. *Annals N. Y. Acad. Sci.,* 1969, *164*, 381–92.

Gengerelli, J. A., and Kirkner, F. J. (eds.) The psychological variables in human cancer. Symposium presented at the Veterans Administration Hospital, Long Beach, Calif., Oct. 23, 1953. Berkeley: Univ. Calif., 1954.

Greene, W. A., Jr. Psychological factors and reticuloendothelial disease. I. Preliminary Observations on a group of males with lymphomas and leukemia. *Psychosom. Med.,* 1954, *16,* 220–230.

———. The psychosocial setting of the development of leukemia and lymphoma. *Annals N.Y. Acad. Sci.,* 1966, *125,* 794.

Greene, W. A., Jr.; Young, L.; and Swisher, S.N. Psychological factors and reticuloendothelial disease. II. Observations on a group of women with lymphomas and leukemias. *Psychosom. Med.* 1956, *18,* 284–303.

Greene, W. A., Jr. and Miller, G. Psychological factors and reticuloendothelial disease. IV. *Psychosom. Med.,* 1958, *20,* 124–44.

Hagnell, O. The premorbid personality of persons who develop cancer in a total population investigated in 1947 and 1957. *Annals N.Y. Acad. Sci.,* 1966, *125,* 846.

Hedge, A. R. Hypnosis in cancer. *British J. Hypnotism,* 1960, *12,* 2–5.

Hoffman, F. C. *The Mortality from Cancer throughout the World.* Newark, N.J.: Prudential Press, 1915.

———. *Some Cancer Facts and Fallacies.* Newark, N.J.: Prudential Press, 1925.

Hughes, C. H. The relations of nervous depression toward the development of cancer. *St. Louis Medicine and Surgery Journal,* 1885.

Hutschnecker, A. *The Will to Live.* New York: Thomas Y. Crowell Co., 1953.

Kavetsky, R. E.; Turkewich, N. M.; and Balitsky, K. P. On the psychophysiological mechanism of the organism's resistance to tumor growth. *Annals N.Y. Acad. Sci.,* 1966, *125,* 933.

Kissen, D. M. Personality characteristics in males conducive to lung cancer. *British J. Med. Psychol.,* 1963, *36,* 27.

———. Psychosocial factors, personality and lung cancer in men aged 55–64. *British J. Med. Psychol.,* 1967, *40,* 29.

———. Relationship between lung cancer, cigarette smoking, inhalation and personality and psychological factors in lung cancers. *Annals N.Y. Acad. Sci.,* 1969, *164,* 535.

Kissen, D. M., and Eysenck, H. G. Personality in male lung cancer patients. *J. Psychosom. Research,* 1962, *6,* 123.

Kissen, D. M.; Brown, R.I.F.; and Kissen, M. A further report on personality and psychological factors in lung cancers. *Annals N.Y. Acad. Sci.,* 1969, *164,* 535.

Klopfer, B. Psychological variables in human cancer. *J. Projective Techniques,* 1957, *21,* 331–40.

Kowal, S. J. Emotions as a cause of cancer: Eighteenth and nineteenth century contributions. *Psychoanalyst. Rev.,* 1955, *42,* 217–27.

La Barba, R. C. Experimental and environmental factors in cancer. *Psychosom. Med.* 1970, *32,* 259.

LeShan, L. A psychosomatic hypothesis concerning the etiology of Hodgkin's disease. *Psychol. Rep.,* 1957, *3,* 565–75.

———. Psychological states as factors in the development of malignant disease: A critical review. *J. Nat. Cancer Instit.,* 1959, *22.*

———. A basic psychological orientation apparently associated with malignant disease. *Psychiatric Quarterly* 1961, *35,* 314.

———. An emotional life-history pattern associated with neoplastic disease. *Annals N.Y. Acad. Sci.,* 1966, *125,* 780–93.

———. An emotional life-history pattern associated with neoplastic disease. *Annals N.Y. Acad. Sci.,* 1966, *125,* 807.

LeShan, L., and Gassman, M. Some observations on psychotherapy with patients with neoplastic disease. *Amer. J. Psychotherapy,* 1958, *12,* 723–34.

LeShan, L., and Worthington, R. E. Some psychologic correlates of neoplastic disease: Preliminary report. *J. Clinical & Experimental Psychopath.,* 1955, *16,* 281–88.

———. Loss of cathexes as a common psychodynamic characteristic of cancer patients. An attempt at statistical validation of a clinical hypothesis. *Psychol. Rep.,* 1956, *2,* 183–93.

———. Personality as a factor in the pathogenesis of cancer: A review of the literature. *British J. Med. Psychol.,* 1956, *29,* 49–56.

———. Some recurrent life history patterns observed in patients with malignant disease. *J. Nervous Mental Diseases,* 1956, *124,* 460–65.

Lombard, H. L., and Potter, E. A. Epidemiological aspects of cancer of the cervix: Hereditary and environmental factors. *Cancer,* 1950, *3,* 960–68.

MacDonald, I. Mammary carcinoma. *Surgery Gynecology and Obstetrics,* 1942, *74,* 75.

MacMillan, M. B. A note on LeShan and Worthington's "Personality as a factor in the pathogenesis of cancer." *British J. Med. Psychol.,* 1957, *30,* 41.

Marcial, V. A. Socioeconomic aspects of the incidence of cancer in Puerto Rico. *Annals N.Y. Acad. Sci.,* 1960, *84,* 981.

Meerloo, J. The initial neurologic and psychiatric picture syndrome of pulmonary growth. *J. Amer. Med. Assoc.,* 1951, *146,* 558–59.

———. Psychological implications of malignant growth: Survey of hypotheses. *British J. Med. Psychol.,* 1954, *27,* 210–15.

Miller, F. R., and Jones, H. W. The possibility of precipitating the leukemia state by emotional factors. *Blood,* 1948, *8,* 880–84.

Mitchell, J. S. Psychosomatic cancer research from the viewpoint of the general cancer field. *Psychosom. Aspects Neoplastic Disease,* 1964, 215.

Orbach, C. E.; Sutherland, A. M.; and Bozeman, M. F. Psychological impact of cancer and its treatment. *Cancer,* 1955, *8,* 20.

Paget, J. *Surgical Pathology* (2nd ed.). London: Longman's Green, 1870.

Parker, W. *Cancer, A Study of Ninety-seven Cases of Cancer of the Female Breast.* New York, 1885.

Parker, C. M.; Benjamin, B.; and Fitzgerald, R. G. Broken hearts: A statistical study of increased mortality among widowers. *British Med. Journal,* 1969, *1,* 740.

Peller, S. Cancer and its relations to pregnancy, to delivery, and to marital and social status, cancer of the breast and genital organs. *Surg., Gynce. & Obst.,* 1940, *71,* 181–86.

———. *Cancer in Man.* New York: New York Internat. Univ. Press, 1952, 556.

Pendergrass, E. Presidential address to American cancer society meeting, 1959.

———. Host resistance and other intangibles in the treatment of cancer. *American J. Roentgenology,* 1961, *85,* 891–96.

Quisenberry, W. B. Sociocultural factors in cancer in Hawaii. *Annals N.Y. Acad. Sci.,* 1960, *84,* 795.

Raef, Y. Psychosomatic aspects of cancer research: A literature survey. *Nat. Fed. Spiritual Healers.*

Rennecker, R. E. Countertransference reactions to cancer. *Psychosom. Med.,* 1957, *19,* 409–18.

Revici, E. *A New Concept of the Pathophysiology of Cancer with Implications for Therapy.* New Haven: Yale Univ. Press.

Reznikoff. Psychological factors in breast cancer—A preliminary study of some personality trends in patients with cancer of the breast. *Psychosomatic Res.,* 1957, *2,* 56–60.

Sacerdote, P. The uses of hypnosis in cancer patients. *Annals N.Y. Acad. Sci.,* 1966, *125,* 1011–12.

Schmale, A. H., and Iker, H. The psychological setting of uterine cervical cancer. *Annals N.Y. Acad. Sci.,* 1966, *125,* 807.

Schneck, J. M. *Hypnosis in Modern Medicine.* Charles Thomas, 1959.

Snow, H. *The Reappearance* (Recurrence) *of Cancer after Apparent Extirpation.* London: J. & A. Churchill, 1870.

———. *Clinical notes on cancer.* London: J. & A. Churchill, 1883.

———. *Cancer and the cancer process.* London: J. & A. Churchill, 1893.

Solomon, G. F. Emotions, stress, the central nervous system, and immunity. *Annals N.Y. Acad. Sci.,* 1969, *164,* 335–43.

Solomon, G. F., and Moos, R. H. Emotions, immunity and disease. *Archives Gen. Psychiatry,* 1964, *11,* 657.

Stephenson, J. H., & Grace, W. J. Life stress and cancer of the cervix. *Psychosom. Med.* 1954, *16,* 287–94.

Stavraky, K. M. Psychological factors in the outcome of human cancer. *J. Psychosom. Res.,* 1968, *12,* 251.

Surman, O. S.; Gotlieb, J. K.; Hochet, T. P.; and Silverberg, E. L. Hypnosis in the treatment of warts. *Arch. Gen. Psychotherapy,* 1973, *28,* 439–41.

Tariau, M. and Smalheiser, T. Personality patterns in patients with malignant tumors of the breast and cervix: Exploratory study. *Psychosom. Med.,* 1951, *13,* 117–21.

Tromp, S. W. Psychosomatischo faktoren under Krebs (insbesondere der lunge und der mamma). *Medizinische,* March 26, 1955, 443–47.

Belief Systems and Management of the Emotional Aspects of Malignancy   155

Trunnell, J. B. Theories of the origin of cancer. Paper read at the Texas conference on psychosomatic implications in cancer, Dallas, Sept. 1956.

Wainwright, J. M. A comparison of conditions associated with breast cancer in Great Britain and America. *Amer. J. Cancer,* 1931, *15,* 2610.

Wallace, R. K.; Benson, H.; and Wilson, A. F. A wakeful hypometabolic physiologic state. *American J. Physiol.,* Sept. 1971, 795.

Wallace, R. K., and Benson, H. The physiology of meditation. *Sci. Amer.,* Feb. 1972.

Weitzenhoffer, A. M. *Hypnotism: An objection study in suggestibility.* New York: Wiley, 1953.

West, P. M. Origin and development of the psychological approach to the cancer problems. *The psychological variables in human cancer.* Berkeley: Univ. Calif., 1954.

West, P. M.; Blumberg, E. M.; and Ellis, F. W. An observed correlation between psychological factors and growth rate of cancer in man. *Cancer Res.,* 1952, *12,* 306–07.

Wheeler, J. I., Jr., and Caldwell, B. M. Psychological evaluation of women with cancer of the breast and of the cervix. *Psychosom. Med.,* 1955, *17,* 256–68.

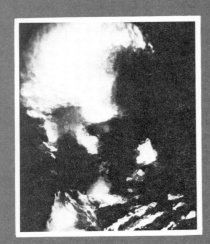

Part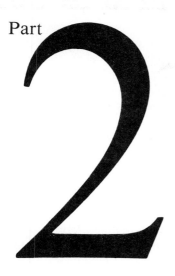

Family, Group, and Organizational Dynamics

Part 1 of this volume portrays death as a life crisis that has powerful physiological, psychological, and behavioral effects upon each of us as individuals. It shows that our ability to cope with grief is related to the internal and external resources available to us. In order to understand fully the dynamics and impact of death, however, we must step back from an individual perspective and take a broader view. We must also comprehend the effects of death on the family, school, hospital, and other organizational settings.

Most of us are not as close to death as we might have been fifty or sixty years ago. At that time most persons died at home in the loving care of family members and close friends. Today, in contrast, we die in institutional settings. We utilize the services of specialists to care for us while we are dying and to bury us when we are dead. Two consequences of this transition are noteworthy. First, opportunities for education about death rarely occur in the home. The responsibility for discussing death therefore falls on schools, colleges, and community mental health centers. Second, hospitals and nursing homes are increasingly being indicted as inhumane care stations.

Part 2 of the book now explores some crucial questions related to these problems of transition. What are the effects of death on the family unit today? How do medical staff view death and dying? What kind of treatment can a terminally ill person expect to receive from medical staff? How can the American funeral be understood as a ritual and ceremony? How are we remembered and eulogized by family members after we die? How do we educate people regarding death and dying? Are some methods of death education more effective than others? Are there ways to humanize our care of the terminally ill?

This section begins with Benjamin Schlesinger's theoretical yet practical view of "The Crisis of Widowhood in the Family Cycle." Though he speaks of the Canadian culture, it is not difficult to generalize his observations to the American sphere. A number of variables are seen as contributing to crisis resolution for the typical family experiencing a death. They include personality factors, age, socioeconomic status, financial assets, and cultural and religious beliefs.

The widow must cope in the three major aspects of life—economic, social, and emotional. They are intertwined, and readjustment is complicated by the presence of children and a social context that may appear impatient to see "recovery." Though Schlesinger focuses on the widow, it should be understood that any widower must also reestablish new patterns of living in each of the three realms.

Family bereavement also affects children in many ways. Children may lose an important role model with whom they identify. They may feel abandoned without understanding why, or they may communicate their anguish nonverbally by "acting out" in school. Schlesinger suggests that children experience three phases during the grieving process. First, a child may angrily protest the death of a parent while trying to regain him or her. Pain, despair, and disorganization are felt next when the reality of death begins to settle in. When the child begins to reorganize his or her life without the loved one, the final stage—hope—is achieved. Strategies for facilitating this process are offered.

Family bereavement may actually begin during a terminal illness itself. At such times, family members are heavily dependent on the medical and paramedical staff. How a medical staff copes with dying patients thus becomes a pivotal matter. A critical review of this literature is presented by Schulz and Aderman.

They suggest that both personality and training cause medical practitioners to see their dying patients as their failures and disappointments. As a result they tend to cope with death by avoiding it. The dying patient is typically neglected by physicians and nurses even though the patient may have a strong desire to be informed about the condition and to discuss it openly. Schulz and Aderman conclude that "although research data suggest that most terminal patients suffer no permanent negative consequences if they are informed tactfully about the true nature of their illness, the majority of physicians adhere to a policy of not sharing their diagnosis with the dying patient." The review is *not* an indictment of professional discipline so much as an indicator that we must focus attention on meeting the sociopsychological needs of such patients.

An institution besides the hospital that attempts to meet the needs of bereaved families is the funeral industry. Using the metaphor of drama or the theatre to understand human behavior in everyday life, popularized by Erving Goffman, Turner and Edgley present an article entitled "Death as Theater: A Dramaturgical Analysis of the American Funeral." They point out that the business from which funeral directors make a living depends on the fixed rate of dying in the local community. Since funeral directors cannot promote business by giving the impression of wanting more people to die, they must find other ways to insure or improve their income. Two ways are: (1) getting a fair share of the existing business from deaths that occur naturally, and (2) merchandising "up" so that the average cost of a funeral increases. In effect, the funeral director's attempt to make money is dependent upon the quality of the "performance" presented to an "audience."

In order to research this "performance on stage," Turner and Edgley unobtrusively observed mortuary practices and funeral services, interviewed funeral directors and staff, and analyzed the content of in-house manuals and advertising materials. We are introduced to new concepts such as "backstage," "frontstage," and "cast of characters," which help describe the conduct of the American funeral. Perhaps the distinction between frontstage and backstage behaviors is most vividly described by Goffman, who notes that "if the bereaved are to be given the impression that the loved one is really in a deep and tranquil sleep, they will have to be kept away from the area where the corpse is drained, stuffed, and painted for its final performance." In effect, this paper elucidates how judicious rhetoric, behind-the-scenes preparations, flexible facilities, control of social settings, and staged impressions are orchestrated to perform a successful funeral.

An exploration of representative research on families and organizational institutions validates numerous theoretical notions described above. In her article entitled "Widowhood and Husband Sanctification," Helena Znaniecki Lopata provides evidence that American widows tend to idealize their deceased husbands, even to the point of sanctification. The wake, funeral eulogy, shiva, and other post-funeral rituals all facilitate sanctification. And the sanctification process facilitates and complements the detachment and reestablishment processes described by Erich Lindemann in chapter 1. Sanctification not only forces the widow to recognize that her husband is dead, but it encourages her to reconstruct him in an immortal, spiritual sense. By so doing she is no longer subject to the feelings of jealousy and resentment that characterize mortal interactions. Grief work in Lindemann's sense is thus enhanced.

Lopata, like Schlesinger, observes that widows face economic, social, and emotional crises. As Lopata points out, income often drops, loneliness is experienced, and housing and relational adjustments must be made. Her paper essentially tests out the following two questions: (1) Do many American urban widows tend to idealize their late husbands to the point of sanctification? (2) Who are the widows who can be located at the polar ends of the husband sanctification tendency?

The process of dying itself is researched and described by Susman, Hollenbeck, Nannis, Strope, Hersh, Levine, and Pizzo in their article "Interactions between Primary Caregivers and Children with Cancer: A Methodology for Systematic Observation in a Hospital Setting." These authors describe (1) the advantages of observation over other methodologies, (2) characteristics of an observational schema, (3) problems encountered in observer agreement, and (4) exploratory approaches to data analysis. In applying their approach to a hospital setting, they have learned that a mother's social interaction with her child may actually decline during the latter part of hospitalization. They have also learned when helpful interventions from caregivers may be most beneficially introduced.

We pointed out earlier that the responsibility for death education is increasingly being absorbed by public institutions as opposed to the home. Methods of death education vary widely but may be polarized along a didactic-experiential continuum. In his study "Comparison between Experiential and Didactic Methods of Death Education," Durlak attempts to assess the relative effectiveness of these two methods on individual attitudes toward life and death. In a workshop conducted at a large southeastern medical center, Durlak collected pre and post data from two groups of workshop participants and a matched control group. One of the workshop groups (didactic group) participated in an educational program emphasizing lecture presentations and small group discussion. In contrast, the second workshop group (experiential) confronted, examined, and shared their own feelings and reactions to grief and death. Role playing, death awareness, and grief exercises were used for this purpose. Results showed that the experiential group showed a significant reduction in fear of death as a result of the workshop, whereas both the didactic and control groups changed negatively over time. Results support the view that an emotional, personal approach to death is an important element in an effective death educational program. The results also justify the inclusion of the structured exercises for death education found in the appendix of this text. Readers are certainly encouraged to use them as a needed adjunct to their educational experience.

As revealing as Durlak's study is regarding the comparison of methodologies, a pressing need exists to provide a systematic model for the practice of death education in our schools and communities. In his article "Death Education: Perspectives for Schools and Communities," Bugen offers a paradigm which suggests that all death educators must plan their efforts according to a definite *goal* or purpose. All instructional variables may then be subsumed under goal in either *target* or *method*. Bugen elaborates on his own role as death educator by operationalizing *goal* as "increasing humanization on a variety of levels."

Bugen presents the triangular model of goal, target and method by relating it to community death education. He urges us as death educators and caregivers to get out of our ivory towers and terminal care stations in order to meet the needs of the typical community citizen. Goals of primary, secondary, and tertiary prevention are each elaborated and exemplified by innovative programs characterizing each. Following a review of these programs, standards of care and practice are outlined for both death educators and professional caregivers. The emerging standards are particularly cogent because the outcomes of our death education efforts are still very much in question.

If one goal of death education is to humanize our treatment of death-related issues, what better setting to focus on exists than the hospital. Terminal care for our dying has received a refreshing breath of vitality through the development of the hospice concept. In their article "Terminal Care—Issues and Alternatives," Ryder and Ross describe the hospice movement and justify its continued influence in institutional care on the basis of both care *and* cost factors. Quoting Cecily Saunders, the founder of the hospice concept, Ryder and Ross help us view such a setting as something "between a hospital and a home which serves as a resting place for travelers and pilgrims. Hospice staff recognize the interest and importance of the individual who must be helped to *live* until he (she) dies and who, as he (she) does so in his own way, will find his own death with quietness and acceptance."

The needs for the hospice appear quite significant in light of (1) our ever changing society and (2) existing professional attitudes and behaviors toward the dying. American culture values youth, beauty, sexuality, and health; it emphasizes the shift from an extended family to a mobile, nuclear family; and it stresses hospitalization over home care. Complementing these trends is a service delivery system that is increasingly technological and overburdened. The plight of the terminally ill in light of these factors is depressing. As pointed out by Shulz and Aderman in chapter 13, the typical medical student's education stresses the idea that death equals failure for both the individual physician and medicine as a whole. The hospice movement questions such an assumption while providing a humanistic alternative.

There is also much we can do to humanize care for the terminally ill within hospital settings. We could increase the patients' decision-making opportunities, for one thing. Sharon Imbus and Bruce Zawacki work within a hospital setting on a burn-care team and are deeply invested in enhancing "Autonomy for Burned Patients When Survival is Unprecedented." Imbus and Zawacki work with patients whose burns are so severe that survival is not only unexpected, but unprecedented. It is the extensiveness of the burns with age that creates this condition. Since most patients lapse into coma after only a few hours of clear consciousness, informed decisions by them must be made soon after arrival at the burn center. These decisions are important because the few remaining hours of clarity remaining to the patient should be his or hers to appropriate, and not anyone else's. Business matters may thus be attended to as well as final good-byes to loved ones. The authors sensitively declare that "truth is the greatest kindness." The essence of bioethics is integral in the above treatment approach and will be addressed more fully in part 3.

Humanistic care for the dying and their families is a practice which must be more broadly based than that found in just hospital or hospice settings. Speaking from his own personal battle with cancer, Orville Kelly documents the need for his grass-roots organization called Make Today Count. When his illness was first diagnosed in 1973, Kelly soon realized that professionals and nonprofessionals alike had difficulty talking about death and dying. His proposal that an organization be created where "open discussion'' was a rule rather than an exception was greeted with strong community affirmation. Make Today Count was quickly founded. In chapter 21 Kelly describes his experiences leading up to the creation of Make Today Count, what happens at a typical meeting, and what benefits might accrue to the participants. We learn that patients, their families, and health care professionals all can utilize the opportunity to share fears, concerns, and frustrations with one another. What can be gained from such an organization? Perhaps Kelly sums it up best when he discloses that he ''has learned the importance of caring, of listening, of touching.'' We all must learn to appreciate the value of life *today*. There may be no tomorrow!

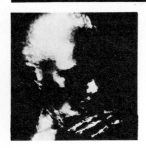

12

Theory

When a family unit experiences death, how do the surviving members cope? What needs emerge as the most prominent and perhaps most difficult to deal with? In particular, what are the key problems of living that widows and children must face as a consequence of the death? Benjamin Schlesinger highlights some of the selected findings in this chapter. The following Appendix exercises are suggested at the completion of your reading:

C. Awareness of Grief Process

D. Awareness of Losses

H. Fantasizing Grief Reaction of Significant Others

K. Planning for Living

The Crisis of Widowhood in the Family Cycle

Benjamin Schlesinger

The 1971 Census of Canada indicated that there were 184,555 female-headed and 38,070 male-headed, widowed, one-parent families in Canada. This group constituted 46.6 per cent of all one-parent families.

We realize that not all of these families have children living at home, and yet social workers will have to deal with the crisis of death in a family almost daily in our country. The author has recently reviewed the literature related to this topic, and the material which follows is a digest of this information.

The Family

The intricate structure of the twentieth-century family with its well defined role patterns and interdependence of parts does not adapt without difficulty to the permanent absence of a family member. If this particular member is either a male or female parent figure and his/her absence from the family structure is caused by death, then the remaining family members will undoubtedly encounter a long and painful series of obstacles.

The family role patterns are ideally based on reciprocal expectations and often unobtrusive but carefully worked out norms prescribe appropriate behavior. Paired relationships between husband and wife, parent and child, sibling and sibling are maintained by means of these guidelines, and the family works out the most suitable division of labor to meet its needs and responsibilities.

While the family may be a unit with mutually dependent parts, it is by no means a closed system. Its nature is such that with a definite degree of selectivity, it interacts with individuals and institutions external to it. It is

This material was first published in *Essence: Issues in the Study of Ageing, Dying, and Death,* vol. 1, pp. 147–155, 1977. Copyright 1977 by Atkinson College Press. It is printed here in slightly modified form by permission.

It is not uncommon for ties with relatives to be weakened.

. . .

only with these characteristics in mind that one can effectively examine the consequences of death upon the family unit. Indeed, many of the behavior patterns of family members, subsequent to a death, can be understood within this drawn framework.

Death and Adjustment

Death may produce a crisis in the family's equilibrium for which there is no ready-made response. The sudden and often unexpected death of a young father with a family will necessitate a reorganization of role responsibilities and status positions. For the widow, alternate patterns of behavior are essential for the new role which she will be expected to play within her family, her kin group, and in her community as well. Children too may find themselves with added responsibilities in an attempt to absorb within the family group the duties of the lost member. Relationships with relatives may change, and the family may seek assistance from clergy, social agencies, or the schools.

A death in a family must be seen as a causal factor which affects and determines the on-going process of family living from the time of the death itself until the dissolution of the family unit. While a death may mean quickly derived solutions for immediate problems, it also means a strain on the emotional and practical aspects of living for a very long time afterward.

The mode which the family chooses to adjust to its crisis will be determined by innumerable variables which relate to the nature of the individuals concerned and the structure within which they have been a part. Personality factors, age, socioeconomic status, and financial assets available to the family, as well as degree of social isolation are important both to the speed with which appropriate functioning is restored and to the characteristics which the newly determined patterns will achieve. It would seem that the personal ability of family members to sustain emotionally satisfying relationships would be crucial at a time when the loss of a loved person is felt so keenly.

Overriding all of these intervening factors are the essential ones of cultural and religious differences.

In some societies cultural mores may provide answers to many of the difficulties which North American widows and their children face. Unlike Western tradition, which urges independence and self-sufficiency for the widow, many ethnic groups absorb the disrupted family into the ranks of the extended kinship group. Young male children may find new status in assuming the vacant position of the dead parent, and widows may find it unnecessary to enter the labor force if relatives assume financial support for the family.

While such traditions may definitely be the case with the members of some Canadian ethnic groups, this is not the usual way in which death is met. It is not uncommon for ties with relatives to be weakened as the mother becomes more involved in earning and providing care for her family. Because we live in an "every man for himself" culture, assistance to the widowed family may be extended in only a limited way once the funeral has passed and the period of mourning has begun.

Differences in religious or philosophical backgrounds greatly affect the mode of adjustment which the family adopts. The death process, like that of birth, engages one in speculation about the spiritual aspects of our existence. If a firmly held belief system is able to provide satisfactory solutions to the bereaved persons' queries, it is probably safe to say that balance within the family is restored with less individual disturbance and confusion.

. . . the often overwhelming expression of condolences and equally impressive offers of usefulness may soon be withdrawn. . . .

The Problems of the Widow

Basically the problems faced by the widow and her family fall into three main categories: economic, social, and emotional. By looking at the component problems of each one of these sections we find that adult and children dependency, poverty, unemployment, and illness frequently occur and aggravate the family disorganization. To be sure, they are also aggravated by the woman's insecure industrial status in the labor force.

The widow may have been away from work for many years. In those years more specialized jobs have emerged and she may find herself insufficiently skilled. As well, it is not uncommon for an older woman to find employers who are less than willing to hire her and the result may be a job which is not satisfying to her expectations and lower in wages than she anticipated.

Socially, the widow finds herself a single woman in friendship interaction with couples. Added to this is the fact that she is now a single woman with children. To be socially active may demand added expenditures for babysitting and housekeeping services—a luxury made difficult if financial resources are budgeted to begin with. Loneliness and apathy may hinder participation in any social encounters. The research of Marris (1958) in England revealed that widows often felt awkward in company, resentful of pity or patronage and easily hurt in their pride in their independence. They found it difficult to spend money on transportation costs needed for visiting and entertainment. Added to these is the problem of sexual satisfaction and the need for sincere emotional affection. Criticism of "affairs" or even of casual dating is very severe following the death of a spouse. While friends may rally to the aid of their friend, pity may prolong the grief period experienced by the widow. Pity on the part of many well-meaning persons can drive a widowed parent into apathy, despair, and isolation.

The result is that emotionally it may be a lonely and isolated existence. While friends and relatives may offer emotional and practical support, we live in a society which values the self-sufficiency of the family unit. Consequently, the often overwhelming expression of condolences and equally impressive offers of usefulness may soon be withdrawn as others turn their at-

> **. . . changes in the woman's personality are a reflection of the intense anxiety faced because of the new, insecure position which she fulfills.**

tention to their own concerns once again. Furthermore, Marris points out that once the shock of bereavement has passed, most of the widows strive to reestablish their independence. Responses to his questioning indicated that they found the continual receipt of kindnesses a constraint because of the obligation which they felt was imposed upon them.

It is not hard to see how the three wide problem areas are interrelated. The success or failure with which a widow endeavors to find solutions to her financial problems will undoubtedly determine the degree to which she must rely on others for support. This, in turn, will aggravate or lessen the intensity of her emotional turmoil and will also affect the desire and means by which she seeks out social contacts. Conversely, the characteristic emotional reactions to bereavement may handicap social adjustment and practical difficulties may intensify the emotional problems.

Given the interdependence of these problems, it is not without reason that many widows face life with ambivalence and conflict. Widows may become restless and active, yet indecisive and lacking all initiative. Practical considerations, particularly where they concern the livelihood of children, force the widow to abandon her grieving and the defenses she may have developed to control her grief. It is with these considerations in mind that we can attempt an understanding of typical reaction patterns of widows.

The responses which may appear to reflect drastic changes in the woman's personality are a reflection of the intense anxiety faced because of the new, insecure position which she fulfills. She is not familiar with all the norm expectations of the male parent role; she is lacking the reciprocal role position which is so fundamental in maintaining the family unit.

The widow may proceed through six phases of her readjustment to the loss. Bereavement may be followed initially by disbelief and consequently numbness. When these short-term effects of the crisis have passed, and the mourning phase begins, the widow may attempt trial and error adjustments, involving herself and her children in the modes of coping heretofore not considered. Slowly old routines will be renewed and necessary new ones adopted. In time, the recovery stage is entered and the family equilibrium is restored.

Such a model as this one is by no means exhaustive of the responses and reactions which may be encountered. Nor is it necessarily followed through by all widows in the order presented. However, while admitting its limitations, it does provide us with a guideline which is useful if we are to examine why particular reactions are commonly found within this group in our population and just how they are dealt with.

Before looking at the handling of reactions there is one very basic assumption which cannot be overlooked. That is, the widow is an acceptable and accepted member of the community. Even if the woman had planned a separation or a divorce prior to her husband's death; even if her attitude toward him was hateful while he was living, the widow is regarded as the unfortunate victim of fate, the pitied mother, and the deserving receiver of sympathy and assistance. This determines, in great part, the form which her reactions will take. It is appropriate that she may mourn outwardly and find initial confusion in her duties as both mother and father. As well, it is "right" for her friends to offer support, both practical and emotional, and to temporarily involve themselves in the family system.

This too is made possible because of the open nature of the system. It has been observed, however, that as the family members begin to reorganize themselves, the system may become more and more closed. In order to satisfy individual and family needs, it may become important to withdraw from family and friends and begin to reestablish a self-sufficient system. Almost as if to complement this process, friends and relatives will be observed to withdraw also, and entrance into the recovery stage is made more inevitable.

Three large problem areas exist for the new widow.

Practically, immediate help with funeral arrangements, caring for the children, legal involvement with the will are almost essential. This is the stage where numbness and disbelief may immobilize an otherwise efficient and able woman. Following the funeral, the most beneficial, practical help may be in assisting the woman to go out and work.

About the house, sons, sons-in-law, or other male relatives may initially assume many of the practical responsibilities which are traditionally so much the domain of the male parent. However, Marris found that for advice, widows turned to their brothers, because they doubted the maturity of their children's judgment.

Emotionally, it is important for the grief to be worked through in all its aspects. Particularly this is so with the feelings of hostility and guilt. Often the widow will feel that such unanticipated reactions cannot be mentioned without expressing disloyalty to the dead person. Yet, when such feelings go unrecognized, mental anguish is prolonged and the children may suffer from behavior which is inconsistent with the mother's behavior prior to the death. The widow must be helped to identify her ambivalence and to understand its natural part in the bereavement process. While a professional person or a clergyman may be called upon to provide the assistance necessary, often a willing and patient friend or relative can be of most help in the immediate period following the death.

In social contexts, relatives and friends tend to assume the predominant function of assisting the widow. Often this is ill-timed and cruelly precipitated by individuals who too hastily assume that the widow is at the recovery stage of the process. In the majority of cases, new social contacts are most successfully initiated by the widow herself. Unlike the divorcee, the widow is less likely to be the prey of "wolves." Particularly if her family unit has been a stable one, she may find that male company is not available until she herself indicates that she is willing once again to participate in social activities. Death does have a stigma which makes association with it awkward and embarrassing for some individuals. As well, traditional mores

In the majority of cases, new social contacts are most successfully initiated by the widow herself.

which dictate a lengthy mourning period, while no longer adhered to by many, do influence the manner in which others interact with the bereaved family.

But the relationships within the family are particularistic in nature. Death of a parent figure not only produces upheaval for the spouse, loss is felt as well by the children. Because they play an integral part in the reshuffling of role responsibilities, we might expect insecurity and bewilderment following the death crisis.

The Child and Widowhood

When the familiar design of family life is disrupted, the child may be deprived of the extra attention and emotional reassurance which a crisis situation necessitates. The young child needs his immediate concerns for care and love provided for and needs support that these will not be taken away from him.

A very young child learns to associate loss with punishment, and consequently it is not unusual for him to associate the fact that "Daddy's not coming home" with any preceding incident in which he perceived himself to be naughty. Concomitant with these feelings may be the association of death with violence. Television and books which capitalize on shooting as a means of death undoubtedly contribute to this.

Like the mother, anger and hostility may be crucial in the child's reaction to grief. However, the reasons are not necessarily the same. The mother's reaction may be understood in terms of her resentment at the insecurity which faces her. The child may simply be reacting aggressively to a force which he perceives to be violent.

But the resultant behavior does vary and aggression is not necessarily the expected response. The following are commonly found behavioral tendencies: denial, bodily distress, guilt coupled with expectations of punishment, replacement of another adult figure in the role of the father, assumption of the mannerisms of the deceased, idealization of the lost parent, anxiety about what else might happen in the future and panic regarding immediate concerns.

The grief of a child is not an easy phenomenon with which to deal. Ambivalence may characterize both his thinking processes and his outward actions. While he probably feels remorseful that a cherished person is dead, he may feel extreme self-pity that he should be picked out for such personal pain. The acceptance of death's finality may account for excessive confusion when he realizes that he can no longer "make up" to the deceased individual. His withdrawal may be tempered with aggressive outbursts; his difficulty in accepting the loss may be overlooked by adults because of his lucid and mature concern regarding the nature of death and its religious implications.

One of the most practical problems involves the absence of a suitable role model for the children. Studies have shown that if a boy loses a mother he may regress to an earlier stage of development. In order to compensate for his loss he may become demanding of attention and whining. In later life he may find difficulty responding to women if his image of them is associated strongly with his loss. The small boy whose father dies will feel the loss of a male person to imitate. A masculine figure is needed in order to learn to temper his feelings of aggressions and love. Similarly for the daughter, those characteristics peculiar to being female may be distorted by the loss of either significant parent.

Because the child may work through the grief process in a largely nonverbal manner, it may be that his reactions are most prominent in school. Bereaved children may feel that effort in the classroom is of little use and may displace their grief onto their work there. In the very young, motivation is often associated with approval and reward, and the loss of a parent who has given particular recognition to the child's performance may be the cause of indifference and apathy. Teachers have found that personality traits that were prominent before the loss of the parent tended to be exaggerated afterward. The shy child became more withdrawn and the antagonistic child more aggressive. The change, however, was less drastic in those who were well-adjusted before the loss.

But many of these dynamics need not occur. Like the widow, it has been postulated that the child moves through a mourning process with certain distinct phases. An understanding of this can be useful in determining the most helpful means of assisting the bereaved child.

Each child experiences three phases in the natural grieving process. The first is protest when the child cannot quite believe that the person is dead, and he attempts, sometimes angrily, to regain him. The next is pain, despair, and disorganization when the youngster begins to accept the fact that the loved one is really gone. Finally, there is hope, when the youngster begins to organize his life without the lost person.

If the remaining parent and others who are involved with the child attempt to help the child proceed to the final stage of this model, then it is probable that they will see acceptance by the child of another significant adult as the ultimate goal. While helping a child who lost a loved one may differ, depending on the phase of grief which is being experienced, the attempt is frequently made to enable the child to work through his feelings so that he is receptive to embarking upon another intimate relationship. Because the family unit is built upon reciprocal relationships, this is of utmost importance.

A constant theme which is evident in the literature concerning death and families is that if we, as individuals and as a society, could ourselves come to terms with death, we could do a better job in telling our children about it.

Like the birth process, death may hold a fascination and bewilderment for children. As well, it is so intricately associated with religious beliefs that the parent may find himself involved in questions of amazing complexity. There are, therefore, both the immediate and ultimate concerns within a child's mind and to which the adult must address himself. This points to the

> . . . if we . . . could ourselves come to terms with death, we could do a better job in telling our children about it.

Recalling happy moments will do much to prepare the child to reinvest the affection he held for the dead person in someone else.

importance of the communication process between parent and child both prior to and following the death crisis in order to remove the possibility of inaccurate and frightening ideas.

Questions should be answered in the spirit in which they are asked. Age is an important factor but so too is the phase of grief which the child is experiencing. Initially, numbness may best be handled in a nonverbal way. Physical and emotional support are essential and will prepare the child for a significant relationship with another adult figure. Disorganization and confusion may best be met with verbal reassurance of love, an acknowledgment of the grief process and the problems which the child is encountering, and, particularly, a working through of the hostile and guilty feelings. It is essential for the child to feel free to express his grief, and the parent who recognizes that this expression may take many different forms will be more tolerant of what may be termed "inappropriate" behavior by adult standards.

To prevent a child from attending a funeral is to exclude him from an important occasion for the entire family unit. Rites and ceremonies have evolved as a means of coping with the sudden overwhelming emotional upsurge that can occur. It is no less so with the child, with the exception of the very young—possibly those under seven years—but added to the therapeutic value which the funeral might have is the very crucial feeling of belonging to and partaking with the family. To deprive him of this is to shake his security. On the other hand it would also be damaging to force an unwilling child to attend a funeral. Such an action could be interpreted by the child as further punishment and reinforce his feelings of guilt over his parent's death.

Guilt feelings should be dealt with as a perfectly reasonable reaction to a death. If the child is able to verbalize his anxieties in this regard, parents should help the child understand that all people try to be good and loving but do not always succeed. Nor does one have to. The important thing is that one does the best he can. It is good to recall those happy moments when the child did make the deceased very happy. Undoubtedly this can best be accomplished when the relationship between the child and adult is intimate and trusting.

Children desire and need an affirmation of life at this time of their lives. Recalling happy moments will do much to prepare the child to reinvest the affection he held for the dead person in someone else. But this is the final phase of the mourning process, and one must guard against impeding the normal mourning process itself. Usually, however, if the child allows himself to find an individual in which he can invest his affection, then this is a good indication that his grief has been worked through.

One danger which must be anticipated and hopefully avoided in the wise dealing of a child's grief are the dependency relations which may develop between a child and his mother. In an attempt to eliminate her own deprivation, a mother may demand more from the child in terms of affection and responsibility. It is easy to visualize how this could be accounted for by the attempt to restore the family balance. But the child who finds he is able to receive complete gratification from one parent will find difficulty in establishing and maintaining relationships for the rest of his life. This emphasizes once again how important it is for the family to remain an open system where children can interact with a variety of adult figures who will give sympathetic attention and understanding to his problems.

The importance of encouraging the *natural* mourning process is reinforced by a brief examination of the effects of the inability to resolve mourning. Distorted mourning reactions, such as continued denial of reality, extended guilt feelings, or prolonged anxiety may result in morbid anxiety over individual health or increasingly hostile reactions to oneself and to others. Poor acceptance of social roles and social responsibility and loss of individual initiative and self-esteem are all implications of an inability to work through a death crisis.

The widow should be encouraged not to deny the support of neighbors in her eagerness to be independent.

Conclusions

While we have tried to show how widows and other adults may assist and encourage the normal grieving process, it may be the case that the mother is herself unable to do this and other adults are not available. Often without outside help, parents in the midst of their own grief cannot properly support the mourning child.

The question at this point concerns the available programs and policies to help the widowed family and the role of the professional social worker or clergyman in working with the widow and her family.

If we assume that the goal of the family is self-sufficiency, then the practical aspect of our help must be with this goal in mind. Arrangements for homemaker service, day-care centers and nursery schools should be readily available. Big Brother Associations and Parents Without Partners organizations are good sources of support for individual family members. However, it would also seem advisable that involvement with the entire family would be beneficial.

Consequently, family therapy and counseling should assume a large part of help for this kind of family. It may not appear to involve more than listening to woes, assistance with practical problems, and the understanding of feelings, but overriding all of these factors is the maintenance of appropriate and sustaining relationships between family members.

The widow should be encouraged not to deny the support of neighbors in her eagerness to be independent. Interdependence within community members in any time of crisis may be considered a singularly helpful support for all family members.

If we as social workers attempt to strengthen those factors conducive to good adjustment to crisis, then we will have done much to establish a healthy outcome in the event of death in a family. Family integration and adaptability, strong parent-child relationships, family-council type of control in decision making, and training of the wife in practical concerns of home management normally left to the male are all goals which should be our priorities. Preventive work is essential if any family crisis is to be overcome with the least amount of disruption to the family unit.

Clarissa Start (1973, p. 124) writes: "Grief teaches you that there are two kinds of people in the world, those who are available and those who are not. You can tell which are open to you by the way they listen when you have sorrow to share."

References

Benjamin Schlesinger. 1975. *The one-parent family: perspectives and annotated bibliography.* Toronto: University of Toronto Press, 3rd ed.
Peter Marris. 1958. *Widows and their families.* London: Routledge and Kegan Paul.
Clarissa Start. 1973. *On becoming a widow.* New York: Family Library.

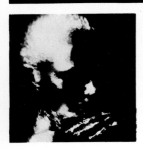

13

Theory

Think back to the last time you were ill. Were there people around who helped you get better? What behaviors and attitudes would you describe as most helpful from caregivers during illness? Would you expect a medical staff to be very effective in dealing with dying patients? Schulz and Aderman take us on a critique of these issues. The following Appendix exercises are recommended:

      A.   Announcing One's Own Death

      B.   Appropriate Death Fantasy

      I.   Life and Death Attitudes: Dyadic Encounter

      L.   Privacy Circles

How the Medical Staff Copes with Dying Patients: A Critical Review

Richard Schulz

David Aderman

This paper examines the attitudes and resultant behaviors which typically characterize the interaction between medical practitioners and the dying patient. The focus will not only be on how doctors and nurses regard death and the dying, but also on the dying patient's feelings about his impending death and the treatment he receives from the medical staff. The aim is to gain some understanding of the plight of the dying patient, to learn whether he is informed of his condition, and to determine how he is treated by the medical staff.

Attitudes and Behavior of Physicians

Numerous researchers have observed that physicians avoid a patient once he begins to die (1–4). To explain this avoidance behavior, researchers have focused either on the physician's training or his personality. Those investigators who are of the opinion that a basic personality structure is responsible for the physician's behavior toward the dying speculate that individuals who become physicians do so because of their inordinate fear of death. Becoming a physician, then, has been interpreted as an attempt to master death (5–7). Kasper agreed with this point of view (8), and added that "part of the psychological motivation of the physician is to cure himself and live forever; he wishes to be a scientist in order to gain mastery over life by treating people as things" (1).

Although not conclusive, some empirical support for self-selection on the basis of personality is found in a study of medical students by Livingston and Zimet (1). These investigators reasoned that medical students high in authoritarianism would be "better defended" against

This material was first published in *Omega: Journal of Death and Dying,* vol. 7, no. 1, pp. 11–21, 1976. Copyright 1976 Baywood Publishing Co., Inc. It is printed here in slightly modified form by permission.

. . . physicians may tend to avoid patients in the process of dying.

unconscious fears and therefore have less overt death anxiety. As a result, these students would function comfortably in specialities where death is relatively common (e.g., surgery). Students low on authoritarianism, on the other hand, would be aware of and made uncomfortable by their death anxiety and as a result choose specialities where death is an uncommon occurrence (e.g., psychiatry). The results supported their hypothesis: Psychiatrically oriented students were less authoritarian and showed higher death anxiety than students oriented toward surgery. The fact that this was true regardless of year of training seems to indicate that medical students decide on a speciality upon entering medical school and that this decision is in part determined by their personality structure.

These personality structures are undoubtedly reinforced by medical training which emphasizes an interaction style between physician and patient described by Lief and Fox as "detached concern" (9). The medical student is advised to be empathic and involved with the patient but, above all, to remain objective. In addition, the specifics of medical training are usually focused at saving lives to the exclusion of dealing with patients who are defined as terminal. As a consequence of both their personality structures and the training they receive, physicians may associate dying patients with failure and disappointment. A patient's death challenges the physician's ability as a healer and sensitizes him to the temporal limits of his own life. It is not surprising, then, that physicians may tend to avoid patients in the process of dying.

Perhaps the most important decision the physician makes when his patient becomes terminal is whether or not to tell the patient about his condition. There already exists a large body of literature advising the physician on this question (2, 3, 10–15), but only a few researchers have actually attempted to determine the extent to which this advice is followed (12, 16).

In an editorial directed at physicians, Lasagna advised physicians not to lie about the terminal patient's condition (13). He also recommended that relatives of the patient should be forewarned. Lirette et al. similarly advised letting the patient know his condition but caution the physician to tell the patient gradually (14). Noyes pointed out that the physician holds the key to providing the patient with a good death, and this is best accomplished by informing the patient of his condition (10). Kübler-Ross focused on the requirements of a "good" death and stressed the physician's role in fulfilling these requirements (2). Through intimate interaction, she argued, the physician can help the patient reach a calm acceptance of his death. Wahl agreed with Kübler-Ross that the physician should acquire intimate knowledge of the patient, but at the same time he cautioned the physician to be selective in choosing those patients to be informed of their condition (11). Although not telling a patient may deprive him of the opportunity for sympathetic communication with physicians and friends, there are some individuals who are too afraid of death to face such information. Those patients who are told, Wahl stresses, should never be told in such a way as to rob them of all hope: "The patient should never be left with the feeling that the physician has played his last card and that nothing further can be done" (11). Evidence supporting the conclusion that patients should be told their condition was reported by Glaser and Strauss (3). After several years of observing patients and medical staff, they found that most patients learned of their condition from cues given by medical personnel, even when they were not specifically told their condition. These cues ranged in subtlety from facial expressions and avoidance behavior to discussions of the patient's condition in front of the patient.

A number of practitioners have addressed themselves specifically to the question of whether or not to tell terminal *cancer* patients of their condition (17–21). Here again, the consensus position is that it is best to be truthful but gentle. Litin argued that it is a patient's legal right to know the truth (17). In Hoerr's opinion, honesty is always the best policy in the long run (18). Desjardins, Wyrsch, and Oken all advocated a "play it by ear" policy. In most cases a patient should be told, they advised, but one should let the patient be the guide as to how much and in what way the information is to be conveyed (19–21).

It should be noted that, with only few exceptions, the advice given above comes from medical practitioners, primarily doctors, and is therefore directed at colleagues. One would expect then that medical doctors would be likely to adhere to such advice. The evidence on the behavior of physicians indicates, however, that this is not the case. Fitts and Ravdin found that of four hundred and forty-two physicians sampled by a mail survey in the Philadelphia area, over two-thirds reported that they infrequently or never disclosed the diagnosis of terminal cancer (16). A similar nationwide mail survey of over four thousand physicians revealed that 22 percent never told while 62 percent sometimes informed the patient of incurable cancer (22). In a recent study reported by Caldwell and Mishara, seventy-three medical doctors at a large metropolitan Detroit, Michigan private hospital were asked to participate in a research project on the attitudes and feelings of medical doctors (32). Although the majority of physicians consented to participate when originally approached, sixty of the seventy-three doctors refused to complete the interview once they found out the questions dealt with their attitudes toward dying patients. All of the thirteen doctors who completed the interview agreed that the dying patient has the right to know that his diagnosis is terminal, but only two of those thirteen admitted to actually telling their patients of a terminal diagnosis. This inconsistency between attitude and behavior may reflect the fact that physicians find the task of actually informing the patient psychologically too difficult for them and/or not their responsibility.

In a more comprehensive study, Oken endeavored to find out not only how physicians behave in regard to informing the cancer patient but also to discover what reasons they gave for their behavior (12). Oken sent a questionnaire to two hundred and nineteen members of the medical staff of Michael Reese Hospital, a private nonprofit teaching hospital in Chicago. Ninety-five percent of the questionnaires were returned and 30 percent of

> . . . of four hundred and forty-two physicians sampled by a mail survey . . . over two-thirds reported that they infrequently or never disclosed the diagnosis of terminal cancer.

. . . nurses
having more
experience with
death were more
likely to avoid the
dying and felt
more uneasy
discussing death
with dying
patients than less
experienced
nurses.

those cooperating were subsequently interviewed. Consistent with previous findings, about 90 per cent of Oken's respondents indicated that they did not tell patients their diagnosis. Those that did tell were found to employ euphemisms for incurable cancer such as "growth," "hyperplastic tissue," "lesion," "mass," or "tumor." The primary reason offered for telling those few patients who were told was concern for the patient's financial responsibility. That is, physicians thought it important for some patients to have the opportunity for planning their financial affairs. Primarily emotional reasons were given for not telling the patient: "Knowledge of cancer is a death sentence, a Buchenwald, a torture"; "the cruelest thing in the world"; "like hitting the patient with a baseball bat" (12).

Oken attempted to find out where physicians acquired their policies of not telling. Only 5 percent mentioned medical school or hospital training as the major source, whereas the great majority, 77 percent, listed clinical experience. Oken reasoned that if experience did indeed determine the physician's policy, then young doctors should have listed experience less frequently as a determinant of their policy; however, young doctors were just as likely as old doctors to list experience as the determinant of their policy. Oken concluded that the physicians' claim that their policy is based on experience was far from accurate. Further probing showed that more often than not a physician's policy was based on "opinion, belief, and conviction, heavily weighted with emotional justification" and not on critical observation (12).

Oken's respondents also voiced substantial opposition to the idea of changing their policy on informing patients. Eighty percent felt that policy change in the future was unlikely, although over half felt that they could be swayed by research. A sizable minority stated that they "wouldn't believe it, or 'it couldn't be true,' if research suggested a policy different from their own" (12). Ten percent of the group objected even to the suggestion that research be carried out in this area.

Attitude and Behavior of Nurses

Although the literature on medical staff other than physicians is sparse, some data on the behavior of nurses toward the dying is available. A study similar to Oken's was carried out by Pearlman, Stotsky, and Dominick (23). These investigators interviewed sixty-eight nursing personnel in a variety of institutions, from state hospitals to nursing homes, and found that those nurses having more experience with death were more likely to avoid the dying and felt more uneasy discussing death with dying patients than less experienced nurses. Lawrence LeShan (reported by Kastenbaum and Aisenberg [4]) recorded nurses' avoidance of terminal patients. Using a stop watch, LeShan measured how long it took nurses to respond to bedside calls and found that it took them significantly more time to respond to terminal patients than to less severely ill patients. Apparently, experienced nurses had learned to cope with death by avoiding or denying it, a behavioral pattern not unlike the one found among physicians. Like the physicians in Oken's study, the experienced nurses also advocated experience with dying patients as the best means for learning how to deal with them. The less experienced nurses, on the other hand, stressed the need for courses and seminars on managing the dying patient as the best means for learning how to deal with death.

What do nurses tell a patient when directly confronted by his thoughts on death? Kastenbaum tried to answer this question by asking two hundred attendants and nurses at a geriatric hospital how they responded to patients' statements about death (e.g., "I think I'm going to die soon," or "I wish I could just end it all") (24). Kastenbaum found five general categories of responses.

Responses to Patients' Death Statements

Reassurance.   "You're doing so well now. You don't have to feel this way."

Denial.   "You don't really mean that . . . You're not going to die. Oh, you're going to live to be a hundred."

Changing the Subject.   "Let's think of something more cheerful. You shouldn't say things like that; there are better things to talk about."

Fatalism.   "We are all going to die sometime, and it's a good thing we don't know when. When God wants you, He will take you."

Discussion.   "What makes you feel that way today? Is it something that happened, something somebody said?"

The most popular response was some form of avoidance, either fatalism, denial, or changing the subject. The majority, 82 percent, evaded any discussion of the patient's thoughts or feelings. "The clear tendency was to 'turn off' the patient as quickly and deftly as possible" (24). Two reasons were given for this behavior. One, nurses wanted to make the patient happy, and felt that the best way to do this was to get him to think about something else. Two, nurses wanted to protect themselves. Most admitted feeling very uncomfortable talking about death, saying that it "bugged" them or "shook them up" to talk about it.

The inability of nurses to deal with the dying patient is also documented in Jeanne C. Quint's book, *The Nurse and the Dying Patient* (25). She analyzed the training that nurses receive which could bring about this avoidance behavior and concluded that, because the young nurse is made to feel very concerned about making mistakes, she learns to defend herself by concentrating on routines and rituals that tend to alienate her

> . . . she learns to defend herself by concentrating on routines and rituals. . . .

**. . . dying
patients are at
some level aware
that they will not
recover. . . .**

from the patient she is caring for. The solution, of course, is to provide professional training early in the nurse's career that will enable her to adequately handle the dying patient.

It should be apparent now that there is a great disparity between the advice offered by some practitioners regarding the treatment of terminal patients and the behavior of most physicians and nurses. The next section examines the terminal patient's feelings about how he is treated by the medical staff and the consequences of such treatment for his psychological well-being.

Patients' Desire for Information About Their Illness

Kübler-Ross and Glaser and Strauss argue that the terminal patient acquires information about his condition even if not directly informed. Data presented below tends to refute this (2, 3). A sizable proportion of terminal patients appear to remain unaware of their condition until the end, although it is sometimes difficult to separate what the patient knows from what he is willing to accept. Most patients are probably best classified as being in a condition of uncertain certainty that Avery Weisman has called "middle knowledge" (4). That is, dying patients are at some level aware that they will not recover, but they vacillate between knowing and not knowing this.

Although few researchers have attempted to specifically determine how aware the dying patient is of his condition, research on the patient's attitude toward the medical staff and the treatment he receives is more abundant. In his study of healthy nonpatients, psychiatric patients, somatically ill patients, and the dying, Cappon asked each group whether or not they would like to know if a serious illness was terminal (26). The majority of subjects, regardless of medical status, responded yes. Of the four groups, however, dying patients desired this information least (67 percent). Eighty-one percent of the somatic patients desired such information, while 82 percent of the psychiatric patients and 91 percent of the nonpatients said they would like to know if a serious illness was terminal. Dying patients were also less interested than the other groups in information revealing "when he will die" and "how he will feel on dying."

Cappon concluded from his findings that physicians should be cautious and not give more information than is wanted. Apparently unaware of the literature showing that physicians only rarely inform the patient of his condition, he advised that physicians, as nonpatients, should recognize that "what they think *now* they themselves would want to know may not hold later when they become ill" (26).

It is unfortunate that in his study Cappon did not report data on whether or not the dying patients knew their condition was terminal when they filled out his questionnaire. One might expect different attitudes toward death and varying desires for information as a function of such knowledge. It could be that Cappon's dying patients were less curious about what it's like to die because they already knew. Hinton's work in part addresses itself to this question (27).

Hinton and his collaborators repeatedly interviewed two groups of patients residing in the same hospital. One group of one hundred and twenty-one patients was selected on the basis that they had a fatal illness, with death expected within six months. A second group consisted of matched controls. These patients entered the hospital at the same time that dying patients did, were the same age, had an illness affecting the same system, and were under the same physician's care. A control patient was always interviewed on the same day as the dying patient. The structure of the interview was left open to the interviewer, provided he collected information on age, sex, marital status, social class, strength of religiosity, level of physical distress, depression, anxiety, and the patient's awareness of dying. Where possible, patients' responses were systematically categorized and analyzed using a chi-square analysis.

Since control patients did not differ from dying patients on any of the demographic variables (e.g., sex, age, social class, etc.), Hinton felt justified in attributing differences on the psychological variables to degree of illness. A cursory analysis showed that physical distress as measured by pain, dyspnoea (difficulty in breathing), nausea, malaise, or cough was greater for the dying patients than the nondying controls. This is hardly surprising given that dying patients were physically more deteriorated. Dying patients were also significantly more depressed and anxious and were, of course, much more likely to perceive themselves as terminal than nondying patients.

Looking at relationships between dependent measures, Hinton found that awareness of the possibility of death was significantly related to a mood of depression. Over 60 percent of the dying patients who showed awareness of death expressed mild or moderate depression. These same individuals were, however, not significantly more anxious, although the results were in that direction. Awareness was also related to greater physical distress and longer illness.

Depression and anxiety were both related to religious faith, but not in the same way. Those with strong religious beliefs showed the least amount of anxiety but the most depression, while individuals with no religious faith were least depressed and only slightly more anxious than strong faith individuals. Patients with some Christian beliefs were high on both anxiety and depression. Perhaps these patients were anxious about their lack of faith and at the same time depressed in the realization that religion really had little to offer. Hinton was unable to offer an explanation for these results or for most of his other findings. His use of univariate instead of multivariate analysis methods undoubtedly hindered his explanatory efforts.

Both Hinton and Cappon concluded that the dying patient is better off not informed about his condition. Thirty-three percent of Cappon's dying

. . . individuals with no religious faith were least depressed and only slightly more anxious than strong faith individuals.

. . . the
conclusion that
dying patients
more often than
not desire
information about
their condition is
better justified by
the data. . . .

subjects expressed a desire not to be told, while Hinton showed that dying patients aware of their condition were more depressed and slightly more anxious than nondying patients. Neither study is, however, convincing in its conclusion. Cappon, for instance, based his conclusion on the fact that fewer dying than nondying patients desired information about terminal illness. Yet well over half (67 percent) still wanted to know. In addition, Cappon did not report whether these responses came from dying patients who already knew they were dying or from patients who perhaps only suspected it but were afraid to find out. In any case, the conclusion that dying patients more often than not desire information about their condition is better justified by the data than the conclusion offered by Cappon.

Hinton can be criticized on similar grounds. He assumed a causal relationship between awareness of condition and depression. His basic argument was that knowledge of condition leads to depression, which is undesirable; therefore, patients should not be informed. His data also showed, however, that depression was significantly higher in those patients who had endured longer illnesses and greater physical distress. Furthermore, as was indicated earlier, awareness of dying came more often to those who had greater physical distress and longer illnesses. Thus, awareness, depression, physical distress, and longer illness were all positively related in dying patients. Given these relationships, one can just as logically argue that physical distress or longer illness result in depression and awareness of dying; or, perhaps even that depression results in longer illness, greater physical distress, and awareness of dying. Many reasonable causal chains are possible, and none can be definitively ruled out given the data presented in this study. Fortunately, other data on this issue are available.

Kelly and Friesen found that of one hundred cancer patients eighty-nine favored knowing their diagnosis (28). One hundred clinic patients who did not have cancer were asked if they would like to know the results of an examination that revealed cancer, and the great majority (82 percent) said, yes. Similar results are reported by Samp and Curerri, who surveyed five hundred and sixty cancer patients and their families and found that 87 percent felt that a patient should be told (29). Subjects who had cancer in these studies were aware of their diagnosis before these surveys were taken. These results are, therefore, slightly suspect since "patients cannot permit doubts about the wisdom of the policy of those whom they need to trust so desperately" (12).

In a recent interview study, Kalle Achté, a Finnish psychiatrist, focused on how one hundred cancer patients acquired the information that they had terminal cancer (30). Forty of the patients had been spontaneously told of their condition. Twenty-nine had asked for a diagnosis and received a frank answer, and thirty-one were reluctant to find out anything about their condition, although six of these patients suspected it was cancer. The majority of the patients (85 percent) had suffered from intense anxiety and depression upon learning the true nature of their illness, but in most cases these symptoms dissipated in a short time.

None of the patients who were spontaneously informed were critical of the act of informing, but a small number did criticize the manner in which they were told, describing the physicians' behavior as tactless and insensitive. Patients who had inquired about their diagnosis were most favorable toward physicians. The remaining patients avoided all discussion of the disease with the interviewer.

This study, then, lends support to the position that the majority of patients desire to be told and suffer no permanent negative consequences as a result of being informed of their condition. It should be noted, however, that subjects who were informed were not randomly selected. This self-selection process may have attenuated the potential negative effects of informing individuals of their condition. The crucial study, where subjects are randomly assigned to information or no information condition, has not been carried out. The dependent measures in such a study would include blind assessment of psychological and physical well-being of the patient.

. . . it is hoped that social-psychological aspects of medical practice will become an important part of the education of medical practitioners.

Conclusion

Alban Wheeler has argued that the dying person is a deviant in the medical subculture (31). Much of the research reviewed above supports this view. The dying person elicits aversive attitudes from his audience and these attitudes often result in avoidance behaviors on the part of physicians and nurses. Future research should be aimed at further documenting medical staff interactions with dying patients as well as investigating ways in which attitudes of practitioners might be changed, should that be necessary. One possible approach to changing the attitudes of practitioners might be to convince medical and nursing schools to focus on the social-psychological aspects of death and dying as part of their curriculum.

With the increased availability of reports such as this, it is hoped that social-psychological aspects of medical practice will become an important part of the education of medical practitioners.

References

1. P. B. Livingston and C. N. Zimet. Death anxiety, authoritarianism and choice of speciality in medical students. *Journal Nervous Mental Disease,* 140, pp. 222–230, 1965.
2. E. Kübler-Ross. *On death and dying.* Macmillan, New York, 1964.
3. B. G. Glaser and A. L. Strauss. *Awareness of dying.* Aldine, Chicago, 1965.
4. R. Kastenbaum and R. Aisenberg. *The psychology of death.* Springer, New York, 1972.
5. C. W. Wahl. The physician's management of the dying patient. In J. Masserman (ed.), *Current psychiatric therapies.* Grune and Stratton, New York, 1962.
6. H. Feifel and J. Heller. Normalcy, illness and death. *Proceedings of the Third World Congress of Psychiatry.* University of Toronto Press, Toronto, 1960.
7. H. Feifel, S. Hanson, and R. Jones. Physicians consider death. *Proceedings of the 75th Annual Convention of the American Psychological Association, 2,* pp. 201–202, 1967.
8. A. M. Kasper. The doctor and death. In H. Feifel (ed.), *The meaning of death.* McGraw Hill, New York, 1959.
9. H. I. Lief and R. C. Fox. Training for "detached concern" in medical students. In H. I. Lief and N. R. Lief (eds), *The psychological basis of medical practice.* Harper and Row, New York, 1963.

10. R. Noyes, Jr. The art of dying. *Perspectives in Biology and Medicine,* 14, pp. 432–447, 1971.
11. C. W. Wahl. Should a patient be told the truth? In A. H. Kutcher (ed.), *But not to lose.* Frederick Fell, New York, pp. 104–107, 1969.
12. D. Oken. What to tell cancer patients. *Journal American Medical Association,* 175, pp. 86–94, 1961.
13. L. Lasagna. The doctor and the dying patient. *Journal Chronic Disease,* 22, pp. 65–68, 1969.
14. W. L. Lirette, R. L. Palmer, I. D. Ibarra, et al. Management of patients with terminal cancer. *Postgraduate Medicine,* 46, pp. 145–149, 1969.
15. The doctor and the dying patient, R. H. David (ed.). *Symposium on the doctor and the dying patient.* University of Southern California School of Medicine Postgraduate Division of the Department of Psychiatry and Gerontology Center, 1971.
16. W. T. Fitts and I. S. Ravdin. What Philadelphia physicians tell patients with cancer. *Journal American Medical Association,* 153, pp. 901–904, 1953.
17. E. M. Litin. What shall we tell the cancer patient? A psychiatrist's view. *Proceedings of Mayo Clinic,* 35, pp. 247–250, 1960.
18. S. O. Hoerr. Thoughts on what to tell the patient with cancer. *Cleveland Clinic Quarterly,* 30, pp. 11–16, 1963.
19. A. V. Desjardins. What the physician should tell a patient who is affected with a malignant lesion. *Journal Main Medical Association,* 30, pp. 16–17, 1960.
20. J. Wyrsh. Should we inform the patient about the cancer diagnosis? *Schweiz Medizinische Wochenschrift,* 92, pp. 1577–1588, 1962.
21. D. Oken. The physician, the patient, and cancer. *Illinois Medical Journal,* 120, pp. 333–334, 1961.
22. D. Rennick. What should physicians tell cancer patients? *New Medical Materia,* 2, pp. 51–53, 1960.
23. J. Pearlman, B. A. Stotsky, and J. R. Dominick. Attitudes toward death among nursing home personnel. *Journal Genetic Psychology,* 114, pp. 63–75, 1969.
24. R. Kastenbaum. Multiple perspectives on a geriatric "death valley." *Community Mental Health Journal,* 3, pp. 21–29, 1967.
25. J. C. Quint. *The nurse and the dying patient.* Aldine, Chicago, 1967.
26. D. Cappon. Attitudes of and toward the dying. *Canadian Medical Association Journal,* 87, pp. 693–700, 1969.
27. J. M. Hinton. The physical and mental distress of the dying. *Quarterly Journal of Medicine,* 32, pp. 1–21, 1963.
28. W. D. Kelly and S. R. Friesen. Do cancer patients want to be told? *Surgery,* 27, pp. 822–826, 1950.
29. R. J. Samp and A. R. Curreri. Questionnaire survey on public cancer education obtained from cancer patients and their families. *Cancer,* 10, pp. 382–384, 1957.
30. K. Achté and M. L. Vauhkonen. Cancer and the psyche. *Omega,* 2, pp. 45–56, 1971.
31. A. L. Wheeler. The dying person: A deviant in the medical subculture. Paper presented at the annual meeting of the Southern Sociological Society, Atlanta, Georgia, April, 1973.
32. D. Caldwell and B. L. Mishara. Research on attitudes of medical doctors toward the dying patient: A methodological problem. *Omega,* 3, pp. 341–346, 1972.

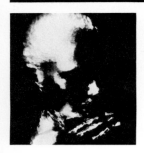

14

Theory

When you die, what kind of funeral would you like to have? Are you willing to make those arrangements today, or is that commitment a bit too threatening to face right now? Turner and Edgley are creative in describing how a typical American funeral is "staged." When you have completed this reading, the following Appendix exercises should enhance your understanding and sensitivity in this area:

        A.   Announcing One's Own Death

        G.   Funeral Fantasy

        J.   Mortuary Form

        N.   The Final Rite of Passage: A Technological Update

They told me, Francis Hinley, they
  told me you were hung
With red protruding eye-balls and
  black protruding tongue
I wept as I remembered how often you
  and I
Had laughed about Los Angeles and
  now 'tis here you'll lie;
Here pickled in formaldehyde and
  painted like a whore,
Shrimp-pink incorruptible, not lost but
  gone before.

Evelyn Waugh
The Loved One

Death as Theater: A Dramaturgical Analysis of the American Funeral

Ronny E. Turner

Charles Edgley

Introduction

The notion that life is rather like a theater, of actors playing their parts to audiences, sometimes within the bounds of roles, and sometimes with considerable distance from them, is an ancient metaphor recently resurrected by social psychology as a device for analyzing behavior. Although sometimes associated almost exclusively with the pioneering work of Erving Goffman,[1] the dramaturgical point of view[2] is more precisely traced to the prolific writings of literary critic Kenneth Burke. . . . Burke, like the pragmatists before him, stressed that the cause of understanding social behavior is best served by beginning with theories of action rather than theories of knowledge. He further claimed that all investigation proceeds through the use of metaphor and that human social life is best seen through the metaphor of drama. "Men relate as actors playing roles to create satisfactions which only other human actors can give them" (Duncan, 1962:112). Our study uses the dramaturgical metaphor to understand some of the relationships and interactions that comprise the American funeral.

The study is based on unobtrusive observations of and information obtained from fifteen mortuaries in three cities. Funeral directors were interviewed, "in-house" manuals on how to successfully perform a funeral were subjected to content analysis, and both national and local advertising material were studied. Only funeral services performed in mortuary chapels (a growing trend) were studied; however, the techniques we describe are probably also applicable to services held in churches of various denominations. No memorial services in which the deceased had been cremated were included in our observations, and all of the funerals we observed were open-casket.

This material was first published in *Sociology and Social Research*, vol. 60, no. 4, pp. 377–392, 1976. Copyright 1976 the University of Southern California. It is printed here in slightly modified form by permission.

1. Goffman's work which seems to us to be most influenced by a dramaturgical conception of social life includes: *The Presentation of Self in Everyday Life* (1959); *Behavior in Public Places* (1962); his essays on "role-distance" in *Encounters* (1963); and his numerous writings on mental disorder, especially *Asylums* (1961); *Interaction Ritual* (1967); and "The Insanity of Place," appendix to *Relations in Public* (1970). . . .
2. We take dramaturgy to be a metaphor, perspective, and strategy for viewing life, not as life itself.

The Nature of Funeral Directing

Funeral directors and allied members of their team may be seen as actors whose job it is to stage a performance in such a way that the audience (the bereaved family and friends) will impute competence, sincerity, dignity, respect, and concern to their actions. Given the one-shot nature of the funeral service, and the impossibility of doing it over in the event of mistakes, the funeral director must necessarily be concerned with those aspects of his business which will lead the audience to be impressed favorably by his effective staging of the show. As in any other performance, the concern is likely to be with whether the show comes off or falls flat, and consequently, to use Goffman's phrase, the expressions given off must be arranged in such a way that the images and impressions formed are favorable ones.

From the standpoint of the sociology of work, the funeral director is in a unique business.[3] He draws his living from a relatively fixed resource: the death rate in a community. He cannot increase the amount of business available to him by increasing the number of deaths in the community, and he must be very careful of how he advertises lest someone gain the impression that he wants more people to die. (One does not, for example, see funeral homes sponsoring such risky events as the Indianapolis 500). His choices for increasing the flow of money, then, are limited and center basically around two options: (1) Getting more than his share of the business from deaths that do occur in the community; and (2) merchandising up, so that the average cost of a funeral rises. In short, his opportunities to make money stem from his . . . ability to stage dramas which are meaningful to his audience and will leave them with an impression favorable enough to contribute to the all-important "reputation" which funeral homes find is in many respects their most marketable, if not tangible, quality.

Role-Distance: The Sacred and the Profane

The necessities of his work are, however, made more difficult by another aspect of the relationship between the funeral director and his audience which has been pointed out repeatedly by various studies: the amount of social distance that exists both between him and his clients and between the object of his work (death), and the public he undertakes to perform before. He deals with objects which are both sacred and profane—simultaneously loved and loathed. As a result, the funeral director often attempts to separate the body work from the directive work, thereby putting distance between himself and his traditionally assigned role. Sometimes this is accomplished when he dresses differently for embalming and for directing; at other times role-distance is accomplished by simply hiring separate functionaries to do the body work so that he can concentrate on staging the show without being seen as someone who has been contaminated by contact

3. Robert Habenstein (1955, 1963) has extensively researched funeral customs the world over and has documented a sociological and historical account of the American undertaker, mortician, or funeral director. He describes and analyzes funerals in different regions of the United States, funeral practices of various ethnic groups, and the organizational and business aspects of the profession.

In his work, Habenstein (1955) suggests that the funeral is comparable in many ways to a performance on stage. This research extends and exploits Habenstein's suggestion of a theatrical or dramaturgical metaphor to understand the ritualized behavior of the American funeral by viewing both the front and backstage preparations and performances.

with the dead. What is separated here by the funeral director is not so much himself from his role, but rather himself from a loathesomeness ordinarily attributed to certain aspects of that role by his audience.[4]

As in other occupations (the medical profession being the most salient example), some emotional detachment from the objects one is manipulating is desirable. Funeral directors and their staff, therefore, tend to separate their own personal identity from the task of embalming bodies. The language and nonverbal conduct in the preparation room, then, demonstrate a type of role-distance which effectively communicates detachment, and sometimes even disdainful alienation from the role one is performing.

Backstage Regions: Preparation and Rehearsal

A successful funeral is a sequence of activities performed by the funeral director and his staff that are later seen by the bereaved as a respectful, appropriate tribute to the life and memory of the deceased. It requires an extensive series of preparations backstage, or behind the scene, that will later be used for the performance. A backregion or backstage is simply the space and the enclosed activities strategically hidden from the audience. It is ordinarily a place, but it may also be constituted simply by the shielding and masking of information in an interpersonal situation so that the audience does not realize certain things which would conflict with the performance as staged. A backstage region, whether a place or an interpersonal strategy, is "bounded to some degree by barriers to perception" (Goffman, 1959:106).

The necessity of backregions is due, obviously, to the fact that preparations for performances, if seen, may contradict, alter, qualify, or destroy the impressions fostered frontstage. Because people seem to have a limited capacity for seeing ritual as ritual, and since funerals, like any other drama, are prepared for, the viewing of the preparations may undercut the impressions fostered frontstage. Similarly, those who have worked in the backregions of a restaurant, in the kitchen or afterhours, and have participated in the preparation of food, the classification of customers by the staff, and so forth, may have difficulty seeing the frontstage performances in the same manner again.

Backstage, equipment and props used to produce the performance are stored, the behavior within the area is considered "private," and the scene is protected from public observation by various territorial imperatives socially constructed and enforced: doors, curtains, locks, and "employees only" signs.

The Backstage Setting

What we have said about backstage regions is generally applicable with few qualifications to the dramas of the American funeral. The preparation room, referred to by some morticians as a "medical laboratory," is spatial-

4. Although Goffman in his initial discussion of role distance (1961–b) illustrates the use of the term through examples of frontstage behavior employed to communicate detachment, a comprehensive reading of Goffman's work shows that role-distance can have reference to management of impressions or self whether it be a front or backstage performance. What is backstage to one audience may be frontstage to another. In the case of the embalmer, his use of impersonal language about bodies and treating a corpse as a body rather than a person reveals detachment from the role he is performing or from the loathsomeness ordinarily attributed to certain aspects of the role of embalmer by his audience. Even in the embalming room, the embalmer is onstage whether the audience be the other assistants or he be his own audience, the objective "me" in Mead's (1934) use of the idea.

The social and physical boundaries that separate the preparation room . . . are essential to the ceremonial performances that will be given later.

ly segregated from the funeral chapel, visitation rooms, viewing rooms, offices, and other regions the public frequents. It may be noted that the awesome and sacrosanct qualities of such places may be heightened by successfully identifying them with medicine, a line of endeavor which seems to establish particularly esoteric meanings for the bulk of Americans.

The social and physical boundaries that separate the preparation room from other parts of the home are essential to the ceremonial performances that will be given later. Here the corpse is washed, shaved, sprayed with disinfectant, sliced, pierced, creamed, powdered, waxed, stitched, painted, manicured, dressed, and positioned in a casket. Embalming involves the draining of blood *via* the major arteries while simultaneously refilling them through an injection point in the neck or armpit with fluid. Through the use of other chemicals, the flesh is softened, stretched, shrunk, restored, colored, and even replaced.

Obviously, these procedures would be likely to shock "nonprofessionals" such as the friends and family of the deceased (Goffman, 1959:106). But more than that, such viewing would tend to present the audience with an impression that would contradict that being fostered frontstage. As Goffman notes, "If the bereaved are to be given the impression that the loved one is really in a deep and tranquil sleep, they will have to be kept away from the area where the corpse is drained, stuffed, and painted for its final performance."[5] In the presence of family and friends, the casketed body is never touched by mortuary personnel; they honor a distance of two to three feet from the body. However, the preparation room *is* characterized by handling of the body (a naked body in some procedures) in ways that would appear disrespectful and even inhuman, even if one were unaware of the identity of the deceased. One might respond to all of these by asking just how it is possible to talk about inhumanity when the object is a corpse, and yet it is precisely this "human identity" conception of the enterprise that supports the funeral profession and, indeed, becomes the basic polarity between which the mortician must balance his act. At any rate, the embalming, restoration, and other preparatory procedures requiring manual labor might appear to the layman as morbidly intimate, repulsive, and a violation of dignity, even to the dead. Virtually all the amenities persons accord to each other in everyday life are violated by the attendants who prepare a corpse for the service.

In order to maintain the historically hard-won image as a legitimate professional and counselor rather than an "undertaker," with all of its attendant morbid stereotypes, a funeral director must seclude the backstage by utilizing rhetoric less suggestive of what transpires behind closed doors. Here we come to the interpersonal shielding we discussed earlier, which is at least as important as the barriers formed by physical space. It should be noted that backstage regions are protected not only by the funeral director, but also by others; most people, except some curious sociologists of everyday life, voluntarily avoid areas where they are uninvited. They exercise the

5. The most difficult part of this research, predictably, was gaining access to the backstage regions of mortuaries. Funeral directors, like other performers, are very protective of their back regions and are reluctant to permit anyone to observe the procedures carried out there.

sort of tact regarding settings that constitutes "discretion" (Goffman, 1959:229). In this sense, the audience actively, rather than passively, participates in the distinctions we have drawn. They seem to recognize that part of the meaning of any performance will be diluted with disenchantment if one knows too much.

Even though the specifics of the preparation room are a mystery, most people know enough to choose acceptable ignorance and avoid trespassing into the region. Once again, the audience is a party to the stage production, avoiding asking questions about embalming procedures, and generally managing their behavior in such a way as to suggest they know nothing of such preparations, and want to keep it that way.

There exists quite clearly in the funeral business a backstage language and another entirely for . . . the performance that . . . is being staged.

The Rhetoric of Backstage Regions

Both the technical and the informal nomenclatures which mark the universe of discourse of backstage regions serve a number of functions, but they are sufficiently different from the language characterizing the frontstage production itself that they must be segregated from clients who seek funeral services. There exists quite clearly in the funeral business a backstage language and another entirely for those occasions in which the performance that has been so laboriously prepared is being staged. A superb example of frontstage rhetoric is a sign on the door of the embalming room at one of the establishments we studied:

> REMEMBER
> This preparation room becomes sacred when a family entrusts us with one of its most precious possessions. Keep faith with *them* by conducting *yourself* as though the family were present. The body is dear to them . . . Treat it reverently.

Backstage, however, morticians develop a very different set of behaviors toward their activities. Rather than being a person, the body becomes an object upon which one performs restorative art. And while the deceased is a dearly beloved, Mr. Doe, a father, loved one, etc. during frontstage encounters with the bereaved family, backstage references are to various types of bodies, such as "floaters" (one who has drowned and was not recovered until the body floated to the surface), "Mr. Crispy" (one who burned to death in an airplane crash), a "fresh" or "warm" one (a body received shortly after death), a "cold" one (a frozen body). References to restorative art in the information materials given the public may in fact be referred to in the preparation room as "pickling" or "curing a ham." The use of "bod" instead of "body," especially with younger female corpses, is not uncommon. Joking, singing, the discussion of political issues, and (infrequently) open sexual remarks, racial slurs, complaints about the size of some bodies, profanity, and other rhetoric inconsistent with the frontstage regions are employed as ways of distancing the embalmer from the role he is performing.

Similarly, frontstage references to the burial containers such as casket, gift to the deceased, home, place of rest, and so on, are referred to backstage as coffins, stuffing boxes, tin cans, containers, stove pipes (a cheap metal over wood casket), or brand names given to caskets by manufacturers.

Such role-distance behavior may manifest alienation from the role "but the opposite can well be true: in some cases only those who feel secure in their attachment may be able to chance the expression of distance" (Goffman, 1959:128). Expression of distance may serve also to relax those attending the task and/or convey an atmosphere of "just another job" in what otherwise would be a situation permeated by anxiety and tension. As in other occupations, role-distance behavior can be noted in the many instances where the actor does "two things at once," singing, joking, and using the aforementioned backstage rhetoric while preparing the body.

The preparation room is a scene constructed in such a way as to establish the impression of a sterile medical atmosphere. Even though the backstage crew may humorously refer to themselves as a "bod squad," they more often refer to themselves and their behavior in medical rhetoric, thereby borrowing credence and legitimacy from that professional most esteemed in American society, the medical doctor. The medical atmosphere and terminology is also a part of on-going role-distance; the white surgical garb, the white walls, and the operating table help the practitioner to see and present himself as at least a quasi-medical professional rather than simply a handler of corpses.

Just as theaters have their make-up rooms, the preparation room serves as a setting for the cosmetology that will turn the corpse into the star of the show. As make-up artists, morticians are unsurpassed, and have elevated their skill to a high art. Given the various causes of death and subsequent kinds of bodily disfigurement, "restorative art" is designed to make the deceased look natural and, in a sense, "alive." Cosmetics in the hands of a skilled mortician can cover a multitude of wounds, bruises, ravages of long-term disease and discoloration, and even major forms of disfigurement. (One funeral director told us with pride of a suicide he had reconstructed, even though the man had succeeded in blowing the top of his head off.) When successful, an unblemished star is born for a magnificent final performance.

As with other performers, the actor is not supposed to appear "made up," but rather the make-up is applied to convey "natural" impressions. (One is reminded of the cosmetic company that advertises that women can achieve the "natural look" only by using their new line of cosmetics.) Funeral directors take as a compliment remarks that the deceased looked natural, at peace, younger than before, asleep, etc., apparently because his art is being validated by the very audience at which it is directed. What

. . . the white surgical garb, the white walls, and the operating table help the practitioner to see and present himself as at least a quasi-medical professional.

. . .

might be seen as "art for art's sake" is justified by funeral directors as a vital element in what has come to be known as "grief therapy," a vocabulary of motives (Mills, 1940) which most practitioners in the industry now espouse. Such a set of rationales holds that the viewing of the body by the bereaved is a necessary step in the acceptance of death. It is of interest to note that an economic vocabulary of motives might also apply (open casket funerals usually generate a larger expenditure of money because the interior designations of the casket become significant to the buyer), although it is, of course, never mentioned to the audience. Instead of such economic motives, the following rationale from a handbook on successful funeral practice is presented:

> Perhaps the most important function of the art of viewing the remains is the confrontation of the emotional fact that one is so anxious to deny. Seeing the dead body seems to break through the defenses more effectively and more completely than any other part of the funeral process [Raether, 1971:140].

The change of titles from "undertaker" to "funeral director" has been perhaps the largest single clue to the dramaturgical functions the industry now sees itself as performing.

Frontstage Performances: Bringing off the Show

The change of titles from "undertaker" to "funeral director" has been perhaps the largest single clue to the dramaturgical functions the industry now sees itself as performing. He is indeed a "director," controlling a dramatic production. The staged performance is supported by elaborate backstage preparations of the body, equipment, and props, and the immediate family is rehearsed as to the schedule of events and protocol. In order to preclude any miscues in the performance, the rehearsal covers entrance cues, exit, places to sit, and timing of events; special requests by the family can also be included in the script and program.

The funeral director and his crew continue backstage activities during the funeral service: automobile drivers, pallbearers, ministers, and musicians must all be orchestrated in a smooth and uninterrupted performance. As a skilled director, the mortician is available but largely unnoticed, particularly by the audience of friends and acquaintances who come to pay their respects. He is often acutely sensitive to matters of "promptness, overall courtesy, ushering, and other tasks involving a sizeable number of people" (Raether, 1971:121). His demeanor, of course, establishes a model of appropriate behavior in a funeral setting:

> The funeral director should not strut, nor should he appear to be mousey. His demeanor should show dignity, concern, and confidence . . . [he] should not talk loud, nor should he whisper secretly. He should speak in a subdued voice . . . should not walk around unnecessarily . . . should not snap his fingers or hiss to get attention [Raether, 1971:121].

In addition, he constantly checks the floral pieces for placement, fallen petals, water leakage, and all such tidying is made prior to the family's arrival.

Controlling the Situation: The Cast of Characters

The funeral as a staged performance features a marquee listing a well respected director affiliated with National Funeral Directors Association; a star, the deceased, whose life and attributes comprise the plot; a supporting cast of the bereaved (one of whom usually takes charge of managing details); supporters of the bereaved; ministers; musicians; and pallbearers; and, of course, the audience of friends and acquaintances. The bereaved are themselves supporting actors and actresses, for they too are part of the performance. They are "on-stage" in that their behavior is reviewed and judged by others whose comments on how well the family "held up" at the funeral will later be taken into account. Observations of funerals and especially post-funeral gatherings show that such evaluations comprise much of the conversation, and the bereaved who shows too little emotion for the audience's conception of their relationship to the deceased, or those who show too much when it is known that the relationship did not warrant it are likely to be judged negatively. Mourners are aware of this, and may construct their performances accordingly. Sometimes, in fact, part of the directing task is coaching mourners on how to act.

Cast members must also be controlled: one of the most potentially troublesome of these is the minister. As such, he may, if not carefully managed, act in such a way as to construct a counterreality[6] which can cast doubt on the entire show. Historically, the undertaker was a minor functionary whose role was under the direct supervision of the minister (Vernon, 1970:246–247, Habenstein, 1955). However, with the emergence of the professional "funeral director," the minister has been increasingly shunted to the background, and now it may be properly said that *he* is the minor functionary. The counterreality that the minister may establish is the idea that all of this funeral business is really nonsense because the body is a shell and the "soul" has departed. In addition, he may feel that there is too much emphasis on rituals involving the body, and that these smack of paganism and status-seeking, as well as being a waste of money. The minister may have long years of close association with the family, and if allowed to operate unmanaged, can be a significantly moderating influence on the family's choice. Consequently, trade journals devote occasional space to giving helpful advice on how to control this potentially truculent member of the cast. *Mortuary Management,* for example, suggests the following when a minister comes with the family to make arrangements:

> We tell the family to go ahead and look over the caskets in the display room, and that the minister . . . will join them later. We tell the minister that we have something we would like to talk to him about privately, and

6. We are indebted to Joan Emerson (1970) for the notion of counter-realities.

we've found that if we have some questions to ask him, he seems to be flattered that his advice is being sought, and we can keep him in the private office until the family has actually made its selection (Vernon, 1970:265).

The Funeral Home as Theater and Stage

Seldom are funeral homes space-age in architectural design; rather they present themselves with traditional white columns, Colonial style, or even proudly as older structures. They are usually decorated profusely with flowers, the walkways are carefully landscaped, the grass must be sprayed green during the winter months and of course the interiors are meticulously decorated. Such appearances are ways of establishing other meanings besides the usual ones of death and morbidity. Brightly colored drapes, curtains, and fixtures seem to breathe life; black hues are out, for they conspicuously betray the image of "undertaker." Even the traditional black limousine is no longer fashionable among more modern funeral homes; colors such as grey, white, and blue are now seen as more appropriate to death-free imagery.

Even the traditional black limousine is no longer fashionable among more modern funeral homes; colors such as grey, white, and blue are now seen as more appropriate to death-free imagery.

The stage itself, the funeral chapel, is a model of theatrical perfection; many chapels would make a Broadway star envious. The chapel is usually arranged with ample entrances and exits, and may be served by back doors, halls, tunnels, and passageways that lead from the preparation room without ever trespassing frontstage areas. Equipment and props such as flower holders, religious symbols and decorative roping are used to set the stage for the performance. In addition, the basic stage area is often neutral so that appropriate props can be used to establish the correct symbols for the various religious types of funerals common in our society.

If all of this background is successfully arranged, the funeral director—like other persons responsible for the direction of performances in our society—is in a position to control the kind of definitions that arise in the situation. Having had little opportunity to rehearse for such rituals, the majority of mourners face a highly problematic, tense, and relatively undefined situation. Consequently, monitoring the director's cues become a way of apprehending what the situation calls for.

Despite the best of scheduling, however, the inevitable "mistakes at work" occur.[7] But while every funeral director can unreel a series of atrocity stories about things that go wrong, ordinarily his recovery techniques are successful in salvaging the show. Caskets are rarely dropped, leak, or have their contents spilled onto the floor, especially since the troublesome role of "pallbearer" has been successfully turned into an honorary position, with the actual carrying of the casket done by members of the staff. Expected contingencies such as "excessive" displays of grief are managed smoothly with cues being given to the clergyman who may then minister to the person (Raether, 1971:21).

7. Everett C. Hughes has shown how "mistakes at work" are an inevitable, and therefore routinized, part of any world of work.

Establishing the Mood

> ... the metaphors used in the American funeral continue to be those of sleep, transition to other worlds, and eternal life, rather than death.

A crucial, and therefore precarious, feature of virtually all human affairs is mood. And it is important to remember that actions establish mood. The putting on of certain conduct will lead the reviewer to feel this way or that; and, as we have already shown, the review of the funeral director's show is in many ways the most tangible product he sells.

Probably the single most effective way of establishing the right mood for a funeral is the judicious use of music. Emanating usually from a veiled location, "appropriate" organ music (as opposed to "inappropriate" music such as amplified guitar) is the vital medium through which the atmosphere of the funeral is created. In counsel with the family, the musical selections are planned to set the mood for serenity, beauty, respect, or whatever values are desired. Many mortuaries offer lists of musicians upon which the family can call, and who will perform for a fee; other establishments have their own musicians available for hire. As in other shows, the selection, volume, tone, and timing of the music provide cues for the series of events or acts that are presented. With the aid of a printed program, music cues the audience in sequence: be respectfully quiet; the service is beginning; the choir is about to sing; a prayer is forthcoming; a minister is about to speak; the eulogy is being delivered; it is time for the processional view of the deceased; the service is over—you may leave. Mood management, then, is a major means by which the director controls the situation.

Frontstage Rhetoric and the Denial of Death

Although one of the consensually stated objectives of funerals is the acceptance of death by the family, the rhetoric of the frontstage as well as the social and physical setting of the funeral service itself tends to contradict such claims. Despite the many criticisms and subsequent industry denials and changes in procedure, the metaphors used in the American funeral continue to be those of sleep, transition to other worlds, and eternal life, rather than death. Much of this denial, of course, stems from religious traditions which tend to treat death as a kind of minor nuisance on the way to glory.[8] And there is little in the funeral to contradict such ideas. "Mr. Jones" reposes in a "Slumber room" in a casket whose mattress rivals the posturepedics designed for those of us still alive but suffering from back trouble. The titles and words of songs frequently sung at a funeral ("Death is only a Dream," "Asleep in Jesus," "It is not Death to Die") pointedly do not say "death has occurred, I am sorry" but rather "he or she is still with us."

In addition to this socially established denial of death, funerals serve as morality plays which weave social commentary into the ritual. Eulogies to the deceased will ordinarily contain references to his community service, character, righteousness, and approved identities. Certain behaviors are validated as noble, while others are by implication denounced. The au-

8. This point as well as a number of related ones are discussed skillfully in Ernest Becker, *The Denial of Death* (1974).

dience is thereby advised to take note, for they too will someday be reviewed in such a public ceremony. One comforting aspect of such eulogizing, however, is that the deceased is usually given the benefit of the doubt; the eulogizer selectively parades his various careers. The dramaturgical necessity of such selectivity, of course, makes for considerable juggling of the available facts of a person's life, especially when dealing with those whose lives have been less than sterling. When mentioned at all, such elements will almost always be placed in contexts that were not used while he was alive: recalcitrance being redefined as "independence," or purposelessness as a "restless spirit," for example. Such rhetoric underscores Burke's (1937) contention that all dramas are essentially morality plays with the themes of deviance and respectability playing large parts.

. . . the dramaturgical metaphor offers an interpretive framework that serves to illuminate what is often obscured. . . .

Conclusion

The dramaturgical metaphor we have employed in this paper offers an alternative way of viewing the interactions and relationships comprising the American funeral. Death and dying obviously involve ritual and ceremony; without these, much of what we take for granted among the living such as respect, character, and substance would likely vanish. "Ritual is then theatre: an assured way of communicating significations . . . funerals are dramas of death and living with death—they involve transformation of identity for the living and the dead (Perinbanayagam, 1974:538). Nevertheless, because social relationships involve ritual communication, much of it of a covert nature, care must be taken that performances be given "in character." For the more the audience wishes to see deeper than the appearances of a given situation, the more they wind up concentrating on those very appearances (Goffman, 1959:249).

We also wish to enter a *caveat* regarding our use of a metaphorical argument. To say that funerals may be seen as performances does not suggest that they *are* performances. Rather, the dramaturgical metaphor offers an interpretive framework that serves to illuminate what is often obscured by those perspectives that center on either the structural apparatus of the society in which death occurs or on the alleged psychological characteristics and states of the participants. Dramas can, of course, be viewed as expressions of either psychological or social determinants, but what we have suggested here is that there may be value in viewing them as fundamental realities in their own right. For no matter how standard the ritual expression becomes, each drama must still be brought off on its own with all the attendant opportunities for error. It is this possibility that makes our dramas at once precarious and satisfying.

References

Becker, Ernest. 1974. *The denial of death*. New York: The Free Press.
Becker, Howard. 1963. *The outsiders*. New York: Free Press.
Bowman, Leroy. 1959. *The American funeral*. Westport, Connecticut: Greenwood Press.

Brissett, Dennis. 1968. "The sense of a rubric." *American Journal of Sociology* 74 (July):70–78.

Brissett, Dennis, and Charles Edgley. 1975. *Life as theatre: A dramaturgical sourcebook.* Chicago: Aldine Publishing.

Burke, Kenneth. 1937. *Permanence and change: An anatomy of purpose.* Indianapolis: Bobbs-Merrill.

———. 1945. *A grammar of motives.* Englewood Cliffs: Prentice-Hall.

———. 1950. *A rhetoric of motives.* Englewood Cliffs: Prentice-Hall.

———. 1968. *Language as symbolic action.* Berkeley: University of California Press.

Burns, Elizabeth. 1972. *Theatricality: A study of convention in the theatre and social life.* New York: Harper Torchbooks.

Duncan, Hugh. 1962. *Communication and social order.* New York: Oxford University Press.

Emerson, Joan. 1970. "Behavior in private places: sustaining definitions of reality in gynecological examinations." Pp. 74–97 in Hans Dreitzel (ed.), *Recent Sociology 2.* New York: Macmillan.

Goffman, Erving. 1959. *The presentation of self in everyday life.* Garden City: Doubleday.

———. 1961a. *Asylums.* Garden City: Doubleday.

———. 1961b. *Encounters.* Indianapolis: Bobbs-Merrill.

———. 1963. *Behavior in public places.* New York: Free Press.

———. 1967. *Interaction ritual.* Garden City: Doubleday.

———. 1970. *Relations in public.* New York: Basic Books.

Habenstein, Robert W. and William Lamers. 1955. *The history of American funeral directing.* Milwaukee: Bulfin Printers, Inc.

———. 1963. *Funeral customs the world over.* Milwaukee: Bulfin Printers, Inc. Kuhn, Manford.

———. 1964. "Major trends in symbolic interaction theory in the past twenty years." *Sociological Quarterly* 5 (Winter):61–84.

Matza, David. 1969. *Becoming deviant.* Englewood Cliffs: Prentice-Hall.

Mead, G.H. 1934. *Mind, self and society.* Chicago: University of Chicago Press.

Messinger, Sheldon, et al. 1962. "Life as theatre: some notes on the dramaturgical approach to social reality." *Sociometry* 25 (September):98–110.

Mills, C. Wright. 1940. "Situated actions and vocabularies of motives." *American Sociological Review* (December):904–913.

Perinbanayagam, R.S. 1974. "The definition of the situation: an analysis of the ethnomethodological and dramaturgical view." *Sociological Quarterly* 15 (Autumn):521–541.

Raether, Howard C. 1971. *Successful funeral service practice.* Englewood Cliffs: Prentice-Hall.

Turner, Ronny E., and Charles Edgley. 1975. "Masks and social relations: an essay on the sources and assumptions of dramaturgical social psychology." *Humboldt Journal of Social Relations* 3, No. 1 (Fall/Winter):4–12.

Vernon, Glenn. 1970. *Sociology of death.* New York: Ronald Press.

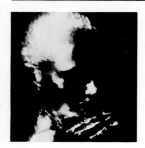

15

Research

Take a moment to recall an old friendship or love you once experienced. What aspects of this relationship do you remember? Primarily the positive moments shared by the two of you? Do you find yourself even exaggerating the good qualities of this person? Helena Znaniecki Lopata explores this tendency to create halos in the following chapter. Two Appendix exercises may help you understand this chapter when you are finished reading it:

        C.   Awareness of Grief Process

        D.   Awareness of Losses

Widowhood and Husband Sanctification

Helena Znaniecki Lopata

Bereaved wives in American society have often been observed to idealize their deceased husbands, even to the point of sanctification. A number of cultural rituals seem to encourage this tendency to purify the deceased in the memory of the survivors. These rituals include the wake, the funeral eulogy, and the shiva (see Berardo 1967, 1968; Marris 1958; Vernon 1970; Turnstall 1966). Sanctification of the late husband may increase the status of the widow at a time when her morale needs boosting. If such an ideal man had married and lived with her, then she must not be as bad a person as her depression makes her feel.

Life prior to the late husband's fatal illness or accident is apt to have been relatively satisfactory for most such couples. At least, the wife was probably adjusted to whatever unhappiness did exist in the relationship. Children are probably grown and established in their own lives, and conflicts over them were not apt to have been frequent at the time of the husband's death. Financial strains, so characteristic of early marriage and parenthood, were probably not pressing most couples.

The death of the husband is apt to introduce several sources of deprivation. Income often drops, loneliness is experienced, housing and relational adjustments must be made. With all these concerns, it would not be surprising for a widow to evaluate her life with her late husband as superior to her current situation. She may even exaggerate this evaluation.

Husband sanctification can perform several functions. Besides making the widow feel important, sanctification may help promote successful grief work. Eric Lindemann (1944) and succeeding psychiatrists have stressed how important it is for the bereaved to work through the grief process. "A widow is faced with two concurrent tasks; she is required, through the processes of mourning, to detach herself sufficiently from the lost object to

Sanctification . . . assists tie-breaking processes and allows the widow to go about her daily living.

permit the continuation of other relationships and the development of new ones; at the same time, she has to establish for herself a new role conception as an adult woman without a partner'' (Maddison and Walker 1967). The grief process often begins with hallucinatory experiences involving the deceased. Widows may even report holding conversations with their husbands at times of decision-making (Marris 1958). Sanctification forces the recognition of death and the reconstruction of the husband in memory as no longer mortal in spirit. Sanctification thus assists tie-breaking processes and allows the widow to go about her daily living. Sanctification moves the late husband into an other-worldly position as an understanding yet purified and distant observer. The widow may then reconstruct old relations or even form new relations and new life-styles.

This tendency to idealize the late husband even to the point of sanctification had been observed during previous investigations by the author (Lopata 1973, 1975a, 1975b). In one study the initial plan had been to gain information regarding the economic, service, social, and emotional support systems of widows in the year prior to the husband's fatal illness. The idealization by many of the widows, however, kept interfering with the picture, and it became apparent that the comments reflected life not as it had been but as it had become reconstructed in the memory of the widow. It became apparent that a study of the phenomenon of husband sanctification itself was needed.

This paper therefore addresses the following questions: Can it be demonstrated that many American urban widows tend to idealize their late husbands to the point of sanctification? What factors influence the degree to which a widow sanctified her late husband? A total of 1,169 widows in the Chicago area—representing when weighted by sample ratios 82,084 women—completed a "sanctification scale" section of a self-administered questionnaire that had two parts. Part 1, a "semantic differential" evalua-

Table 1 Semantic differential evaluation of late husband by Chicago-area widows: Part 1 of sanctification scale

Characteristic (Positive Extreme)	Evaluation of Husband*							Characteristic (Negative Extreme)	Number of Respondents (100%)
	1 %	2 %	3 %	4 %	5 %	6 %	7 %		
Good	76	8	6	5	2	1	2	Bad	79,959
Useful	72	8	9	5	2	2	1	Useless	79,912
Honest	82	6	4	4	2	1	1	Dishonest	80,259
Superior	55	14	13	13	2	2	2	Inferior	78,375
Kind	79	7	5	4	2	2	2	Cruel	79,728
Friendly	79	7	5	5	1	2	2	Unfriendly	80,301
Warm	77	7	6	7	1	1	2	Cold	79,813
Total	74	8	7	6	2	2	2		

*Rows do not all add up to 100 percent due to rounding.

tion, had opposite pairs of qualities to be attributed to the deceased along a seven-point scale: good-bad, useful-useless, honest-dishonest, superior-inferior, kind-cruel, friendly-unfriendly, and warm-cold. Part 2, an evaluation of "life together," consisted of seven statements which each called for a response at one of four levels: "strongly agree," "agree," "disagree," "strongly disagree." The statements were: "My husband was an unusually good man"; "My marriage was above average"; "My husband and I were always together except for working hours"; "My husband and I felt the same way about almost everything"; "My husband was a very good father to our children"; "Our home was an unusually happy one"; and "My husband had no irritating habits."

Table 1 shows that many widows do indeed sanctify their late husbands.

About three-fourths or more of Chicago-area widowed beneficiaries of social security defined their late husbands as having been extremely good, useful, honest, kind, friendly, and warm. "Life together" with the late husband was not idealized as much as was the person (see Table 2). The "life together" segment refers to the family relationship and may contain a current reality component. It may therefore be more difficult to sanctify.

The statement "My husband had no irritating habits" was the most extreme item on the questionnaire and drew disagreement from 44 percent of the widows, 8 percent of whom disagreed strongly. Even here, however, over one-fourth of the widows strongly agreed with the statement. All but five percent of the respondents judged the deceased as having been a very good father, and almost as many judged him as having been an unusually good man.

An analysis of item responses revealed that women who defined their late husbands as superior were not as likely to rank him as friendly, warm, or even useful. Husband's warmth appeared to be related to kindness and

> . . . women who defined their late husbands as superior were not as likely to rank him as friendly, warm, or even useful.

Table 2 Evaluation of life together by Chicago-area widows: Part 2 of sanctification scale

	Level of Agreement				
	Strongly Agree (%)	Agree (%)	Disagree (%)	Strongly Disagree (%)	Number of Respondents (100%)
Husband an unusually good man	64	25	9	2	80,384
Marriage above average	45	37	15	3	80,173
Husband and I always together	50	27	18	5	80,084
Husband and I felt same way about almost everything	35	36	24	5	80,110
Very good father	69	26	3	2	73,704
Ours was unusually happy home	54	30	11	5	79,524
Husband had no irritating habits	28	28	36	8	79,571

friendliness, and honesty, goodness, and kindness were apt to be closely related to each other in the way a widow remembered her late husband.

Results also revealed that a widow who defined her late husband as unusually good also rated the marriage as above average. Being evaluated as a good father, on the other hand, did not necessarily relate to being remembered as a companion in all nonwork activity, to being a sharer of all feelings, or to being absolved of all irritating habits. One gets the picture that the man defined as having been a good father above all had a sex-segregated traditional marriage with his wife and was more apt to irritate her than was the man remembered as having shared an above-average marriage.

The second question addressed in this study concerned the factors which influence the degree to which a widow sanctifies her late husband. Length of widowhood was expected to be an important variable but it proved insignificant in this study; all of our respondents had been widowed over a year. Other variables that proved insignificant influences on husband

Table 3 Gamma associations, percent of first place ranks, strongly-agree judgments, and mean ranks of items on the sanctification scale, by years of schooling, Chicago-area widows*

Scale Items	Gamma	% of Respondents Rating Positive Extreme	Mean Rating
Semantic Differential			**(Range 1–7)**
Good-Bad	.27	76	1.62
Useful-Useless	.18	72	1.68
Honest-Dishonest	.20	82	1.47
Superior-Inferior	.20	55	2.07
Kind-Cruel	.22	79	1.56
Friendly-Unfriendly	.13	79	1.53
Warm-Cold	.22	77	1.61
Life Together			**(Range 1–4)**
Husband unusually good	.30	64	1.48
Marriage above average	.23	45	1.76
Did things together	.06	50	1.80
Felt same way	.02	35	1.98
Good father	.11	69	1.38
Home happy	.11	54	1.67
No irritating habits	.02	28	2.25

*Total N varies somewhat by item: For example, "Good-Bad"

sanctification included current income, number of living children, number of friends, and expressed feelings of loneliness or life satisfaction.

The four variables measured that had the main influence on husband sanctification were age, education, income prior to the husband's fatal illness or accident, and race. These factors also appear to be mutually interdependent. The strongest association was between sanctification and race. For the purpose of this short paper, only the effects of education and race upon husband sanctification will be discussed.

Table 3 contains three sets of data: (1) the gamma association between each item on the questionnaire and years of schooling; (2) the percentage of women in each schooling category who circled the positive extreme for each item on the questionnaire; and (3) the mean ratings for each item for all respondents and for each schooling category.

Both the percentages and the means show significant differences between the least-educated and the rest of the women. The least-educated women were particularly unlikely to rank their husbands as superior,

The four variables measured that had the main influence on husband sanctification were age, education, income prior to the husband's fatal illness or accident, and race.

Years of Schooling											
Less Than 8		8		9–11		12		13–15		16 and over	
%	Mean	%	Mean	%	Mean	%	Mean	%	Mean	%	Mean
58	2.32	77	1.63	78	1.55	81	1.35	80	1.32	78	1.30
56	2.43	80	1.49	73	1.63	76	1.46	74	1.46	72	1.41
71	1.78	84	1.43	80	1.54	84	1.35	86	1.34	92	1.15
39	2.70	56	2.01	56	2.09	58	1.84	61	1.82	68	1.63
64	2.07	80	1.57	82	1.53	83	1.33	80	1.36	84	1.31
66	1.88	85	1.53	84	1.44	80	1.44	78	1.45	81	1.34
60	2.13	79	1.52	77	1.63	82	1.41	80	1.40	80	1.40
42	1.90	63	1.52	69	1.40	74	1.30	67	1.39	73	1.30
31	2.08	36	1.81	48	1.71	57	1.61	47	1.68	54	1.53
38	2.13	58	1.67	54	1.74	55	1.68	34	1.89	43	1.86
29	2.22	44	1.78	34	2.02	40	1.87	26	2.14	32	2.11
54	1.56	78	1.33	69	1.40	75	1.28	69	1.35	60	1.46
36	2.05	60	1.50	64	1.60	59	1.59	49	1.71	45	1.64
20	2.48	34	2.13	34	2.13	29	2.18	28	2.32	18	2.56
14,395		15,342		15,465		21,023		6,640		4,123	

**White widows
. . . appear to
have a stronger
tendency to
sanctify their
deceased
husbands than do
nonwhite widows.**

useful, or good. However, they resembled the most-educated in refusing to agree that the late husband had no irritating habits. They were less apt than most categories to remember sharing activities with him, and they were least apt to remember having an above-average marriage. The least-educated category, like all the other categories of widows, gave their late husbands relatively high credit as a good father. But even here they were least likely to report the positive extreme.

The high-school finishers and college dropouts were very similar to each other both in percentages and in means except that the latter did not so often claim to have done things together with their late husbands or to have felt the same way. There is also a difference in defining their homes as happy and their late husbands as good fathers. The widows who had completed 16 or more years of schooling were least likely to rate their husbands as devoid of irritating habits. They were also below the average in agreeing strongly that their home had been a unusually happy one, that the husband had been a good father, and that the marriage had been above average.

In regard to the influence of race on degree of sanctification by widows, a distinction was made between "white" and "nonwhite"; the majority of respondents in the "nonwhite" category were black. Forty-nine percent of the whites but only 27 percent of the nonwhites scored at the positive extreme of the semantic differential scale while only 10 percent of the whites and 42 percent of the nonwhites scored at the negative extreme. White widows thus appear to have a stronger tendency to sanctify their deceased husbands than do nonwhite widows. The superior-inferior item was the one nonwhites were least likely to score at the positive extreme, and the item on which they differed most from the whites. The gaps between mean scores of the two groups are not so large for the life together as for the semantic differential scale.

There are interesting patterns to these differences between the two groups when we analyze some of the significant variables such as age and education while controlling for race. One expected finding was that the nonwhite widows were less likely to have achieved much schooling. Schooling, however, has much stronger effects on the nonwhites than on the whites. That is, the higher the level of schooling for a nonwhite widow, the more apt she was to sanctify her late husband (gamma = .26), while for whites the association was not so strong (gamma = .09). White widows with less than a ninth-grade education were less likely to sanctify their husbands than women with more education, but comparably educated nonwhite widows were even less apt to do so.

On the other hand, age was a more important influence for whites (gamma = .25) than for nonwhites (gamma = .10) in the semantic differential scale. Age had just the opposite effect on the life-together scale (gamma = .14 for whites, = .23 for nonwhites). The older white women, regardless of their educational level, tended to sanctify a late husband but not the relationship, while the more educated nonwhites tended to sanctify him regardless of their age. Age had less effect on the extent to which whites compared to nonwhites defined positively life together prior to the husband's fatal illness or accident.

Yet another variable which indicates a difference between whites and nonwhites is place of birth (gamma = .38 for nonwhites, .06 for whites). Eighty-eight percent of the nonwhite widows were born outside of Illinois, and these women tended not to be the sanctifying respondents, unless they are relatively educated.

In summary, Chicago-area widows tend to idealize their late husbands to the point of sanctification. Although less likely to idealize their life together prior to his fatal illness or accident, these women were apt to consider him to have been an unusually good father, husband, and man in general. Some went so far as to agree with the statement that he was free from any irritating habits. This is a statement that few wives of living husbands would probably make. Older widows, particularly if they were white, were more likely to idealize the late husband. Education influenced willingness of nonwhites more than of whites to idealize the husband. However, among both groups the least educated were the least idealizing. Some of the least educated even indicated hostility.

References

Berardo, Felix. 1967. Social adaptation to widowhood among a rural-urban aged population. Washington State University, College of Agriculture, Experiment Station *Bulletin* 689 (December).

———. 1968. Widowhood status in the United States: Perspective on a neglected aspect of the family life-cycle. *The Family Coordinator* 17 (July):191–203.

Lindemann, Eric. 1944. Symptomology and management of acute grief. *American Journal of Psychiatry* 101 (July):141–148.

Lopata, Helena Znaniecki. 1973. *Widowhood in an American city.* Cambridge, Mass.: Schenkman Publishing Company, General Learning Press.

———. 1975a. On widowhood: Grief work and identity reconstruction. *Journal of Geriatric Psychiatry,* 8, no. 1:41–55.

———. 1975b. Widowhood: Societal factors in life-span disruptions and alternatives. In *Life-span developmental psychology: Normative life crises.* New York: Academic Press, Inc.

Maddison, D. C., and W. L. Walker. 1967. Factors affecting the outcome of conjugal bereavement. *British Journal of Psychiatry* 113 (October):1057–1067.

Marris, Peter. 1958. *Widows and their families.* London: Routledge and Kegan Paul, Ltd.

Turnstall, Jeremy. 1966. *Old and alone.* London: Routledge and Kegan Paul, Ltd.

Vernon, Glenn M. 1970. *Sociology of death.* New York: The Ronald Press.

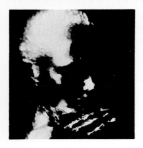

16

Research

The thought of a child dying in a hospital is a disturbing one. Add to this image the picture of a mother or father attempting to interact with their child during this period of time. How much social distance do both child and parent need as a result of the emotional burdens of their situation? If we wanted to understand more about such interactions, how would we go about studying this process? Elizabeth Susman et al. discuss a variety of methods for doing so, and strongly justify the use of systematic observation in such studies. The following Appendix exercises may be useful supplements to this chapter.

I. Life and Death Attitudes: Dyadic Encounter

M. Saying Good-bye to a Loved One

Interactions between Primary Caregivers and Children with Cancer: A Methodology for Systematic Observation in a Hospital Setting

E. J. Susman

A. R. Hollenbeck

E. D. Nannis

B. E. Strope

S. P. Hersh

A. S. Levine

P. A. Pizzo

The human experience includes a lot of acute or chronic illness resulting from disease or accident. To some degree, illness is part of the life of every child. Surprisingly, few investigations have been concerned with how loss of their physical well-being affects children's psychological development.

Studies of life-threatening illnesses have usually been focused on death and dying. Much of the early work in death and dying was based on clinical populations of geriatric patients. Recently research has focused on how the patient, family, staff, and physician cope with the threat of death. Research with children has dealt primarily with either their concepts of death (Koocher 1973) or studies of mourning and orphanhood (Freud and Dann 1970). In a pioneering attempt to quantify elements associated with the experience of dying, Spinetta, Rigler, and Karon (1974) used an interpersonal distance measure to assess feelings of isolation assumed to be present in a child with a fatal illness. The study was interpreted as demonstrating that a sense of isolation from parent and caregivers develops and grows stronger as the child nears death. In contrast to most studies emphasizing the development of thoughts and attitudes about death, the Spinetta, Rigler, and Karon investigation focused on the behavior and emotions associated with *living* with a potentially fatal illness.

Most research in this area assumes that people with a life-threatening illness orient themselves towards death and dying. This assumption may be legitimate for a geriatric population but of questionable validity in a study of children and adolescents. Two conceptual issues need to be addressed. The first is whether a point of view developed for a later stage of the life cycle is applicable for an earlier stage. The second is whether individuals with a life-threatening illness do, in fact, orient themselves toward death and dying.

What is the effect of hospital isolation on specific social behaviors?

The purpose of this chapter is to present a methodology for studying the behavior of children with a life-threatening illness in a cancer treatment setting. Development of such a methodology was in part stimulated by the need to understand whether or not the stereotype of the depressed and withdrawn geriatric patient was applicable to a younger sample. Observation was the methodology adopted to answer the following questions: (1) When illness is life-threatening, what is the nature of social interaction between the child patients and their parents and between the children and their caregivers in the hospital? (2) What is the effect of hospital isolation on specific social behaviors? The observational system used can easily be adapted to answer a variety of research questions in many contexts. (For a more basic presentation of observational methods, a number of recent publications are recommended: Brandt 1972; Cairns, in press; Sackett, in press, a and b.)

This chapter will focus on four issues: (1) the advantages of using observation in a clinical setting; (2) development and characteristics of the observational system; (3) the problem of observer agreement; and (4) exploratory and confirmatory approaches to data analysis.

The Case for Observational Studies

The behavior of individuals hospitalized with a life-threatening illness and the behaviors of his or her family members have not been systematically observed. Methods used in studies of illness have included interviews, rating scales, observations, self-reports, and projective techniques. These methods, however, are susceptible to biases from multiple sources. There are usually no systematic procedures for quantifying data derived from interviews or observations. Ratings by the patient and those close to the patient are subjectively biased by unobservable events. Projective techniques may tap intrapsychic factors within the ill individual, but the information they yield may not accurately represent external events. In contrast to the above techniques, systematic observation allows one to assess behavior directly. Consequently, investigator bias is minimized.

Human auditory and visual sense receptors as well as judgmental abilities are the measuring instruments in observational research (Sackett, in press, a). Such an instrument may be limited in the number of complex discriminations that it can make; however, it can capture complex behaviors in a way not obtained by any psychological instruments. Advantages of observational methodology have been outlined in detail elsewhere (Susman, Peters, and Stewart, 1976).

A strong mandate for use of observation in the study of social interaction has been established in behavioral research (Cairns, in press). A number of advantages have been noted: (a) Direct observation eliminates many biases associated with traditional psychometric instruments. (b) Observational methods have been used extensively to explore the effects of isolation on subhuman primates with the express purpose of finding implications for humans. It might be assumed, therefore, that observation is a useful direct way to study the effects of isolation on humans. (c) The same observational techniques can be applied over a wide range of subjects. Interview and psychometric instruments usually must be standardized on age-appropriate samples for valid data interpretation. Observational data, however, can yield natural frequencies, durations, and sequences of real observable behaviors as they occur in the natural setting. Since we know little about the behavior of individuals in an oncology setting, there was a need to develop a preliminary taxonomy of behavior in that setting. An observational methodology was most appropriate for this purpose.

. . . there was a need to develop a preliminary taxonomy of behavior. . . .

Sample

The sample consisted of children and adolescents with metastatic solid tumors and lymphomas who failed to respond to the usual therapeutic treatments. Because of severe bone marrow toxicity and a significantly increased risk of fatal infection associated with intensive therapy, the National Cancer Institute is studying the utility of "germ-free" isolation rooms to deliver such chemotherapy (Pizzo and Levine, 1977). Children in the study are housed in Laminar Air Flow isolation rooms (experimental group) or in a regular hospital room (control group). For the experimental group, physical contact with others is through plastic gloves, and anyone entering the isolation room is attired in sterile gown, mask, and gloves.

The children in the experimental group generally enter the isolation room one week prior to chemotherapy to rid their bodies of natural bacteria. Chemotherapy is then administered for approximately one week. This chemotherapy is nearly always accompanied by toxicity, especially nausea and vomiting. The remaining period of hospitalization may last four to eight weeks and may be complicated by fever, infection, and other side effects of chemotherapy.

The Observational System

Categories
An observational scheme with mutually exclusive categories was devised to record ongoing behavior of children, their families, and their caregivers. Observational categories were developed in a two-step process. First, narrations of ongoing child-parent and child-caregiver interactions were gathered by naïve observers. These narratives were transcribed and used to develop an extensive preliminary taxonomy of behaviors exhibited in the hospital setting. This first step was important for two reasons: (1) the frequency and range of behaviors was determined, and (2) observers who were unfamiliar with a medical setting were able to begin to cope with the realities

of a cancer ward. Secondly, categories of theoretical interest were added in order to answer specific research questions. For instance, the category *technical information* was added to allow assessment of when and where children are given information about their illness. Categories may all be placed under the four behavior dimensions presented in Table 1. The four dimensions are: *role, behavior, communication, and affect.*

Coding Behavior

Categories were arranged and scored on coding sheets. Categories were listed vertically and time horizontally on the coding sheets. Each observational unit is a 30-second interval. An observational session lasts for 15 minutes, or 30 intervals. Observational sessions were scheduled randomly throughout the day to include four weekday observations and one weeknight observation.

In every interval, behavior of the child and a "significant other" was scored. The "other" may be mother, father, nurse, doctor, or anyone else within the child's immediate environment. It is difficult for an observer to reliably record behaviors for two people simultaneously, and almost impossible to record more than two individuals. When such situations occur, the behavior of only one "significant other" is scored. The person scored is determined by the following hierarchy: father, mother, nurse, doctor, sibling, medical technician, or anyone else in the environment. For instance, if child, mother, and doctor are present, child is the focal person and mother becomes "other." However, interactions between a third person and the child or "other" are coded. For example, if the child is talking to the doctor and the mother is present, the mother is coded as "other" and the child is coded in terms of his or her interaction with the doctor. In brief, the observational system allows for coding sequences of child-other behavior.

For every 30-second interval only one dimension is scored. Further scoring within a dimension is done only in the event of a behavior change

Table 1   Child-other observational categories

Role	Behavior	Communication	Affect
nonsocial	play	no talk	none
initiate	sleep	general conversation	pleasant
reciprocate	vocal	dependency	happy
reciprocate-ignore	passive	technical information	anger
	physical	prosocial	crying
	protest	complain	response to pain
	medical procedure	humor	
		praise	
		nonverbal	
		illness-information	

during that interval—e.g., behavior changes from *physical* to *vocal.* A change in *role, affect,* or *communication* does not constitute grounds for additional coding in a particular time interval. In the event that a subject engages in more than one behavior at a time, behavior is scored according to a predetermined hierarchy. Because of the nature of our research questions, interactional behaviors—e.g., *vocal* and *medical procedure*—are given priority over noninteractive behaviors—e.g., *physical.*

For ill children, deteriorating physical condition is associated with a restricted behavioral repertoire.

Problems of Agreement

Validity of observational data is dependent upon observers collecting reliable data. Considerable theoretical and empirical literature on issues of reliability has appeared in the last decade (Hollenbeck, in press; Mash and McElwee 1974; Taplin and Reid 1975; Yarrow and Waxler, in press). Although reliability is usually discussed in relation to accuracy, stability, and observer agreement, only the problems with observer agreement will be discussed in this chapter.

Estimates of observer reliability are usually reported as "agreement statistics." Hollenbeck has devoted some attention to this area and has outlined advantages and disadvantages of seven observer agreement statistics. An agreement statistic should be chosen based on: (1) its statistical properties, (2) the observational system, and (3) the phenomenon being observed. The last criterion is particularly important in oncology settings. The frequency of observed behaviors can influence agreement among observers. For ill children, deteriorating physical condition is associated with a restricted behavioral repertoire. In our study, the frequency of *passive* or *sleep* behavior was high, and the likelihood of scoring changes in behavior was low. Because of the high probability of agreeing by chance that any one behavior occurred, estimates of observer agreement could be artificially inflated. Kappa is one agreement statistic that takes into account the probability of agreeing by chance. Kappa is defined as the proportion of agreement among observers after chance is removed (Cohen, 1960):

$$Kappa = \Sigma \frac{Po - Pc}{1 - Pc}.$$

Po = observed proportion of agreements

Pc = chance proportion of agreements [$Pc = \frac{K}{1} \Sigma(P_1 * P_2)$

where P_1 and P_2 are the category marginals for observer one and two.]

To illustrate the usefulness of correcting for chance agreement, data from three observer agreement checks are presented in table 2. Kappa is compared to percentage agreement, the most widely used agreement statistic. Table 2 shows the relation between kappa and percentage agreement for a 15-minute observer agreement trial on three different children. The proportions for kappa represent the ratio of kappa to maximum kappa (the maximal value kappa can attain given observed marginal distributions). This ratio represents the amount of agreement between observers after chance has been removed, thus reflecting a more precise measure of agreement. With the exception of the *communication* dimension for S_3, percentage agreement was consistently higher than the kappa ratio. For *affect,* mean percentage agreement was 76 percent. However, kappa for *affect* was virtually zero. This does not necessarily indicate a lack of agreement between observers. Rather, it reflects the fact that *affect* shows little variability and thus there is a high probability of agreement by chance.

Variability in an observational system may be increased by redefining categories to make them more sensitive to subtle changes in *affect* or by increasing the number or length of observational sessions. While these procedures may increase variability, they may also lead to greater disagreement among observers. Another alternative is to eliminate or combine categories with low variability before the data are analyzed. However, it may be important to report low variability behaviors. For example, with hospitalized children, absence of change in *affect* may be an indicator of depression. In summary, both statistical and clinical criteria must be used to evaluate the meaning of low variability behaviors.

Approaches to Exploratory and Confirmatory Data Analysis

Observational data may be analyzed at two levels to answer specific research questions: (1) descriptive and exploratory approaches may be used to identify relations among variables, and (2) the general linear and probability models may be used to confirm hypothesized relationships. To illustrate the use of these two levels of analysis, data from single subjects will be presented. These analyses are also adaptable to multiple subject designs.

Table 2   Ratio of kappa to maximum kappa (Max. K.) compared to percentage agreement (% Agree.) for three 15-minute sessions (S)

Dimension	S_1		S_2		S_3	
	Kappa Max. K.	to % Agree.	*Kappa* Max. K.	to % Agree.	*Kappa* Max. K.	to % Agree.
Role	.64	.85	.50	.62	.48	.63
Behavior	.58	.82	.84	.80	.40	.56
Communication	.63	.97	.75	.76	.28	.23
Affect	.24	.97	−.12	.80	−.13	.52

Descriptive and Exploratory Approaches

Plotting the frequency of behaviors is a useful first step in the analysis of longitudinal data. Such a graphic description provides useful information, but it may also be used to generate hypotheses regarding the nature of interaction. Figure 1 illustrates social and nonsocial interactions between a seventeen-year-old and her mother over an eighteen-day period prior to the child's death. Social interactions include those occurrences of mother's *initiate, reciprocate,* or *reciprocate-ignore* behaviors relative to the child's behavior. *"Nonsocial"* refers to mother being present but interacting with someone other than child or passively sitting by the bedside.

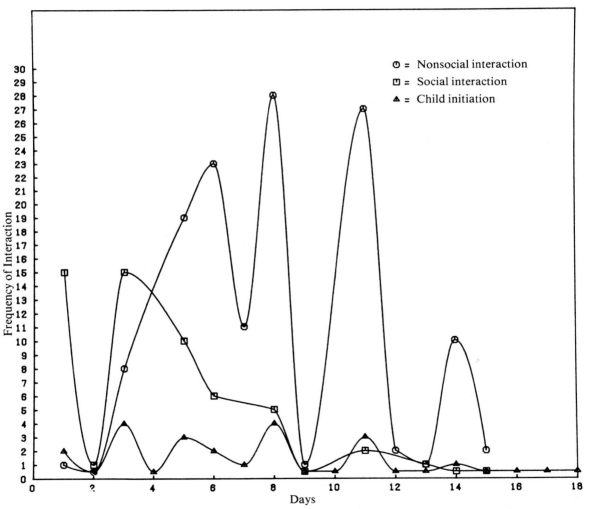

Figure 1 Frequency of mother's social and nonsocial interaction and child's initiations by days of treatment.

Important information can be understood from this profile of mother-daughter interaction presented in Figure 1. Mother's social interactions with her child decreased during the period prior to death. Her nonsocial behavior also decreased. That is, she interacted less with the child when she was present. During the first half of the observation period, 57 percent of mother's behaviors were social compared to seven percent in the last half of the period. Mother was also absent more often as the child's physical condition deteriorated. From this cursory view of interaction, one might conclude

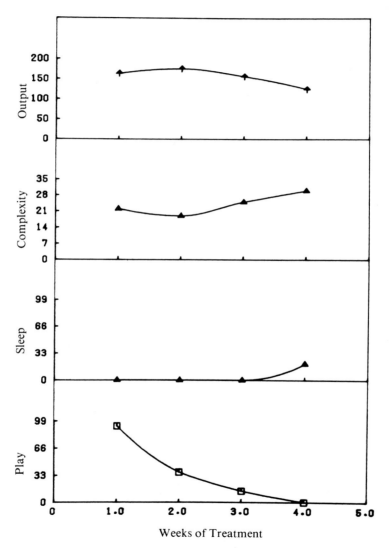

Figure 2 Frequency of child's play and sleep behavior and two summary indices, complexity and output, by weeks of treatment.

that the frequency and quality of adult physical and verbal contacts decreases as the child approaches death. This latter conclusion is consistent with earlier clinical observations (Binger et al., 1969).

It must be remembered, however, that the mother's interactions are likely to be influenced by the child's deteriorating medical status. That is, the child may be less likely to initiate interactions with mother. Figure 1 shows that the child's initiations decreased during the course of treatment. What might be interpreted as the mother's need to distance herself from her dying child may reflect the child's overall lack of social responsiveness rather than retreat by the mother. The need to assess reciprocal influences of parent-child socialization is highlighted in this example of interaction.

Other methods for extracting information from exploratory data analysis have been suggested by John Tukey (1977). For instance, longitudinal data may be collapsed across time periods to identify trends in behavior. Figure 2 shows an adolescent's *play* and *sleep* collapsed over weeks as well as two summary measures of behavior.

Complexity and Output
"Complexity" and "output" are two measures that assess qualitative changes in behavior. Complexity consists of the number of unique behavior codes scored each week, e.g., *initiate, vocal* or *dependency;* or *initiate, vocal, protest, response to pain.* Complexity allows one to answer the question of whether behavior becomes more or less varied over time, given the limited amount of stimulation in the setting. Output consists of active behaviors—*play, vocal, physical,* and *protest.* Rather than showing increases or decreases in specific behaviors, this measure allows one to address questions of quantity of behavior change over time. In Figure 2, *complexity* increased while behavioral *output* declined. Figure 2 also reveals that as "play" decreases, sleep increases over the five-week period. Although the child became less active, behavior became increasingly complex because vocalizations and affect became more varied.

The stability of the measures in this illustration may appear misleading because of the few points plotted. The summary measures, however, are based on approximately 2,000 behaviors. Exploratory graphic tools, such as those highlighted here, are useful for generating hypotheses to be tested by traditional statistical techniques as well as for describing trends in the data.

Confirmatory Approaches
To confirm trends identified above, the general linear model may be used to examine longitudinal behavior changes. Theoretical rationale might initially be used to divide behavior into time periods. For example, does the frequency of social interaction for the mother-child dyad change significantly during two phases of treatment—chemotherapy and onset of complications? The time periods here would represent the period during which chemotherapy was received and the interval following its presentation. Analysis of variance for single-subject designs (Shine and Bower, 1971) might then be

> . . . the frequency and quality of adult physical and verbal contacts decreases as the child approaches death.

**Sequential
analyses have the
potential for
identifying those
interactions
leading to
comfort and
support for the ill
child.**

used to confirm hypotheses. Time period (phase of treatment) would represent the between-subjects factor and trials (days) would represent the within-subjects factor.

Data presented in Figure 1 were used in the analysis. Results indicate a decrease in mother-child social interaction over phases of treatment, F $(8,4) = 4.15$, $p < .07$. The degrees of freedom for the experimental error term is determined by number of trials. In the same manner that number of subjects increases the probability of statistical significance in a factorial design, the number of trials increases the probability of statistical significance in a within-subject design. If there is a large number of trials, then time series analysis is a more appropriate tool for assessing longitudinal change. Glass, Willson, and Gottman (1975) provide an excellent overview of time series analysis and its applicability to observational research.

Sequential Analysis
The traditional approaches to developmental research have assumed only that parents influence children's behavior. Children, however, can also influence parent behavior. As techniques for observation and data analysis become more sophisticated, it becomes more possible to investigate these interactional relationships. Sequential analysis is one that can be used to draw suggestive causal inferences about the direction of influence among parent and child behaviors. Sackett (in press, b) has developed one such method that determines the probability of each observed behavior following the presentation of a predetermined criterion behavior.

The following example illustrates the potential use of sequential analyses for identifying behavioral change. One might ask, "What child behaviors follow the onset of mother's vocalization as a criterion behavior?" All child behaviors following mother's vocalizations could then be recorded during the first nine days of treatment. The event sequential analysis would allow one to look for the probability of all behavior following the criterion—i.e., mother's vocalizations—and also to look for the most probable behaviors that follow that behavior (lag 1), and follow the next behavior (lag 2) and the next (lag 3), until the sequence cannot be examined further. The extent to which parent-child behaviors depend upon one another can thus be recorded.

Although there are many unresolved methodological problems in sequential analysis designs, many potential uses also exist for assessing patterns of interactions among children and caregivers. This analysis can be repeated for any interactional dyad to determine sequences of behaviors—e.g., what is the likelihood that certain child behaviors follow certain nurse or doctor behaviors? This is the first attempt we are aware of to empirically demonstrate sequences of caretaker-patient behavior in an oncology setting. Sequential analyses have the potential for identifying those interactions leading to comfort and support for the ill child.

Summary and Conclusions

Observational studies of children with a life-threatening illness have the potential for generating data with theoretical and practical implications. Contrary to previous research, which deals primarily with thoughts and attitudes of the ill patient in the context of death, the emphasis in this chapter has been on parent-child *behavior* as it occurs in a cancer treatment setting. Outcome of illness was a secondary factor. Our focus was on changes in daily behaviors of the patients and those in their environment over a prolonged period of hospitalization. This is not meant to reflect an interest in planning for life while denying death, but rather an interest in understanding how children and their families cope with life while facing death. Observational methodological problems were discussed in relation to the need for careful assessment and monitoring of observer agreement. Exploratory and confirmatory data analytic models were proposed for evaluating the frequency and sequential dependencies among observed parent-child behaviors.

Observational studies have the potential for generating hypotheses which can then be structured into theoretical statements regarding the impact of illness on psychological development. Observational studies also have the potential for generating practical knowledge. Empirically demonstrating patterns of behaviors that lead to comfort or distress for the child and family can provide a basis for designing intervention programs to accomplish specific humanitarian goals. Earlier it was suggested that a mother's social interactions with her child declined during the second week of hospitalization. At that point intervention might have assisted the mother in accepting her disengagement or in becoming re-engaged, which might have been an additional source of comfort for the child. Interventions that can enhance the quality of social interactions and lead to the development of coping strategies for children and caregivers would be a valuable contribution to the care of children with life-threatening or less severe illnesses.

References

Binger, C. M., et al. 1969. Childhood leukemia: Emotional impact on patient and family. *New England Journal of Medicine* 280:414–418.

Brandt, R. M. 1972. *Studying behavior in natural settings.* New York: Holt, Rinehart and Winston.

Cairns, R. B. *Social interactional analysis: Methods and illustrations.* Hillsdale, New Jersey: Lawrence Erlbaum Press, in press.

Cohen, J. 1960. A coefficient of agreement for nominal scales. *Educational and psychological measurement* 20:37–46.

Freud, A., and S. Dann. 1970. An experiment in group upbringing. In F. Rebelsky and L. Dorman (eds.), *Child development and behavior.* New York: Alfred A. Knopf, Inc.

Glass, G. V., V. L. Willson, and J. M. Gottman. 1975. *Design and analysis of time-series experiments.* Boulder, Colorado: Colorado Associated University Press.

Hollenbeck, A. R. Problems of reliability in observational research. In G. P. Sackett (ed.), *Observing behavior* (vol. 2). Baltimore: University Park Press, in press.

Koocher, G. P. 1973. Childhood, death, and cognitive development. *Developmental Psychology* 9:369–375.

Mash, E. J., and J. D. McElwee. 1974. Situational effects on observer accuracy: Behavioral predictability, prior experience, and complexity of coding categories. *Child Development* 45:367–377.

Parke, R. D. Interactional design. In R. B. Cairns (ed.), *Social interactional analysis: Methods and illustrations.* Hillsdale, N. J.: Lawrence Erlbaum Press, in press.

Pizzo, P. A., and A. S. Levine. 1977. The utility of protected environment regimens for the compromised host: A critical assessment. In E. B. Brown (ed.), *Progress in hematology* (vol. 10). New York: Grune and Stratton.

Sackett, G. P. Measurement in observational research. In G. P. Sackett (ed.), *Observing behavior* (vol. 2). Baltimore: University Park Press, in press (a).

———. The lag sequential analysis of contingency and cyclicity in behavioral interaction research. In J. Osofsky (ed.), *Handbook of infant development.* New York: Wiley, in press (b).

Shine, L. C. and S. M. Bower. 1971. A one-way analysis of variance for single-subject designs. *Educational and psychological measurement* 31:105–113.

Spinetta, J. J., D. Rigler, and M. Karon. 1974. Personal space as a measure of a dying child's sense of isolation. *Journal of Consulting and Clinical Psychology* 42:751–756.

Susman, E. J., D. L. Peters, and R. Stewart. 1976. Observational child study: An empirical analysis of recent trends and directions. Paper presented at the Fourth Biennial Southeastern Conference on Human Development, Nashville, Tennessee.

Taplin, P. S., and J. B. Reid. 1975. Effects of instructional set and experimenter influence on observer reliability. *Child Development* 44:547–554.

Tukey, J. W. 1971. *Exploratory data analysis.* Reading, Mass.: Addison-Wesley.

Yarrow, M. R., and C. Z. Waxler. Observing interaction: A confrontation with methodology. In R. B. Cairns (ed.), *Social interactional analysis: Methods and illustrations.* Hillsdale, N. J.: Lawrence Erlbaum Press, in press.

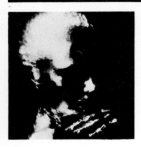

17

Research

There are many ways to learn about death. Certainly experiencing an actual death is one way. More and more, however, people are choosing to learn through a formal death education class or workshop. These formal approaches usually emphasize either didactic lecture or experiential sharing. Which of these two approaches do you think is more effective in changing attitudes toward life and death? Joseph Durlak has investigated this question and offers a possible answer. When you have completed this chapter, the following two Appendix exercises are recommended:

I.   Life and Death Attitudes: Dyadic Encounter

K.   Planning for Living

Comparison between Experiential and Didactic Methods of Death Education

Joseph A. Durlak

Although 20,000 death education and training programs have been offered in the United States (1), there are few systematic investigations of the effectiveness of these various programs. For example, Murray (2) found a reduction in death anxiety for nurses involved in a death education course, but there was no control group against which to compare and measure the significance of obtained findings. Subsequent to an academic course on death and dying, Bell (3) reported that college students changed significantly more than did controls in frequency of thinking about death and interest in death-related discussions. However, there were no significant inter-group differences or within-group changes in students' feelings and attitudes toward death. Aside from using college students, which limits the generality of findings, Bell (3) offered no evidence in support of the reliability and validity of his specially constructed death questionnaire measures.

This report improves upon the shortcomings of previous studies in that it attempts to examine the impact of a death and dying workshop on individual attitudes toward life and death. Pre- and postquestionnaire data were obtained from workshop participants and a nonparticipant control group. Two widely used death scales (4, 5) were used in conjunction with Crumbaugh and Maholick's Purpose in Life Test (6) as outcome measures. Due to changes in workshop format on two occasions, it was also possible to examine the differential effects of an educational approach emphasizing didactic versus experiential components. This latter aspect of the experimental design was considered important from a research standpoint. Although several authors have implied that an emotional, personal approach to death is more effective than didactic presentations in death education and training programs (7–11), there is no empirical data supporting these claims.

This material was first published in *Omega: Journal of Death and Dying,* vol. 9, no. 1, pp. 57–66, 1978. Copyright 1978 Baywood Publishing Co., Inc. It is printed here in slightly modified form by permission.

Method

Instruments

Test packets were prepared containing an information facesheet, a series of questions assessing concern and contact with death, and four psychometric scales appearing in randomized order. The data relevant to the death concern and contact measures are not reported here. The information facesheet sought the respondent's age, sex, marital status, occupation, religious affiliation, and a self-rating of religiosity along a 4-point scale (1 = nonreligious, 2 = somewhat nonreligious, 3 = somewhat religious, 4 = religious; cf. Feifel and Branscomb [12]).

The four psychometric scales consisted of Templar's Death Anxiety Scale (5), Lester's Fear of Death Scale (4), Crumbaugh and Maholick's Purpose of Life Test (6), and the Marlowe-Crowne Social Desirability Scale (13). The Lester and Templar scales are two widely used research instruments that have been developed with considerations of reliability and validity in mind. The Purpose in Life Test is an attitude scale that measures the degree to which a person experiences a sense of meaning and purpose in life. Crumbaugh and Maholick (6) have presented evidence that the instrument is a reliable and valid operational measure of the existential concepts of meaning and purpose in life as proposed by Frankl (14, 15). Frankl theorizes that true meaning and purpose in life are associated with an individual accepting and finding meaning in suffering and, ultimately, death. Death actually becomes a factor in life's meaningfulness. Previous research has supported Frankl's theory in this regard (16–18). The Marlowe-Crowne Scale was included within the test packets to measure the possible influence of social desirability response parameters on questionnaire scores.

Respondents

A total of 51 individuals who participated in five successive workshops completed the test packets from 1–3 days before and from 1–3 days after attending the workshop. A 19-member nonparticipant control group completed pre-post testing during a comparable time period. The workshop group was divided into two experimental groups consisting of 19 participants from two didactically oriented workshops (didactic group) and 32 participants from three experientially oriented programs (experiential group). The total sample averaged 32 years of age; 67 percent were female; 43 percent were married; mean religious self-rating was 2.58 (midway between "somewhat nonreligious" and "somewhat religious"); 38 percent were nurses; 14 percent physicians; 24 percent paramedical staff; 9 percent administrative and secretarial employees; and the remainder consisted of other hospital personnel. Experimental and control groups did not differ on the above characteristics.

All respondents completed the materials voluntarily and anonymously after being told that individual attitudes toward death and dying were being studied.

Death and Dying Workshop

The death and dying workshop under study is part of a continuing education training program at a large southeastern medical center. The workshop is held monthly from September to June, publicized throughout the hospital, and open to every hospital employee. It is an eight-hour small-group experience conducted for four hours on each of two successive weekday mornings and is attended by eight to sixteen participants selected from a waiting list to represent a cross-section of hospital personnel (physicians, nurses, ward medics, laboratory technicians, etc.). A psychiatric nurse, psychologist, general physician, and two chaplains lead the workshop and assume personal responsibility for separate presentations during the two-day program.

The psychologist and one chaplain simultaneously decided to change the nature of their presentations in two of the five workshops from an experiential to a didactic focus. This change made it possible to compare the differential effects of workshop programs that emphasized didactic versus experiential components. In didactic presentations, the chaplain spoke about helping patients to deal emotionally with impending death, and the psychologist talked first about personal feelings regarding death and then about emotional reactions involved in mourning and bereavement, including anticipatory grief. The didactic presentations also included a discussion of social factors influencing the treatment of dying and grieving persons, psychological styles of adaptation of death, and the frequent denial of the reality of death.

During the other three workshops the chaplain and the psychologist used an experiential rather than a didactic focus with the groups. The chaplain led the group in two hours of role-playing similar to that described by Barton and Crowder (7). Roles involving caregivers and dying and grieving persons were described on separate index cards and volunteers were solicited. Participants frequently exchanged roles as both actors and observers shared their feelings in each situation.

In his experiential presentation, the psychologist began with a fifteen-minute discussion of emotional aspects of grief and bereavement. He then asked group members to perform Berman's death awareness exercises (19), in which each individual is asked to imagine that he has only 24 hours to live and then is asked to share first with one other group member and then with the entire group how he would spend his last day. As noted by Berman (19), this exercise produces strong affective reactions among participants and leads to intense personal discussions concerning anxieties, insecurities, and fears about death and dying.

After reactions to this exercise were shared and processed, the group was asked to participate in a grief-related exercise. Participants were divided into small (two to four person) groups and asked: (a) to relate their past personal experiences in which someone close to them had died; and (b) to imagine how they would feel and react if the person closest to them was going to die soon. One of the five workshop leaders monitored each

> . . . each individual is asked to imagine that he has only 24 hours to live and then is asked to share . . . how he would spend his last day.

The experiential workshop . . . sought to provide participants with both a cognitive *and* emotional encounter with death while the didactic program emphasized only the former component.

small group discussion in this exercise, which, similar to the death awareness exercise, aroused strong emotional reactions among group members. Experiences and feelings discussed in each of the small group discussions were shared with the total group.

The presentations of the other workshop leaders did not change during the five monthly workshops. The nurse began the workshop with video-taped interviews of dying patients and their spouses followed by a group discussion and a didactic presentation of Kübler-Ross's work (20). After a short break, the physician spoke about the need for honest and direct communication with dying patients and problems encountered by medical staff in this regard. He also indicated the general lack of training for medical personnel in the psychosocial aspects of dealing with terminal illness. The first part of the psychologist's presentation ended the first half of the workshop.

On the second day the psychologist completed his presentation and the two chaplains presented their material. The second chaplain concluded the workshop by discussing theological and philosphical concerns of dying patients and their families.

In summary, the primary difference between the didactic and experiential workshops lay in the methodology rather than the content of instruction. Each program dealt broadly with such topics as emotional reactions to grief and death and communication with the terminally ill. However, during a critical three and one-half-hour time period in which the psychologist and one chaplain led the workshop, the didactic group learned about grief and death through lecture and small-group discussion—a method of instruction that continued the didactic emphasis of other workshop experiences. This same time frame was spent differently in the three experiential workshops. Here participants were assisted to confront, examine, and share their own feelings and reactions to grief and death. Role playing and personalized death awareness and grief exercises were used for this purpose. The experiential workshop thus sought to provide participants with both a cognitive *and* emotional encounter with death while the didactic program emphasized only the former component.

Table 1 Pre- and posttest scale correlations for the total sample

	SDS	DAS	FOD	PIL
SDS		− .14	− .06	.01
DAS	− .30*		.24*	− .59**
FOD	− .11	.33**		− .49**
PIL	.00	− .54**	− .36**	

Note The upper half of the matrix contains pretest and the lower half posttest correlations. SDS = Social Desirability Scale, DAS = Death Anxiety Scale, FOD = Fear of Death Scale, and PIL = Purpose in Life Test.
*p <.05
**p <.01

Results

Table 1 presents the pre- and posttest scale correlations for the total sample. Correlational data indicated that social desirability response parameters were a relatively unimportant influence on questionnaire scores. Only the posttest relationship between the Death Anxiety and Marlowe-Crowne scales reached significance and this correlation was small in magnitude ($r = -.30, p < .05$). The Purpose in Life Test was significantly and negatively correlated with both death scales ($r \geq -.36$). These data replicate previous findings regarding the relationship between "purpose in life" and death-related concerns and feelings (16–18). The significant pre- and posttest correlation ($r = .24$ and .33, respectively) indicated some, but not a major, degree of measurement overlap between these two instruments. The significance of this finding is discussed later.

One-way analyses of variance were performed on pretest questionnaire scores to assess initial comparability of groups. No significant differences between groups were found. To study the effects of the workshop experience, scores on each life and death questionnaire were subjected to a 2 × 3 analysis of variance with groups (experiential, didactic, and control) as a between-subjects main effect and time of evaluation (pre- and post-) as a repeated measures, within-subjects main effect. Duncan multiple-range tests with significance set at the .05 level were applied to inspect mean differences following significant F ratios.

All F tests were nonsignificant for scores on the Purpose in Life Test. A significant main effect for time ($F = 14.06, df = 1/67, p < .001$) and a significant group by time interaction ($F = 12.15, df = 2/67, p < .001$) appeared in the analysis of scores on the Templar scale. Post hoc mean comparisons indicated the didactic group differed significantly from the experiential but not the control group. The latter two groups did not significantly differ from one another.

Analysis of scores on the Lester scale also yielded a significant main effect for time and a significant group by time interaction ($F = 24.76, df = 1/67, p < .001$, and $F = 113.27, df = 2/67, p < .001$, respectively). Duncan tests indicated that the experiential group differed significantly from the other two groups, which did not differ from one another.

Table 2 presents the pre- and post- group means on the life and death questionnaires. Inspection of group means indicated that the pattern of results differed on the two death scales. On the Templar scale, scores increased over time for all groups, but the experiential group demonstrated the smallest and the didactic group the greatest amount of change. On the Lester scale, however, whereas scores rose for the didactic and control groups from pre- to posttesting, scores declined over the same time period for the experiential group.

In summary, results indicated that the experiential workshop decreased participants' fears and concerns about death while only slightly heightening

> . . . results indicated that the experiential workshop decreased participants' fears and concerns about death. . . .

their anxieties about death. In contrast, the didactic workshop had negative effects since participants reported greater fears and anxieties about death at the end of the workshop than when they began it. Controls showed slight negative changes on these death measures over time. No changes appeared in purpose in life scale scores for any of the groups.

Discussion

Results suggest that a death education program with experiential exercises to assist individuals in confronting and sharing their personal feelings about death and dying was significantly more effective in changing attitudes toward death than an educational workshop not containing such components. These data lend empirical support to the view that an emotional, personal approach to death is an important element in an effective death education program (7–11). Current findings therefore encourage further investigations on the value of experiential exercises within the context of other death-related educational and training paradigms.

Although this research is a step forward in the systematic evaluation of death education programs, there are several experimental limitations. The death and dying workshop studied here was conducted in a hospital setting by a multidisciplinary teaching staff for an 8-hour period with small groups of voluntary, heterogeneous participants. These findings may not be replicated in other settings if any of the factors differ, such as group composition and workshop length.

Table 2 Pre and post means and standard deviations for experiential, didactic, and control groups on the life and death questionnaire

| Groups | Measures | | | | | |
| | FOD | DAS | PIL | FOD | DAS | PIL |
		Pre			Post	
Experiential						
M	5.56	6.40	106.03	4.92	6.78	107.78
SD	1.01	2.28	14.71	0.72	2.89	15.24
Didactic						
M	5.38	6.57	106.42	5.73	7.68	106.42
SD	0.87	2.34	15.52	1.13	2.05	17.69
Control						
M	5.39	6.63	104.31	5.56	7.26	103.95
SD	0.92	3.56	19.38	0.89	3.23	13.89

Note FOD = Fear of Death Scale; DAS = Death Anxiety Scale; PIL = Purpose in Life Test.

In addition, program evaluation was confined to immediate, self-report measures of death attitudes and feelings. The durability of obtained changes and their relation to subsequent behavior was not assessed. Although several thanatologists believe that positive modifications in caregivers' death-related feelings and attitudes does improve the care given to dying and grieving persons, the direct connection between attitudes or feelings and behavior has not been demonstrated empirically.

Current outcome data illustrate the difficulties involved in attempting to assess attitudes and feelings toward such broad concepts as life and death. For example, in retrospect, it was perhaps naive to assume that significant changes on the Purpose in Life Test would occur as a result of the death workshop. According to Frankl (14, 15), acceptance of death is but one aspect in the development of personal meaning and purpose in life. Modification of death attitudes may not necessarily affect the larger construct of purpose in life, although the reverse may be true. However, the significant negative correlations that were obtained in the present study between the Purpose in Life Test and Lester's Fear of Death Scale replicate previous findings (16–18) and suggest the utility of the former measure in future death research.

Problems of interpretation also arise with findings on the two death scales. Although the present study found a significant but low correlation between the Lester and Templar death scales, other studies have reported nonsignificant correlations between these scales, indicating that these two instruments are not measuring the same dimensions (21, 22). Krieger, Epsting, and Leitner (22) developed a threat index for use in death research and reported significant positive correlations among their threat index, Lester's death scale, and a direct, specific, self-report of fear of death, but Templar's scale was significantly associated only with the latter measure. The authors interpreted these findings to mean that Lester's scale is more a measure of the conceptual meaning death holds for individuals, including the elements of fear and threat, than it is a measure of death anxiety per se.

There is both theoretical and empirical support for the view that individual reactions to death are multidimensional. For example, Ray and Najman (23) report data to indicate that anxiety about death and acceptance of death may coexist within individuals. Therefore, current data for the experiential group that reflect a reduction in test scores on the Lester scale concomitant with a rise in scores on the Templar scale over time are plausible. Nevertheless, much further work is needed to determine the exact components of death-related concerns that are being assessed by different measuring instruments.

It is unclear exactly how workshop experiences exerted changes in reactions to death, but some speculations can be offered. Personal consideration of death and dying appears unsettling, and the context in which individuals approach death affects personal reactions to the topic. Controls who merely completed pre- and post- questionnaires displayed negative

> . . . anxiety about death and acceptance of death may coexist within individuals.

changes on scales measuring death anxiety and death fear, but didactic group members who were involved in a more intense, personal exposure to death-related topics demonstrated even greater negative changes. In contrast, experiential workshop experiences seemed to minimize anxious reactions to death and to positively affect concerns and fears about death.

It is believed that positive changes occurred in the experiential group because participants benefited from a nonthreatening atmosphere in which they could "work through" their death-related feelings. Workshop leaders observed that although the experiential exercises produced a significant ventilation of personal fears, anxieties, and insecurities about death and dying, the sharing of these reactions was beneficial to individuals in recognizing and resolving these feelings. Individuals were relieved that others shared similar feelings about death, and they felt supported in coming to terms with the personal meaning death had for them. Future research attempting to evaluate the above (and other) speculations regarding factors responsible for changes in death-related feelings and attitudes would be useful.

In summary, current findings and implications must be offered tentatively due to limitations in the experimental design and the lack of strong, pervasive program effects. Nevertheless, even on an exploratory basis, this research represents a more objective assessment of effects than is currently available in most other death programs. It is hoped that this report will encourage further systematic investigations of other death-related educational programs.

References

1. Somerville, R. S. 1975. Book review. *Journal of Marriage and the Family* 37:1042–1044.
2. Murray, P. 1974. Death education and its effect on the death anxiety level of nurses. *Psychological Reports* 35:1250.
3. Bell, B. D. 1975. The experimental manipulation of death attitudes: A preliminary investigation. *Omega* 6:199–205.
4. Lester, D. 1967. Fear of death of suicidal persons. *Psychological Reports* 20:1077–1078.
5. Templar, D. I. 1970. The construction and validation of a death anxiety scale. *Journal of General Psychology* 82:165–177.
6. Crumbaugh, J. C. and L. T. Maholick. 1964. An experimental study in existentialism: The psychometric approach to Frankl's concept of noogenic neurosis. *Journal of Clinical Psychology* 20:200–207.
7. Barton, D. and M. K. Crowder. 1975. The use of role playing techniques as an instructional aid in teaching about dying, death, and bereavement. *Omega* 6:243–250.
8. Bloom, S. 1975. On teaching an undergraduate course on death and dying. *Omega* 6:223–226.
9. Kopel, K., W. O'Connell, J. Paris, and P. Girardin. 1975. A human relations laboratory approach to death and dying. *Omega* 6:219–221.
10. Simpson, M. A. 1975. The do-it-yourself death certificate in evoking and estimating student attitudes toward death. *Journal of Medical Education* 50:475–478.
11. Weiner, H. B. 1975. Living experiences with death—A journeyman's view through psychodrama. *Omega* 6:251–274.
12. Feifel, H. and A. B. Branscomb. 1973. Who's afraid of death? *Journal of Abnormal Psychology* 81:282–288.
13. Crowne, D. P. and D. Marlowe. 1960. A new scale of social desirability independent of psychopathology. *Journal of Consulting Psychology* 24:349–354.
14. Frankl, V. E. 1963. *Man's search for meaning.* New York: Washington Square Press.

15. Frankl, V. E. 1965. *The doctor and the soul.* New York: Knopf.
16. Blazer, J. A. 1973. The relationship between meaning in life and fear of death. *Psychology* 10:72–73.
17. Durlak, J. A. 1972. Relationship between individual attitudes toward life and death. *Journal of Consulting and Clinical Psychology* 38:463.
18. Durlak, J. A. 1973. Relationship between attitudes toward life and death among elderly women. *Developmental Psychology* 8:146.
19. Berman, A. L. 1972. Crisis interventionists and death awareness: An exercise for training in suicide prevention. *Crisis Intervention* 4:47–52.
20. Kübler-Ross, E. 1969. *On death and dying.* New York: The Macmillan Company.
21. Berman, A. L. and J. E. Hays. 1973. Relation between death anxiety, belief in afterlife, and locus of control. *Journal of Consulting and Clinical Psychology* 41:318.
22. Krieger, S. R., F. R. Epsting, and L. M. Leitner. 1974. Personal constructs, threat and attitudes toward death. *Omega* 5:299–310.
23. Ray, J. J. and J. Najman. 1974. Death anxiety and death acceptance: A preliminary approach. *Omega* 5:311–315.

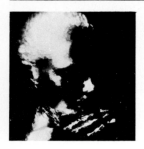

18

Practice

How might a death education class be set up and what can participants like you expect to gain from such an experience? Would you expect it to change your attitudes about dying, or perhaps living? Is it realistic to think that you may leave such a class more capable of coping not only with your own feelings about death but with the feelings of others also? How do we educate our communities to mobilize resources in this area? These issues and others are explored here by Bugen. The following Appendix exercises may be useful when you complete this chapter:

I.   Life and Death Attitudes: Dyadic Encounter

K.   Planning for Living

O.   Values Grid

Death Education: Perspectives for Schools and Communities

Larry A. Bugen

It has been said that death is un-American, for it is contrary to life, liberty, and the pursuit of happiness. Such a political attitude suggests that death and dying might best be left to legislators. In fact, Texas passed at least four bills during the 1977 legislative session that dramatically reflected the current interest in death issues. These mandates included: (1) a right-to-die bill, (2) a death-by-injection bill, (3) a Sudden-Infant-Death-Syndrome (SIDS) bill authorizing funds for autopsies and family counseling, and (4) a bill legalizing Laetrile, a drug claimed to combat cancer. Each of these innovations regarding death requires an educational program for the public. But the education is not likely to come from the legislators.

Death education presently lies instead in the hands of psychologists, sociologists, health educators and, yes, even English professors. It is regrettable that presentation of death-related issues is still relatively unknown in professional education. Liston (1975), for example, reviewed the Cumulative Index Medicus for the years 1960–1971 and failed to turn up one article documenting instruction concerning death and dying for medical students. A vastly different picture is seen at the college level, where course offerings have proliferated to at least 1,000 throughout the United States (Shneidman, 1976). Just the opposite picture is presented outside the United States. Leviton (1977) reports that countries such as Sweden, Canada, West Germany, and Great Britain maintain "no significant effort to develop death education in their public school or university sectors." Death education abroad seems to exist *only* in medical education.

The rapid growth of death education in this country since 1970 appears to be due to a number of interesting factors. (1) Emphasis on consumer awareness has made many individuals wary of the carcinogenic elements in their food and immediate environment. Almost daily, consumers are told about a new threat to their health. (2) Renewed emphasis on health and physical fitness is feeding into our ever-present interest in longevity. (3) Death continues to be a much discussed topic in the media, particularly the press and television. (4) Tragic cases of figures such as Karen Quinlan have dramatized issues of living and dying and challenged the public's responses and ability to face them. (5) The inner sanctums of the medical kingdom and the conspiracy of silence that has characterized death and dying, particularly in institutional settings, are being invaded and exposed to public view by such things as malpractice suits. The net effect of these societal forces is not so much increased acceptance of death as confrontation—acceptance that it is an entity to be reckoned with.

An Instructional Model for Death Education

The proliferation of death education courses mentioned above warrants our presenting an instructional model. The model offers a framework for evaluating the present diversity of offerings. It could also be a guide for future development.

Leviton (1977) uses six dimensions to characterize the present array of courses. (1) The *target audience* may be elementary, high school, or university students. (2) The *target domain* may be an emphasis on feelings or cognitive processes. (3) *Number of students.* (4) The *endorsing discipline* may include health education, psychology, etc. (5) The *methodology* may involve lectures, small-group discussions, role-playing, films, guests, etc. (6) *Goals* may include therapy, knowledge, social reform, or professional preparation. These six dimensions are certainly key elements in any death education venture. The relationships between these elements, however, must be clarified in order for us to truly capture the present innovations in the field and in order to do this, we must put our values squarely on the line and take a stand.

I believe the great diversity present today in death education can be tied together with a simple diagram (see figure 1). All death educators must begin their efforts with a definite *Goal* or purpose. All instructional variables may then be classified under either *Target* or *Method,* which both follow neatly from goals. In my own course at the University of Texas at Austin my overriding goal is to humanize death and dying. Now humanization is a very amorphous goal! One minute I think I have my finger on it; next minute I don't.

Certainly we see signs of increasing humanization on several levels. On the individual level, we strive to alleviate pain and suffering. On the community level, we have created hospices, and some funeral homes have begun to recognize the need for grief counselors. On the societal and social systems level, we are attempting to curtail sensationalism in the media regarding death, and we are passing important new legislation which increases rather than decreases our options.

The humanization that is our major goal seems to have three components. The first is to help students increase their personal ability to confront their own fears and concerns regarding death or bereavement. Can they discuss these concerns with one another or with loved ones? Can they clarify their values, goals, beliefs, and life plans? Do they have the skill to reach out and help others who find themselves in the role of bereaved or terminally ill? Personal effectiveness is many-sided. My own research suggests that personal effectiveness as just defined can be enhanced but that personality traits such as ''death concern'' may be too enduring to be modified by even the most intensive death education efforts.

The second component of humanization involves identification, creation, and maintenance of humanistic resources within our communities. Where does the ordinary citizen, consumer, or student of life go to find out about living wills, funeral prepayments, right-to-die prerogatives, donor facilities, and rap groups or counseling groups dealing with death-related issues? Where does a terminally ill or bereaved person go to meet with others in similar circumstances? Where does one find a physician willing to let one participate in decisions regarding treatment? Where are the specialists in grief? We have employment counselors, marriage counselors, retirement counselors, and sex counselors. Where are the grief counselors? When abortions were legalized, a need for abortion counselors arose. With the creation of legislation concerned with our right to die, similarly, counseling resources for the community appear necessary. Where will the funds be coming from, and who will be doing the educating?

The third component of humanization is eloquently summarized by the brief statement of Kastenbaum (1977, p. 220): ''Patients, families and staff *all* have legitimate needs.'' It is true that physicians are trained to intervene best on a technical level. It is true that nurses and other support staff are short-handed and overwhelmed with excessive daily tasks. It is true that pa-

Where does the ordinary citizen . . . go to find out about living wills, funeral prepayments, right-to-die prerogatives, donor facilities, and rap groups or counseling groups dealing with death-related issues?

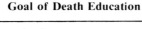

Goal of Death Education

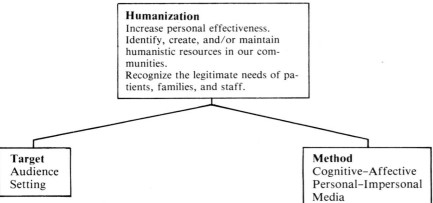

Figure 1 Goal of death education. Model for death education instruction proposed by Bugen and reflecting goals determining target and method.

tients and families sometimes desire *not* to make decisions or not to communicate with others. And it is also true that the wishes of the terminally ill person and his or her family must be taken into account. The family must know that they can discuss emotional and other caregiving needs with the staff. Similarly, the staff must have a mutual support network that encompasses *both* technical and social emotional issues. We need advocates in hospitals, medical schools, nursing homes, and other institutional settings to help make these needs realities. Community and institutional settings may then be the most important centers for innovations in death education in the coming years.

I urge that any educational course or seminar involving death and dying issues make humanization its goal. Which of the three components is emphasized will depend upon the target population. Psychology students, to be of therapeutic assistance to others, will need to confront their own fears, understand the human grief process, and learn and practice helping skills. Health educators, while being concerned with all three parts of the goal, may concentrate on learning about and helping to develop educational resources and community programs. Medical students and nursing students should be exposed to all three components but may spend most of their time learning to recognize and respond to the legitimate needs of all persons who meet as members of a hospital network system.

It would probably be a mistake to conceive of death education purely in terms familiar to psychology majors, sociology majors, medical students, etc. Classes are likely to be heterogeneous, as my own is, composed of students in anthropology, art, nursing, premed, psychology, health education, and sociology. Attempting to meet the needs of each of these students requires highly varied content and activities, which I'll briefly address under method. A class blended of these varied disciplines creates a dynamic atmosphere and parallels the real world.

With our goal for death education clear and our audience defined, we must decide on the methods to be utilized. All death education efforts can be profiled along a cognitive-affective dimension. At one extreme, only lectures and didactic presentations are used to impart knowledge. At the other extreme, structured exercises are used to promote personal and interpersonal development for the participants. Methods most used in death education fall somewhere between these two extremes. Death, dying, life, and living all affect our total selves. Our thoughts, emotions, and behaviors are all inextricably intertwined in dynamic interplay. To focus only on cognitive development at the expense of exploring feelings or rehearsing helping behavior is to miss an opportunity at total integration. I believe the really innovative programs in death education approach the individual on all these levels. Which end of the continuum is emphasized will depend on the goal and the target population. A community workshop designed to acquaint the public with funeral options or health care alternatives may focus on audiovisual or lecture presentations, although small group discussions would also be needed. Death education directed toward psychologists and social workers may tend toward experiential components, although the presentation of didactic material will certainly be necessary. My own course balances both, with lecture, audiovisual, or guest presentation the first half of a class session, and experiential exercises the second half.

I believe decisions regarding size of class, background of instructor, location, and frequency and duration of classes all depend on where you orient the presentation along the cognitive-affective continuum. If the goal is only to transmit information to the average consumer, there can be much leeway in each of those elements. But the more the presentation emphasizes the affective domain, the more carefully planned each of the elements must be.

I begin my first class session each semester by announcing that both cognitive and experiential components will be incorporated in the class. I cover the desired readings and mention the anticipated visits to the funeral home and cemetery and our exposure to terminally ill patients, grieving parents, and to one another in small groups. At the end of the orientation session I expect to lose 5 percent of the participants. I believe I have the ethical responsibility to warn the participants ahead of time of my methods so that their choice to be a part of the experience is an informed one. I have taught the course over fifteen weeks and also over a three-week intensive summer session, and have learned to limit class size to twenty-five, especially for a three-week summer session. During this time there seems to be no getting away from death and dying. Class extends for three hours, reading averages another two hours, and entries into journals average another hour. Emotions ranging from anger and depression to joy are all commonly reported by the end of the second week. Their support groups become vital to class members, as evidenced by very high cohesion scores. I make sure that the intensity of their explorations into death and dying is matched by the intensity of their explorations into life and living. I usually end my classes with life planning and a picnic and barbecue. Frisbees, beach balls, and balloons are all pleasant symbols of my class coming to an end.

What effects should we expect from death education courses?

What Are the Effects of Death Education?

Do participants in death education courses emerge from the experience with all concern about death obliterated? Are they able to express their fears more openly? Will they feel confident about helping others who find themselves in bereaved or terminal roles? What effects should we expect from death education courses? Are some effects more preferred than others?

For the most part, the above questions have not been asked until very recently. Readings in other courses may often include such phrases as ''Numerous investigations have found that . . .'' It is regrettable that such a statement cannot be applied to the domain relating to death education effects. Death educators have likened themselves to early explorers who mere-

One of the most important things death education can teach us is to appreciate the variety of life's losses that involve the grieving process.

ly describe new terrain. Descriptions of courses abound. Leviton (1975), Leonard (1976), Barton (1975), Jeffrey (1977), Bloom (1975), and Somerville (1977) have all provided detailed analyses of method, procedure, purpose, and materials that might be used in the teaching of death and dying.

We urgently need to understand the results of our efforts in this field. Leviton (1977, p. 260) stated that "the need for research to determine more fully the effects of death education courses is obvious. We need to know what is happening to our students, under what conditions, and for how long. Most of the research accomplished thus far in the field of death education has been essentially descriptive, although a few investigators have used sophisticated experimental design."

Results have generally been inconclusive in the few studies that have attempted to assess death education effects (Bell 1975). One difficulty appears to be inadequacy of the measurement instruments. In one study designed to investigate the effects of thanatology instruction on attitudes and fears about death and dying, Silberman (1977) concluded that the measurement instrument she was using, the Collett-Lester scale, was not reliable enough for use with high school students.

A second reason for inconclusive results is that the effects are not necessarily testable at a particular time. For instance, Leviton (1977, p. 235) has pointed out that how one actually feels and behaves when death comes forcefully into one's life cannot be tested until the event actually happens.

A third difficulty is that measures of state are, by their nature, sensitive to change and measures of trait assess enduring characteristics. Bugen (1977) used Dickstein's Death Concern Scale as a pre- and postmeasure to assess change as a result of a death and dying seminar. An overall test-retest reliability of r = .77 was obtained at the end of the fifteen-week course. Students with high, average, and low death concern were all equally unchanged in their level of concern following both didactic and experiential instruction. Bugen concluded that death concern, as measured by Dickstein's scale, was a relatively stable characteristic and would not be sensitive to change as a result of courses of this kind.

Whether students learn to cope more effectively as a result of thanatology instruction is a point that death education should be more concerned about (Bugen 1977). The real issue, according to Hart (1976), is "how people cope with loss and what the implications are of that loss in terms of the learning process and in terms of the emotional well-being of the youngster. That is what death education is all about" (p. 407). One of the most important things death education can teach us is to appreciate the variety of life's losses that involve the grieving process. Divorce, marriage, graduation, and retirement all have components of loss and require coping skills to pass through the crisis.

A study conducted by Bugen (1979a) assessed increase in coping capacity of college students who completed a death and dying seminar. The test instrument was developed by asking students as part of a final exam to indicate what they got out of the seminar. The responses were then set up with a seven-point Likert Scale, from "strongly agree" to "strongly disagree" and presented to a subsequent class as a thirty-item "Coping with Death Scale." The items, listed below, are diverse but can be divided into two categories: coping with self, and coping with others. Coping with self includes statements relating to increased understanding, knowledge, and expression of emotions, such as items 10, 11, and 14. Coping with others includes statements relating to increased abilities to communicate with and/or help the bereaved and terminally ill, such as items 23, 26, and 30.

Coping with Death Scale

Directions: Please consider EACH of the following items carefully. Each item represents a *perspective* or *coping strategy* relevant to death and dying. As you read the items consider how you feel NOW.

1. Thinking about death is a waste of time.
2. I have a good perspective on death and dying.
3. Death is an area which can be dealt with safely.
4. I am aware of the full array of services from funeral homes.
5. I am aware of the variety of options for disposing of bodies.
6. I am aware of the full array of emotions which characterize human grief.
7. Knowing that I will surely die does not in any way affect the conduct of my life.
8. I feel prepared to face my death.
9. I feel prepared to face my dying process.
10. I understand my death-related fears.
11. I am familiar with funeral prearrangement should I prefer to use it.
12. Lately I find it OK to think about death.
13. My attitude about living has recently changed.
14. I can express my fears about dying.
15. I can put words to my gut level feelings about death and dying.
16. I am making the best of my present life.
17. The quality of my life matters more than the length of it.
18. I can talk about my death with family and friends.
19. I know who to contact when death occurs.
20. I will be able to cope with future losses.
21. I feel able to handle the death of others close to me.
22. I know how to listen to others, including the terminally ill.
23. I know how to speak to children about death.
24. I may say the wrong thing when I am with someone mourning.
25. I am able to spend time with the dying if I need to.
26. I can help someone with their thoughts and feelings about death and dying.
27. I would be able to talk to a friend or family member about their death.
28. I can lessen the anxiety of those around me when the topic is death and dying.
29. I can communicate with the dying.
30. I can tell someone now, before I or they die, how much I love him or her.

Students completed the "Coping with Death Scale" at the beginning of a three-week seminar and again at the completion of the course. They reported significant increases in their abilities to cope on 23 out of the 30 items on the questionnaire. The most significant changes were reported for items 2, 4, 5, 10, 11, 12, 15, 21, 23, 26, 27, 28, and 29.

A matched control group, which did not experience the entire death and dying seminar, did not report these kinds of changes. As encouraging as the above findings are, it is important to stress that they are self-reports by the students, without actual experiences being involved. Whether a student will actually "be able to talk to a friend or family member about their death" needs to be behaviorally assessed at the proper time.

Death Education for the Community

The most neglected target area for death education is the local community. We must get out of our ivory towers and terminal care stations and face our local communities—the Uncle Harrys and Aunt Marys. Education for living and dying needs to include this group.

A death-education week could be proclaimed, and promoted by local TV, radio, magazine, and newspaper features. One-day symposia could be devoted to special topics such as "the cost of dying" or "life-planning workshops." Such community efforts should emphasize prevention of hardships and stress later on. Persons are usually forced to make irrevocable decisions at times when they are least able to cope—usually when they are experiencing a great deal of stress. Community death education could, using established preventive public health principles, help reduce stress and encourage decision making under more rational circumstances. The same purpose underlies living wills, right-to-die legislation, and prefuneral arrangements.

Prevention of mental and physical health disorders related to death and dying can be thought of in three ways. *Primary prevention* seeks to promote mental health and/or forestall distress. Efforts are usually directed toward education before the onset of a crisis. *Secondary prevention* is directed toward shortening the duration, impact, and negative aftereffects of disorder. Efforts are usually directed toward early detection and early treatment interventions. *Tertiary prevention* attempts to minimize impairments or disorders that are essentially irreversible. These concepts can be of great help in organizing community death education.

For example, primary prevention at the community level is represented by the Value of Life Project sponsored by the Texas Conference of Churches. The project is a joint effort of educators, scientists, and religious leaders to (a) encourage examination of new attitudes in medicine, law, and ethics toward problems raised by rapid advances in life science technology (such as life-sustaining equipment and test-tube pregnancy), and (b) stimulate statewide programs to improve educational resources available in local communities. Groups of citizens and professionals in over eighty Texas communities work together in raising public consciousness regarding bioethical issues. These groups also assess needs and concerns of their local communities and the local resources available to meet those needs.

The Value of Life Project culminated in a statewide conference in December 1976. Well over eighty communities within the State of Texas sent representatives to Dallas to address the following twelve critical issues:

1. Distribution and allocation of health care resources—the political, economic, and social considerations.
2. Health care delivery to poverty areas—problems posed by socio-economic conditions, ethnic traditions, language differences, and availability of services.
3. Humanizing the health care system—concern for the individual, patient family, and health care professionals.
4. Death and dying—approach to terminally ill patients, family, and friends and impact on health care professionals.
5. To save or let die—using extraordinary procedures to prolong life.
6. Moral issues in birth decisions—parenting, prenatal care, abortion, etc.
7. Mental and physical health care for the aging—institutions, family resources, governmental programs, etc.
8. Human experimentation—human dignity, informed consent.
9. Chronic illness and physical handicaps—economic, social, and psycho-emotional effects.
10. Behavior control—effects of environmental, chemical, and psycho-surgical methods.
11. Mental retardation—as an effect of prenatal neglect, genetic accident, and malnutrition.
12. New possibilities in human reproduction—fertility awareness, genetics modification, and research.

Response to the conference was excellent; however, the true test of success must be measured by the continuity and program planning that follows. The representatives attending the conference must organize their communities in regard to the above issues. Programs must be implemented and evaluated. Such a task is sure to face roadblocks along the way. Professionals and lay persons may choose to avoid such controversial issues. Program planning and implementation may be jeopardized through lack of funds. For instance, grant support for primary prevention efforts is particularly difficult to find. Finally, the difficulty of establishing clear goals and actual results in the area of bioethics will make evaluation difficult.

An example of secondary prevention at the community level is a *"Widow-to-Widow Program"* described by Silverman (1976). Available statistics indicated that young widows and widowers have an extraordinarily difficult recovery period following the death of a spouse. During the first year following bereavement they have a high risk of developing emotional,

> **. . . young widows and widowers have an extraordinarily difficult recovery period following the death of a spouse.**

Silverman's program is to develop *and* maintain an ongoing relationship with the widows in order to help them work through the different stages of grief.

physical, and psychological disorders that need treatment. Silverman created a program designed to (a) ease the distress of the bereaved, (b) support them through their grief process, and (c) lessen the possibility of their developing emotional disorders.

The pilot program began with five widows recruited to work as "aides" in a target community in the Boston area. They obtained from death certificates, located in the bureau of vital statistics, the names of all new widows under the age of sixty within their target community. Additional information on race and religion was obtained from funeral directors.

One widow aide writes to each new widow on personal note paper. She offers condolences and, explaining that she is also a widow, proposes a time when she might visit. The aides help the new widows find jobs and sort out finances, but most important, they offer friendship. They visit back and forth in each other's homes, explore each other's experience with widowhood, and often eat dinner and socialize together. Group meetings to which all new widows are invited are also organized. Silverman's program is to develop *and maintain* an ongoing relationship with the widows in order to help them work through the different stages of grief. All available resources are used to accomplish this goal.

The widow aides were women without any special educational background. They were selected because they (a) had personal skills with people, (b) were active in their communities, (c) represented the dominant religious and racial groups in the community, and (d) lived in or near the community in which they worked.

Perhaps the essence of the Widow-to-Widow program is the conviction that the mental health clinic is *not* the locus for preventive work. Prevention is better achieved through the efforts of those individuals and agencies which deal continuously with people as they pass through the normal phases of a life cycle. Community involvement here is vital.

An inspiring example of tertiary prevention is provided by Yalom and Greaves (1977) in their *Group Therapy with the Terminally Ill*. With the aid of a patient with metaplastic cancer, Yalom began a group for other patients with metastatic carcinoma. The explicit purpose of the group was to counter the anguishing isolation that dying patients experience by providing an opportunity for sharing, open communication, and opportunities to be helpful. A second purpose was to teach professional caregivers effective psychotherapeutic techniques for other populations as well.

Patients came on their own initiative from the community or were referred from such organizations as the American Cancer Society's Reach to Recovery program. Eventually physicians began to refer patients to the group when they realized that its purpose was to improve the quality of life rather than to focus on dying.

Presence was the most significant help provided by the group. Persons facing death feel anxious, cut-off, and shunned by the living. The group offered them sustaining relationships and thereby helped ease the loneliness that accompanies dying.

Although psychiatrists, psychiatric residents, social workers, and guidance counselors were available to help the average group of seven or eight, the members themselves were the prime agents of help. They telephoned and visited members in despair, they shared books and coping techniques, and they role-played methods of asking doctors questions. Yalom concludes that "the therapy group has become a key support system for many patients and has enabled them to cope more effectively with enormous stress that invariably accompanies metastatic carcinoma." In addition, it is apparent that this form of community intervention helps minimize negative psychological side effects to illness. Such groups are a rich resource to the community.

> . . . "the therapy group has become a key support system for many patients. . . ."

Emerging Standards

Standards of care to guide those working with the terminally ill have been elucidated by Kastenbaum (1977). And standards of instruction to guide death educators have been expounded by Leviton (1977). In order to function ethically in either arena, professionals are obligated to become aware of and practice these standards.

Patient care standards proposed by Kastenbaum are as follows:

Basic premise: patients, family, and staff all have legitimate needs and interests.
A. Patient-oriented standards
   1. The terminally ill person's own framework of preferences and lifestyle must be taken into account.
   2. Remission of symptoms is a goal of treatment.
   3. Pain control is a goal of treatment.
   4. The living will or similar document will be respected as part of the total health care package.
   5. Efforts should be expended toward increasing a patient's sense of security within his or her setting.
   6. Leave-taking opportunities should be provided with the people most important to the patient.
   7. A patient's final moments should be made as meaningful as possible.
B. Family-oriented standards
   1. Family should have opportunities to discuss death, dying, and related emotional needs with the staff.
   2. Family should have opportunities for privacy with the dying person, both while alive and while newly dead.
C. Staff-oriented standards
   1. Caregivers should be given adequate time to establish meaningful relationships with the dying patient.
   2. A mutual support network should exist among staff which allows for discussion relating to technical and social/emotional needs.

These guidelines are standards to aim for. They will not be achieved overnight. All persons involved in health care delivery systems—in institutions or caregiving agencies—need to be educated and supported in their efforts toward planned change. Consultants with special expertise and sensitivity with regard to death and dying issues may become a new breed of catalysts. They surely have not arrived yet, but the groundwork has been laid.

Finally, criteria for selecting death educators need to be defined. Should death educators be psychologists? Is it necessary to experience a death in order to be a death educator? Should death educators be "licensed to practice"? Five standards proposed by Leviton (1977) are presented below.

1. The death educator must have come to terms with his/her own death feelings and be aware of their influence on the total personality.
2. The death educator must be knowledgeable about the appropriate subject matter.
3. The death educator must be able to use the language of death naturally, especially in the presence of the young.
4. The death educator must be familiar with psycho-thanatological developmental events throughout life, and possess an understanding of the concomitant difficulties.
5. The death educator must be cognizant of important social changes and their impact on the attitudes, practices, laws, and institutions concerned with death.

In addition to Leviton's five points, the following two are strongly recommended:

6. The death educator must be aware of his or her goals and potential emotional impact and should select target audiences and methods of instruction accordingly.
7. The death educator should identify local community resources and integrate them into the structure of the course.

Standards can never be static or established with once-and-for-all finality. Standards must be advocated and disseminated vociferously. There are agencies and work groups that help in this process, like the Forum for Death Education and Counseling located in Arlington, Virginia. Besides formulating a code of ethics for death educators and counselors, the forum is also available as a resource to help meet the needs of health caregivers. This is the kind of action profile that must accompany the development of standards and the process of death education within the community.

References

Barton, D., J. Flexner, J. Van Eys, and C. Scott. 1975. Death and Dying: A course for medical students. *Journal of Medical Education* 47:945–951.

Bell, B. 1975. The experimental manipulation of death attitudes: A preliminary investigation. *Omega* 6:199–206.

Bloom, S. 1975. On teaching an undergraduate course on death and dying. *Omega* 6:3, 223–225.

Bugen, L. 1979a. Coping: Effects of death education. *Omega,* in press.

———. 1979b. Death education effects upon death concern stability. *Psychological Reports,* in press.

Hart, J. 1976. Death education and mental health. *Journal of School Health* 46:7, 407–412.

Jeffrey, D. 1977. Death education: Teaching a course on death and dying. Paper presented at the 85th Annual Convention of the American Psychological Association, August 27.

Kastenbaum, R. 1977. *Death, society and human experience.* Saint Louis: C. V. Mosby.

Leonard, V. 1976. Death education in the helping professions. *Australia Journal of Social Issues* 11:2, 108–120.

Leviton, D. 1975. Education for death or death becomes less a stranger. *Omega* 6:3, 183–191.

———. 1977. Death education. In H. Feifel (ed.), *New meanings of death.* New York: McGraw-Hill.

Liston, E. H. 1975. Education on death and dying: A neglected area in the medical curriculum. *Omega* 6:193–198.

Shneidman, E. 1976. *Death: current perspectives.* Palo Alto, California: Mayfield.

Silberman, N. 1976. Effects of thanatology instruction on attitudes and fears about death and dying. Unpublished manuscript. University of Wisconsin, Oshkosh.

Silverman, P. 1976. The widow-to-widow program: An experiment in preventive intervention. In E. Shneidman (ed.), *Death: current perspectives.* Palo Alto, California: Mayfield.

Somerville, R. 1977. Audiovisual materials on aging, death, sex roles. *The Family Coordinator* (January):86–88.

Yalom, I. and C. Greaves. 1977. Group therapy with the terminally ill. *American Journal of Psychiatry* 134:4.

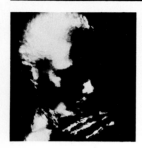

19

Practice

Do you believe that our grandparents or great-grandparents experienced the dying process any differently than we will? If so, how has changing society contributed to this shift? Claire Ryden and Diane Ross explore this shift and suggest organizational alternatives to a dilemma we all shall face. The following Appendix exercises are recommended:

    A.   Announcing One's Own Death

    B.   Appropriate Death Fantasy

Terminal Care: Issues and Alternatives

Claire F. Ryder

Diane M. Ross

As the aim of contemporary medicine moves more clearly to diagnosis and cure, the criterion of rehabilitation potential has been a deciding factor for reimbursable services under Title XVIII of the Social Security Act. However, with the increasing ability of medical technology to prolong life past its natural point, with slight chance of recovery, the prevailing criterion has been questioned. The definition of skilled care in skilled nursing facilities, as published in the September 24, 1975, Federal Register, is that:

> The restoration potential of a patient is not the deciding factor in determining whether a service is to be considered skilled or nonskilled. Even where full recovery or medical improvement is not possible, skilled care may be needed to prevent, to the extent possible, deterioration of the condition or to sustain current capabilities. For example, even though no potential for rehabilitation exists, a terminal cancer patient may require skilled services as defined . . .

Such emphasis is characteristic of an increasing interest in death and dying, by the public as well as health professionals, that has triggered greater attention to the care of the terminally ill generally and the needs of individual dying patients and their families. These needs, ranging from relief of physical pain to emotional support, require services that are not readily met in a conventional hospital or skilled nursing facility. Because the aim of treatment is "to preserve life and to relieve distress, to palliate, to maintain comfortable existence as long as possible" (1), many health professionals have proposed removing terminal patients from a traditional institutional setting. Consequently, these professionals have attempted to create programs in home care and in inpatient facilities specifically geared for terminal patients and their families. These innovations will require a

This material was first published in *Public Health Reports,* U.S. Department of Health Education, and Welfare, vol. 92, no. 1, pp. 20–29, January/ February 1977. It is printed here in slightly modified form by permission.

With the aging thus removed from the nuclear family, the succeeding generations became desensitized to death of the old.

change in federal policy, and, in fact, will demand long-term legislative change, which, in turn, must take into account:

1. The attitude of community leadership, health professionals, and the public to deny the reality of death and needs of the patient and family.
2. Inadequate services to meet the needs of the patient and family.
3. Inadequate financing mechanisms.
4. Inadequate information regarding cost effectiveness of alternatives to traditional institutional care for the terminally ill patient.

Our Changing Society

Basic to our failures in the care of "the terminally ill is the fact that American society in its preoccupation with perpetual youth, beauty, sexuality, and strength has typically disguised, avoided, denied, and embellished death" resulting in alienation of the dying (2a). This isolation has been encouraged by a change in societal institutions, most prevalent of which is the change in family structure, a metamorphosis that followed economic evolution from the extended family to the modern nuclear family. Within the extended family, the processes of the life cycle were an accepted and natural part of daily life, with birth and death on a continuum in nature. Ill persons were cared for in their homes by their families, and the burials of those who died were attended by all members of the family.

With the emergence of industrialization and urbanization, the family ceased to function as the sole support of the individual, resulting in mobility and a schism between occupation and home. The extended family was whittled down as the middle-class young gravitated toward the suburbs and left the old and the poor isolated in urban centers. With the aging thus removed from the nuclear family, the succeeding generations became desensitized to death of the old. In addition, the establishment of hospitals isolated the ill. Therefore, because people rarely saw death, they could avoid it, and in doing so, feared it (2a).

Concurrent with technological changes that altered the family structure were those that altered morbidity and mortality rates. From 1900 to the present, the life expectancy at birth has increased substantially, from 47 to 70 years. However, along with changes in overall death rates came changes in causes of death. Infant and maternal mortality rates have sharply declined, and infectious diseases have been replaced by heart disease and cancer as leading causes (67 percent) of U.S. deaths. Concomitantly, these degenerative diseases are classified as long-term or terminal illness in that the prognosis given indicates a time limit on a person's survival. Thus, a new problem in the health field is the care of persons with lingering illnesses (3).

Professional Attitudes Toward Death and Dying

The present orientation of the medical profession is not in caring for patients afflicted with degenerative diseases but in curing them. Technological breakthroughs in medicine have perpetuated a phenomenon found among health professionals as well as in the society at large, a phenomenon referred to as "death denying." Until recently, this attitude was reflected in the training of physicians and nurses. Recurrent in the medical student's education was the idea that "every death corresponds to a failure, either of the individual physician, or more commonly, of medicine, as a whole" (4a). The student becomes desensitized to death symbols—blood, bone, corpses, and the characteristic stench—and through transference may become desensitized to death itself (4b). In his dedication to the ideals of the scientific community, the physician responds with "vigorous application of laboratory diagnostic tests, technological gadgetry, and heroic therapy in order to prolong life" (4c). Therefore, whereas 50 years ago the physician was considered a member of a consolatory profession, science has now given him omnipotent powers to keep the vital functions of a body operative by artificial means long after the natural course of disease has vitiated these functions.

Thus, the new orientation of physicians reduces . . . the problem to the question: When does death occur? Much of the current literature deals with ethical and legal questions surrounding the point of death and delineates problems that occur when the prolongation of life past its natural point preempts death as a natural process. We are now at the point where considerations of quality of life are secondary to concern about the length of life. Quality of life is a subjective assessment, but when applied to the terminal patient . . . it takes on specific meaning. One can debate whether survival amid tubes and respirators is life at all.

Technological breakthroughs in medicine have perpetuated . . . a phenomenon referred to as "death denying."

Where People Die

As mentioned previously, the home no longer provides a person with an extensive support system. In light of this, it is not surprising that the death rate in institutions has risen considerably over the past decades. Although national statistical studies pertaining to deaths in institutions as opposed to deaths at home are scarce, some state and local data are available. From 1949 to 1958, a 10 percent national increase occurred in institutional deaths, including those in general hospitals, mental hospitals, and nursing homes. New York City statistics reveal an increase from 53,746 institutional deaths in 1955 to 64,083 in 1967, representing a 7 percent increase, and a 7 percent decrease in deaths at home, from 25,598 in 1955 to 21,222 in 1967 (3). Furthermore, there is evidence that this latter figure has decreased rapidly in more recent years.

Paradoxically, a survey of deaths from cancer between 1969 and 1971 in south-central Connecticut showed that 67 percent of these patients had expressed a desire to die at home as opposed to the 20 percent who did die at home. . . . Those in the upper socioeconomic level were more successful in meeting their desires, as were many in the low socioeconomic group, although for disparate reasons. The upper income group had the advantage of personal control, private health insurance, and monetary resources to aid in keeping the patient home. However, the low socioeconomic group and lower-middle class were successful because of reimbursement for care services under Medicaid, as well as support supplied by a cohesive extensive family. The report of this survey, prepared for the National Cancer Institute, identifies the upper-middle class as unique:

> In the upper-middle class, the resources of Medicaid are not available and Medicare is only available for patients over 65. It should also be noted that visiting nurses are most effective in a family situation where there are several primary caregivers to relieve one another from the emotional and physical burdens of the care. In the upper-middle class family, it is our observation that when the family caregiver is a man, he usually keeps on working, ergo the necessity for some form of institutionalization where the upper-middle class has better insurance coverage.

Since 70 percent of institutionalization for the terminally ill pertains to the general hospital, the burden of care is placed largely on the hospital staff (5). However, the organizational structure of the hospital makes care routinized rather than individualized, and is, therefore, frequently inappropriate to the needs of the dying patient. The large teaching hospital's primary functions are diagnosis and treatment of patients with acute illnesses. In contrast, the chronic illness hospital or wing, which houses a large population of dying patients, . . . has difficulty in attracting funding and quality staff. The hierarchy for patient care in a general hospital is (a) acute illness, (b) chronic illness, and (c) terminal illness (6).

The medical staff adheres to this hierarchy in its orientation toward care. As more demands of physical care of those with acute curable illnesses are met, the psychological and emotional needs of the incurable are more often neglected. Physicians tend to view cure as their triumph and death as their failure; they therefore attend to dying patients as prescribed only by duty. Nurses tend to "pull away" from dying patients and to focus more on the diagnostic and curative aspects that are implicit in their trained professional approach to patients (7). According to Sheldon and associates (8):

> . . . conceptual limitations include an inability to perceive and interact with the psychological and social needs of patients and their families, a lack of effective communication among physicians, nurses, and other ward personnel, and a failure to appreciate the emotional and psychological difficulties that characterize the medical staff's reaction to patient problems.

Patients suffering from cancer are often shuttled from one specialist to another, which results in further fragmentation of care rather than an integration of services encompassing the physical, social, and emotional needs of the patient.

Pain is . . . treated with the use of psychopharmacological agents. These agents often replace staff contact, which, in the case of the dying patient, is already minimized. The psychological experience of the patient and family "is deadened by the use of narcotic and analgesic drugs which reinforce the collusion of avoidance rather than enhance the experience of death" (9). The drugs aid in meeting the goal of patient manageability, essential in a busy hospital.

Terminal patients also die in nursing or convalescent homes, many of which are classified as skilled nursing facilities. These facilities are often not oriented to meet the needs of the dying patient, focusing on physical rehabilitation or restoration rather than on the total needs of the patient. In a 1975 survey of 77 nursing homes (10), a majority indicated that they removed deceased patients as clandestinely as possible so as not to disturb the other residents—a practice that seeks to deny death by making it a covert issue.

The result of the institutionalization of dying patients is a phenomenon of "social death" prior to biological death. . . .

Social Death Versus Biological Death

The result of the institutionalization of dying patients is a phenomenon of "social death" prior to biological death. . . . Once the patient has been labeled terminal and the physician has given up hope for recovery, the institution treats the patient as a dying body with little concern for his individuality or humanness. Sudnow (11), in his study of a county hospital, observed:

> When a physician abandons hope for a patient's survival, the nurses establish what they refer to as a "death watch," a fairly severe form of social death in which they keep track of relevant facts concerning the gradual recession of clinical life signs. As death approaches, the patient's status as a body becomes more evident from the manner in which he is discussed, treated, and moved about. Attention shifts from concern about his life, possible discomforts, and the administration of medically prescribed treatments to the mere activity of the events of biological leave-taking.
>
> In a patient who has not yet passed into a death coma, suctioning the nasal passages, propping up pillows, changing bed sheets, and the like occur as part of the normal nursing routine. As blood pressure drops, and signs of imminent death appear, these traditional nursing practices are regarded as less important, the major items of interest become the number of heartbeats and changing condition of the eyes. On many occasions nurses' aides in the county hospital were observed to cease administering oral medications when death was expected within the hour.

When social death precedes biological death in this manner, the needs of the dying patient essentially become secondary to institutional routine. What are these unique needs and how are they met? Hospice, Inc., New

Haven, Conn., in a study of cancer deaths between 1969 and 1971 in the South Central Health Planning Region in Connecticut summarized these needs (5):

> (1) the noxious symptoms of the illness, (2) the need to be with family and friends in familiar surroundings, (3) involvement in decision-making, (4) honest and frequent communication, (5) a need to maintain one's identity and role, (6) freedom from heroic measures which become more of an obstacle to the quality of life than even the disease, (7) need for a staff which understands and helps the patient work through anger and depression in coming to terms with dying, and (8) unattended bereavement which results in physical and/or psychological impairment to the survivors.

In a 1975 symposium on the terminally ill, Dr. Balfour Mount, medical director of the Royal Victoria Hospital's terminal patient ward in Montreal, Canada, noted that each need is interconnected and that all needs essentially signify relief from pain. Although all else is secondary to physical pain and must be dealt with before any other consideration, a hospital environment often limits the definition of pain to somatic. An expanded definition would include mental, financial, interpersonal, and spiritual aspects of pain. The dying patient may experience a sense of isolation, especially in a hospital setting, because of a lack of comfort and communication with medical personnel and family. Physicians, in avoiding the reality of death and projecting their fears onto the patient, often choose not to disclose the prognosis of impending death to the patient. Hence, an aura of deceit and covertness hampers the patient's ability to cope with his situation and to take care of unfinished business.

Coping with Dying and Death

The coping process involves several stages, the transition from one to another being facilitated by a neutral uninvolved party, be it physician, nurse, social worker, professional counselor, member of the clergy, or understanding volunteer. The stages, as outlined by Ross (12), are (a) denial, (b) anger, (c) bargaining, and (d) acceptance, each with its unique reactions and communication patterns. The patient experiences these various emotions in regard to his finiteness, successes, failures, family, all tied together into a package of fear, guilt, and an intense desire, on the part of many, to remain independent. The concerns of dying patients, of course, vary with age—the young girl feeling alienated from companions, the mother worried about the burden on her family and the safety of her children, the successful businessman concerned about his finances—all essentially emphasizing the need to retain a unique identity. This realization of individuality is in conflict with the treatment of only the physical discomfort of the deteriorating body rather than the whole human being with a past and a present.

The mental anguish of a person approaching death is intrinsically bound to interpersonal communication with those who are close to him, usually the family. In actuality, the needs of the family are so closely interwoven with the patient's needs that to deny the former is to hinder the patient's process of acceptance. Indeed, often the family must experience the same mental stages as the patient's. Communication is enhanced by a realistic, honest expression of feeling through which both the patient and family are relieved of guilt. Often a "game" is played between spouses that consists of hiding knowledge of impending death from each other. Until both parties can communicate and share this knowledge, progress toward mutual acceptance of the inevitable is halted. Again, each patient and family unit's problems and the manner in which they are most appropriately handled are unique.

Financial considerations are an undeniable aspect of the problems of coping with terminal illness. According to a Department of Health, Education, and Welfare Report of the Task Force on Medicaid and Related Programs (cited by Pollack 13), "the catastrophically ill are at almost any income level where insurance benefits (including the most liberal major medical coverage) do not cover the cost of sustaining expensive, long-term illnesses." Generally, those under 65 years of age are not eligible for Medicare and those above a certain income level (specified by each state) are not covered by Medicaid. A study by Cancer Care, Inc., in 1973 (14), revealed that the median cost incurred by the families of cancer patients was $19,055, which is 2 2/3 times more than the median family income of $8,000. Such universal inability to meet the high cost of hospitalization, surgery, and other treatment strikes hard at the nerve of the patient's guilt, as he may feel personally responsible for the foregone education of a child or the general depletion of the family funds for the future. Financial difficulties may trigger maladjustments as family members may be forced to adopt new roles; for example, housewife turned sole supporter.

Of course, the spiritual needs of a patient are an individual matter. Each person copes with religion or the absence of religion in his own way. Although some attempt to deal with death as the cessation of existence of the mind and body, many patients need to view their death in a religious context, either in relation to a deity or to nature, or both. There are as many perceptions of death as there are people, including concepts such as an indestructible soul, continuation with nature, reunion with Christ, or continuity through survivors. Each patient should be encouraged to express his feelings about death.

The ultimate culmination of a dying person's needs is dignity of personhood in living and in death. . . . "Death with dignity" . . . implies [to some] accepting death, [to] others, . . . dying in the fashion in which one lived; for example, a hostile person would die with the grudge he carried with him through life. Nevertheless, the crux of dying with dignity is in retaining one's individuality, be that in acceptance or denial, anger or serenity, without the humiliation of unnecessary life-prolonging machines.

> . . . the crux of dying with dignity is in retaining one's individuality, be that in acceptance or denial, anger or serenity, without the humiliation of unnecessary life-prolonging machines.

Although the concerns of the patient cease with the end of his life, the problems of the family linger; in fact, they often intensify with the patient's death. The length and pattern of bereavement are contingent upon the relationship of the survivor to the deceased and the degree to which communication channels were open during the dying process of the patient, relating to identification with the patient, working through ambivalent feelings, and the satisfaction of mutual dependency needs (15). Hospital environments seldom are conducive to laying the groundwork for a normal bereavement period as relatives are rushed in and out at prescribed visiting hours, children are not allowed to visit patients, and there are incidents of the family being pushed into the hallways while the patient is pronounced dead by a hurried physician who is not capable of dealing with the emotional reaction of the family.

The Hospice Concept

In attempts to deal with all these very special needs of the dying patient and his family, various plans in the United States and Canada have adopted the paradigm of caring for the total patient and family needs with the ideals set forth in the hospice concept. This concept is used in two British facilities which serve as prototypes. Saunders (16), medical director of the largest of these models, St. Christophers' Hospice in London, speaks of the goals of this concept as individualization of death and relief of distress:

> The name hospice, "a resting place for travellers or pilgrims," was chosen because this will be something between a hospital and a home, with the skills of the one and the hospitality, warmth, and the time available of the other and beds without invisible parking meters beside them. We aim, above all, to recognise the interest and importance of the individual who must be helped to *live* until he dies and who, as he does so in his own way, will find his "own" death with quietness and acceptance. A staff who recognise this as their criterion of success will not find this work negative or discouraging and will know that it is important, both in its own right and also in all the implications it holds for the rest of medicine and, indeed, the rest of life.

St. Christopher's Hospice is a 54-bed inpatient facility for people who are in the advanced stages of neurological and malignant diseases. The foremost concern is the relief of the symptoms that often become so closely interwoven with mental anguish. Common problems in addition to pain are nausea and vomiting, constipation, diarrhea, anorexia, and anticholinergic effects. It is essential that the patient be as symptom-free as possible, so that the dying does not derive from the symptoms rather than the disease. Tension and anxiety can result from the common practice of withholding medication until the pain has become incapacitating. Furthermore, this may cause the patient to become dependent, not only on the drug but on the person who administers it. St. Christopher's Hospice makes a practice of giving a fixed dosage continually in anticipation of the pain so that the patient never knows the severe potential of the pain. A common pain killer used for this purpose is Brompton's Mixture, a concoction of heroin, cocaine, alcohol, and fruit syrup—understandably, the possibility of addiction is not of concern. In addition, steroids are used to enhance the sense of well-being, to improve the appetite, to relieve pain and lower the narcotic dose, to reduce inflammation, and to alleviate weakness. In short, great care is given to the relief of pain and, in turn, to relieve mental anguish and to facilitate awareness of the experience of living until death.

The importance of living until death as a positive fulfillment necessitates an interdisciplinary staff. Each aspect of care is essential to meet the goal of total patient and family unit, including physical, mental, interpersonal, and spiritual elements. As the primary evaluator and prescriber of a medication regimen, the physician is an essential member of the hospice team. His concern for the patient's mental and physical comfort moves him to open channels of communication. As Cotter observes (17):

> In ways unique to the relationship with each individual patient, caring enables the doctor to discern the patient's desire to discuss the future course of his illness, the nearness of his death, and the circumstances which may surround it, as well as the ways in which his family may best be supported in bearing this knowledge.

This sharing allows both the patient and family to discuss matters openly and permits them to "say goodbye," which studies have revealed as important. The physician is essentially in an omnipotent position to help this exchange or to "inflict wounds by his own thoughtlessness or need to hurry away from something that is very hard to witness" (18).

In the hospice, the nursing staff must be sensitive to the elements of human dignity. They must be aware of individual differences and responses in personal care because many patients have become quite helpless, and the nurses must convey feelings of compassion and understanding for the person's integrity and retention of uniqueness. The nurses must relay any changes in the patient's condition to the physician, so that appropriate adjustments may be made in medication as well as to the patient's daily needs for food and fluid intake, oral hygiene, and body positioning. Cotter points this out (17):

> Taking time to explain procedures, to honor preferences, to respect privacy and modesty, to consult with the patient concerning his feelings and his needs, to involve him in social and recreational activities and in small celebrations reflect the nurse's recognition of the patient's personal worth and convey to him the certainty that he still matters, that he has not been "written off" as finished.

The emphasis on religion in this therapeutic community takes on a new meaning of the spiritual. At St. Chrisopher's, a church-based institution, there is an involvement of clergy and other church-based personnel whose

In the hospice, the nursing staff must be sensitive to the elements of human dignity.

vocation is founded in such work. However, there is an active application of McMurray's definition of religion that "it is the field of personal relationships between people prepared to give themselves to each other in the context of a common life" (19a). The religious commitment of St. Christopher's is thus manifested in its very existence as a community of vulnerable, caring, and involved people, including professionals, volunteers, patients, families, and visitors.

Although substantial attention is given to inpatient care within the physical structure of St. Christopher's, where 400 patients die each year, 10 to 15 percent of the patients are discharged home for a period of time before death. The staff realizes the value of home care by allowing the patient to feel a part of his family and to return to a relative degree of normalcy, however limited and temporary.

In essence, St. Christopher's Hospice has successfully combined the art of medicine . . . with the science of medicine, to assuage the pains of patients as they approach death and . . . [to help] families. The prevailing ideology is succinctly summed up in Saunders' assessment (19b): "There is a stage when the treatment of a hemorrhage is not another transfusion, but adequate sedation, or someone who will not go away but will stay and hold a hand."

An American Model

In an attempt to fill the existing gap in the health care system regarding services for the terminally ill, various facilities and organizations have incorporated the ideals of St. Christopher's Hospice. The most successful U.S. model to date is Hospice, Inc. of New Haven, Conn. Under a National Cancer Institute grant, a 44-bed inpatient facility for cancer patients is being planned. Using St. Christopher's Hospice as a model, Hospice, Inc. services are meant to (5):

(1) provide medical care for the continuing control of symptoms such as pain, nausea, anorexia, etc.; (2) concentrate on bedside nursing to provide comfort, close attention to easing physical distress, slow lengthy encounters that allow for the patient's care, interpersonal interactions, attention to feeding, emotional support, etc.; (3) focus on the family unit and allow the patient and family to use the assets of their life-style to cope with the situation; (4) include the patient and family by being very careful to develop good open communications; (5) involve the community by including volunteers, many of whom are widows or widowers, in varied activities from assisting with patient care to gardening, assisting in the day-care center, helping in the business office; (6) provide spiritual care through ecumenical services, discussion groups, and through an atmosphere of love and concern; (7) include an outpatient and inpatient program to provide a comprehensive program to meet different patient/family needs; (8) have a carefully constructed facility which fosters a spirit of friendliness, encourages individuals to participate in life, and is more homelike than hospitals; and (9) have built-in supports for staff and volunteers so that they can carry on a demanding work.

Since March 1974, Hospice, Inc. has serviced 85 families through its home care program, guided by the philosophy that, it is hoped, will continue through completion of the inpatient facility—that the patient should be maintained in the home as long as possible before being institutionalized. The program is under the medical direction of Dr. Sylvia Lack, who heads a staff consisting of two part-time physicians, six registered nurses, two licensed practical nurses, a social worker, a director of volunteers, and an admissions registrar. Consultant staff includes a clinical pharmacologist, a psychiatrist, a radiologist, and a physical therapist. In addition, there are 50 volunteers who had been carefully screened and given extensive orientation before they were assigned to specific patients. The home care program is coordinated with hospitals in the vicinity and includes medical and nursing consultation and family counseling and pain consultation and services on a 24-hour-a-day basis. All staff members are available on call, through an answering and paging service—an essential element, not only for complete service but for the confidence of the patient and family unit of care. Eligibility for participation requires residence within a specific geographic area and is contingent upon a referral from a primary care physician who is involved throughout the duration of the patient's illness.

> **Studies have revealed that people prefer to die at home. . . .**

The success of Hospice, Inc. has established the program as a national demonstration center and has encouraged other medical and nursing personnel to investigate possibilities for establishment of similar programs in their respective geographic locations. One such program operates under the title Hospice of Santa Barbara, Inc., a nonprofit voluntary agency incorporated in December 1974. Since September 1975, it has been operating as an information and referral service for those terminal patients and their families who suffer from uncontrolled pain of a physical, psychological, social, or spiritual nature. No special plans have been made as yet regarding an inpatient facility, because the present focus is on the home care program, which started on a pilot basis on December 1, 1975. The program was certified as a home health agency with contracts with two visiting nurse associations for the provision of skilled nursing care. The personnel of Hospice of Santa Barbara include a medical social worker, a part-time physician, a part-time pharmacist, a medical records librarian, and an executive director.

Other Care Programs

This emphasis on home care must not be underplayed. Studies have revealed that people prefer to die at home or, at least, remain at home for as long as possible, for they often feel lonely and isolated within a sterile institutional setting. Within this framework, an increasing number of institutions which do not care for the terminal patient within the facility, for monetary or other reasons, nevertheless do provide home care services. In addition to being psychologically preferred by many patients, it appears

. . . many institutions have incorporated the ideals set forth by St. Christopher's Hospice within a conventional hospital setting. . . .

from informal statements that the cost factor for home care is well below that of hospitalization. For example, Dr. Balfour Mount . . . claimed that his hospital's home care program saves the equivalent of $100,000 per year as compared to the cost of hospitalization. Jack Lally of the Cardinal Ritter Institute of St. Louis, Mo., a home health agency, cited the following comparative figures based on the actual cost of home care for 140 terminally ill patients for about 4 months in contrast to what the cost would have been for varying patterns of care for that same period in 1972:

Source of care	Cost
Home	$ 94,000
Hospital	1,768,000
Nursing home	350,000
Home and last 2 weeks in hospital	162,000

Although it is apparent that home care is both economically and psychologically feasible, it is not adequate by itself—rather, it is most effective when used in conjuction with some type of facility, be it hospital, nursing home, or hospice. There often comes a point when a family is no longer able to keep the patient at home for medical or emotional reasons. In fact, there is often an interplay throughout the illness between institutional and home care. This shuffle between hospital, home, and nursing home poses a problem in reimbursement policies under Medicare in that admission to a skilled nursing facility after a prolonged stay at home must be preceded by a 3-day hospital stay before reimbursement can be made.

As the movement for hospices has grown, many institutions have incorporated the ideals set forth by St. Christopher's Hospice within a conventional hospital setting, as a separate ward for the terminally ill. Lamerton cites Saunders' support for a separate unit of care (20):

> A unit for patients with advanced or terminal cancer does not have the challenge of diagnosis nor difficult decisions to make concerning radical treatment. It does not have the interest and encouragement of cure and only rarely of remission, but it is easier for its workers to look at their patients as people, to spend time with their relatives and concentrate on the relief of distress whenever it appears. Above all, it should be easier for them to give a patient the kind of unhurried attention he needs so greatly.

This is the philosophy behind the Life Acceptance Program in the Pinecrest Hospital of Santa Barbara, Calif. Within this unit, which has a fairly rapid turnover, there are from 6 to 12 patients at any one time. Two problems exist: (*a*) because of staffing needs and other undefined logistical reasons, the unit is required to include stroke rehabilitation; this presents a conflict since the rehabilitative needs of the stroke patient are quite divergent from the needs of terminal patients, who have no rehabilitative potential; and (*b*) frequently physicians do not assess patients as terminally ill until they are semicomatose, thus giving the staff a brief and inadequate 48 to 72 hours to get to know a patient and his family. Because such care for patient and family is not begun until the patient is transferred to this special ward, fragmented care results.

A strong argument is made by Lamerton against the isolation of the dying in a general hospital (20):

> I do not see a special terminal ward within a general hospital as a good solution, either. Those nurses who did not want to do this kind of work would dread being posted to the ward and would not be the right people to work in it. Matron (or do I mean the chief, principal senior, or nursing officer?) would be overheard to say, "I can't help it, we have three nurses off sick in the acute surgical ward; they'll just have to be brought from the Dead End." Consequently, the terminal unit would be permanently understaffed.

Another case is made against the segregation of the terminally ill in the philosophy and practice of Veterans Administration programs for these patients. Their policy is that such isolation is highly detrimental since the patient is thus labeled as dying or "hopeless." Others have verbalized this objection, which appears to be valid when viewed within the context of a society that has not, on the whole, considered death a natural process. With this in mind, indeed such labeling can be deleterious.

Thus, the third alternative to employing the hospice concept is the hospital that does not segregate its terminally ill but caters to their special needs. One such plan is used at the Harrisburg (Pa.) Hospital, a 450-bed general hospital, where the success is attributed to one nurse, Joy Ufema. She, dubbed the "death and dying specialist," claims that the hospice concept is more dependent on an administrative commitment than on an edifice. Working as the patient's advocate, she has developed the skill of listening, allowing the patient to make his own decisions by asking: What do you need? Whom do you need? When do you need it? She then proceeds to satisfy these needs, with the help of a very cooperative social service department and the patient's family.

The Harrisburg model is used by hospitals that have some plans for a terminal unit, but for financial and logistical reasons, the plans remain long range. There are indications that some members of hospital staffs, often a member of the clergy, are attempting to attend to dying patients in a unique way. Rev. Leroy Joesten, pastoral care director of Lutheran General Hospital, Park Ridge, Ill., in a personal communication, described the staff's orientation:

> It is important to say that our hospital's approach to care of the dying is to deal with it in the total context of care and treatment of a disease. Hence, each of our medical and surgical units functions from a multidisciplinary model directed at "total patient care." This total care attempts to address terminal care needs for patients, family, and staff as well as curative and palliative care needs.

. . . the third alternative to employing the hospice concept is the hospital that does not segregate its terminally ill but caters to their special needs.

. . . building hospices may benefit only a minority . . . while simultaneously diverting attention from demands that need to be met within hospitals.

The key to this type of care is a commitment by the entire staff—administration, medical, nursing, and social service. However, the feasibility within the framework of a general hospital is dubious because, as previously discussed, hospitals are routinized for the purpose of curing the acutely ill. Catering to dying patients' needs is often at the risk of disrupting patterns that, perhaps, were created for efficient and effective treatment of those with rehabilitative potential. The individual needs of terminal patients seemed to be best tended outside such an environment.

Cost Factor

The case for the viability of a hospice as a freestanding facility can be argued on two fronts: (*a*) care effectiveness and (*b*) cost effectiveness. Thus far, most of the literature has dealt with the effective care factor. It has been shown that the present orientation of medical personnel, hospitals, and nursing homes . . . is incompatible with hospice ideals. The cost factor has only been estimated without the aid of a formalized study. Lack (21) projects a cost of $105 a day in New Haven for a hospice room in 1977–78, the planned completion date for the inpatient facility. This figure should be compared with an estimated $190 a day in a general hospital in that vicinity, at that projected time. The cost differential is attributed to a hospital's overhead costs due to "the operating rooms, the specialized care areas, the machines for extending life beyond its natural term" (21). Although services that are integral to patient assessment and treatment will be included, such as a pharmacy with a full-time pharmacist to provide the pain-control medication needs, diagnostic radiology, oxygen, suction systems available at every bed, and a small laboratory to conduct the most frequently administered testing procedures, Hospice, Inc., of New Haven will rely on neighboring hospitals for services such as chemotherapy, palliative radiation therapy, and surgical units, if necessary.

The cost factor also includes the price of erecting special structures. Hospice's 1975 annual report quotes $1,325,000 for planning and building the facility. The consideration to be made is whether the amount saved over general hospitalization costs merits the high cost of building new facilities when there is a plethora of beds in existing community hospitals. In a 1975 lecture in Branford, Conn., Mount cited a possible impracticality in reference to St. Christopher's Hospice, which serves 54 patients within a 6-mile radius: "This does not encompass even half the target population and leaves 70 percent of the patients in need dying in institutions." Thus, . . . building hospices may benefit only a minority of those in need while simultaneously diverting attention from demands that need to be met within hospitals.

Summary and Conclusion

The most desired goal for patients and concerned health professionals is home care for the terminally ill. The familiar surroundings and faces help to relieve the psychological suffering encountered in the dying process and allow freer communication channels between patient and family. However, it is apparent that during some point in the last weeks of life the patient may require closer medical supervision for pain relief, or the family may not be able to continue care once the patient has reached a certain phase, thereby warranting some type of institutionalization. The present choices are, basically, acute-care hospital or nursing home, but, as presently structured, these settings are too often inappropriate to satisfying needs of the terminal patient and family unit. An innovative yet long-awaited alternative is . . . the hospice concept, which aims at anticipatory pain relief as well as . . . psychological . . . terminal care.

No extensive cost effectiveness study has yet been undertaken comparing hospital and hospice costs, taking into account the cost of planning and construction. . . . Such a study would have implications for possible legislative changes regarding the 3-day hospitalization requirement for Medicare reimbursement. If . . . the cost of hospitalizing for 3 days before hospice care is greater than direct admittance to the hospice, it should not be classified as a posthospital extended-care benefit for Medicare purposes but rather as a separate category of care facility that would need to be defined.

Because the development of hospices is a long-range goal and hospices may be able to serve only a portion of the target population, short-term goals should focus on ameliorating conditions for the terminally ill within existing hospitals and long-term care facilities. To do this, an extensive educational program should be organized in medical schools and in institutions, not only to teach methods of pain control and how to deal with dying patients, but also to enhance the concept of death as a natural process. Instruction dealing with psychological management should be an integral part of the training of physicians and nurses, as should continuing education of the same content for hospital staff.

As stated by Schoenberg and Carr (2b):

> Many university and teaching hospitals hold "death conferences" when a patient dies in order to determine if any additional efforts could have been expended in order to prolong the life of the individual patient. An appropriate parallel would be a "life conference" preceding death to determine what steps should be taken to assist the patient, family, and hospital personnel in managing the painful feeling of grief, guilt, depression, anxiety, and anger.

Of course, some professionals perhaps have a greater affinity than others for working with dying patients and their families. These people should be engaged as specialists in terminal care and be responsible for in-

The most desired goal for patients and concerned health professionals is home care for the terminally ill.

tegrating efforts for a system of continuity of care. The result, it is hoped, would be an increased ability on the part of health professionals to recognize the unique and individual needs of these patients within an acute-care hospital. Although all hospital staff should be sensitized to problems in terminal care, the most effective management should probably take place in a separate ward where all staff would be specialists. Such a ward should be an appendage to the hospital in structure only and operate under a different routine and set of regulations that are more applicable to terminal care than to acute care. In short, the goal is to use existing facilities and expedite proper and appropriate care as a hospice within a hospital until such time that hospices are established in geographic areas where they are able to serve a large enough segment of the target population to be cost-effective.

Because Medicare primarily covers people over age 65, a definite gap exists between reimbursement policies and the reality of occurrence of terminal illness, inclusive of all degenerative diseases. A large number of these diseases occur in people under 65, including children. The costs of care are so exorbitant that these illnesses are correctly categorized as "catastrophic" in regard to the devastating effect on patient and family, emotionally and financially. Legislative policy should parallel the need of a large segment of the population who are unable to meet the costs incurred by a long illness that ends in death. Just as patients with end-stage renal disease are eligible for reimbursement under Medicare, so should those afflicted with other catastrophic illnesses. The combined efforts of legislative change, educational programs, and realistic institutional changes . . . should aim at overcoming the defense mechanisms in the presence of death—denial, withdrawal, and avoidance—which manifest themselves in present institutional and professional practices.

References

1. Weisman, A. C. Psychosocial considerations in terminal care. In *Psychosocial aspects of terminal care.* Columbia University Press, New York, 1972, p. 163.
2. Schoenberg, B., and Carr, A. C. Educating the health professionals in the psychosocial care of the terminally ill. In *Psychosocial aspects of terminal care.* Columbia University Press, 1972; (*a*) p. 9, (*b*) p. 13.
3. Lerner, M. When, why, and where people die. In *The dying patient.* Russell Sage Foundation, New York, 1970, pp. 12–16.
4. Rabin, D. and Rabin, L. Consequences of death for physicians, nurses, and hospitals. In *The dying patient.* Russell Sage Foundation, New York, 1970; (*a*) p. 174, (*b*) p. 175, (*c*) p. 181.
5. Nelson, R. J. Hospice: An alternative solution to the problem of caring for the dying patient. *Colloquy,* March 1974, pp. 22–23.
6. Olin, H. S. Failure and fulfillment: Education in the use of psychoactive drugs in the dying patient. In *Psychopharmacologic agents for the terminally ill and bereaved.* Foundation of Thanatology; distributed by Columbia University Press, New York, 1973.
7. Glaser, B. G., and Strauss, A. *Awareness of dying.* Aldine Publishing Co., Chicago, 1965, p. 86.
8. Sheldon, A., Ryser, C. P., and Krant, M. J. An integrated family oriented cancer care program: The report of a pilot project in the socio-emotional management of chronic disease. *J. Chronic Dis.* 22: 743–755, April 1970.
9. Klerman, G. L. Drugs and the dying patient. In *Psychopharmacologic agents for the terminally ill and bereaved.* Foundation of Thanatology; distributed by Columbia University Press, New York, 1973, p. 15.

10. Koff, T. H. Social rehearsal for death and dying. *J. Long Term Care Admin.* 3: 42–53, summer 1975.
11. Sudnow, D. Dying in a public hospital. In *The dying patient.* Russell Sage Foundation, New York, 1970, p. 194.
12. Ross, E. K. *On death and dying.* The Macmillan Company, New York, 1969.
13. Pollack, J. Observations on the economics of illness. In *Proceedings* of the Fourth National Symposium on Catastrophic Illness in the Seventies. Cancer Care, Inc., New York, 1971, p. 26.
14. Cancer Care, Inc. *The impact, cost and consequences of catastrophic illness on patients and families.* New York, 1973, p. 54.
13. Maddison, D., and Raphael, B. The family of the dying patient. In *Psychosocial aspects of terminal care.* Columbia University Press, New York, 1972, pp. 188–209.
16. Saunders, C. Terminal patient care. *Geriatrics* 21: 70, 74, December 1966.
17. Cotter, Z. M. Institutional care of the terminally ill. *Hosp. Prog.* 52: 42–48, June 1971.
18. Saunders, C. *The management of terminal illness.* Hospital Medicine Publications, Ltd., London 1967, p. 23.
19. Saunders, C. The patient's response to treatment. In *Proceedings* of the Fourth National Symposium on Catastrophic Illness in the Seventies. Cancer Care, Inc., New York, 1971; (*a*) p. 35, (*b*) p. 39.
20. Lamerton, R. C. The need for hospices. *Nursing Times,* Jan. 23, 1975, p. 156.
21. Lack, S. Death with dignity at home. *Washington Post,* Nov. 16, 1975.

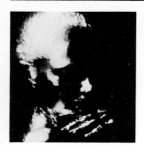

20

Practice

I magine being burned so extensively that your chances for survival are almost nil. What would you expect from the medical team responsible for caring for you? Imbus and Zawacki face this dilemma daily as members of a health care delivery team. When you have completed this chapter, the following Appendix exercises may be particularly helpful:

      A.   Announcing One's Own Death

      B.   Appropriate Death Fantasy

      F.   Euthanasia Exercise

Autonomy for Burned Patients when Survival is Unprecedented

Sharon H. Imbus

Bruce E. Zawacki

No burn is certainly fatal until the patient dies; the most severely burned patient may speak of hope with his last breath. Unable to prophesy, and unwilling to strip the patient of any hope he may cherish, we therefore prefer to diagnose burns as "fatal" or "hopeless" only in retrospect. Every year, however, several patients are admitted to our burn center with injuries so severe that survival is not only unexpected but, to our knowledge, unprecedented. Although difficult to face, the problems that these patients present must be anticipated and not simply ignored.

The surgical literature gives little attention to these patients except for brief phrases allowing an occasional glimpse into a particular surgeon's philosophy.[1-3] The literature on death and dying, voluminous since Kübler-Ross's work,[4] offers rich background but says little about the unique situation of our patients who, after their injury, often have only a few hours of mental clarity in which to respond to their predicament. Several recent articles about withholding intensive care seem to ignore or incompletely answer the problem of obtaining the patient's informed consent. In some of these discussions, the authors simply assign to the physician what we believe to be the patient's ultimate right to decide whether he will or will not receive a particular form of therapy.[5-7] One suggests, perhaps unconstitutionally, that "certain competent patients" may be excluded from such decision making "when, in the physician's judgment, the patient will probably be unable to cope with it psychologically."[8] Still others, who recognize patient primacy in such decision making, offer no practical suggestion how it is best honored in practice.[9]

Our approach, developed empirically over several years, is based on our conviction that the decision to begin or to withhold maximal therapeutic effort is more of an ethical than a medical judgment. The physi-

This material was first published in *The New England Journal of Medicine,* vol. 297, no. 6, pp. 308-311, August 11, 1977. Copyright 1977 The Massachusetts Medical Society. Reprinted by permission.

. . . the patient may give or withhold his consent to receive a particular form of therapy . . . before communication and competence are seriously impaired by intubation or altered states of consciousness.

cian and his colleagues on the burn-care team present to the patient the appropriate medical and statistical facts together with authoritative medical opinion about the available therapeutic alternatives and their consequences. Thus informed, the patient may give or withhold his consent to receive a particular form of therapy, but it is his own decision based on his value system, and it is arrived at before communication and competence are seriously impaired by intubation or altered states of consciousness.

Definitions and Methods

The patient whose management this paper addresses is characterized by some combination of massive burns, severe smoke inhalation, or advanced age. Such a patient's condition is designated by ''1'' on the Bull Mortality Probability Chart[10] and ''0'' in the National Burn Information Exchange Survival Analysis Diagrams,[11] both indicating nonsurvival from the indexes of age and percentage of body-surface area burned. Furthermore, our staff members cannot, from their own experience, our burn-unit statistics, or references from the literature, recall survival in a similar patient.

To allow the patient maximal clarity of thought in decision making, several points must be communicated to the paramedic teams in the field and to local hospitals who transfer burned patients to our burn center immediately after injury: no administration of morphine or other narcotics before arrival; prompt fluid resuscitation; oxygen administration in treatment of possible carbon monoxide intoxication; avoidance of tracheostomy or endotracheal-tube insertion unless absolutely necessary to preserve the airway and maintain ventilation; and rapid transportation to the burn center.

Upon admission of a patient for whom survival seems in doubt, the burn center's most experienced physician is consulted, day or night, to evaluate the patient. His assessment, combined with a social and family history, is presented to all involved team members. Standard works are rechecked to determine if there has ever been a precedent for survival.

When the diagnosis is confirmed, the physician and other team members enter the room. Family members are not invited into the room to ensure that the decision of the patient is specifically his own. In an attempt to establish a relation with the patient, the attending physician or resident under his guidance tries to assume the role of a compassionate friend who is willing to listen. Hands are often held, and an effort is made to look deeply into the patient's eyes to perceive the unspoken questions that may lie there. Nonverbal cues are watched for closely. The presence of the burn team serves to witness and validate the patient's desires and requests, gives consensus to the gravity of the situation and supports the physician member of the team in this delicate, painful task.

At times, when the question of impending death does not spontaneously arise, suggestions such as ''You are seriously ill'', ''You are sicker than you have ever been" or "Your life is in immediate danger" may be made, always in a caring, gentle way.

Some patients will not respond because of coma or mental incompetency. In those circumstances, the burn team and the family confer, again in a compassionate, concerned relation. All attempts are made to determine and do what the patient would be most likely to want if he were able to communicate.

A few patients will hear but not listen because of a need to deny their predicament. In general, such denials, if persistent, are considered an expression of a strong desire to live, and the patients are treated accordingly with maximal therapeutic effort.

A large majority of patients, however, understand the gravity of their situation and make further inquiries. The very frequent question—"Am I going to die?"—is answered truthfully by the statement, "We cannot predict the future. We can only say that, to our knowledge, no one in the past of your age and with your size of burn has ever survived this injury, either with or without maximal treatment." At this point, those who interpret this diagnosis of a burn without precedent of survival as an indication to avoid heroic measures typically become quite peaceful. Regularly, they then try to live their lives completely and fully to the end, saying things that they must say to those important to them, making proper plans, reparations and apologies and, in general, obtaining what Kavanaugh refers to as "permission to die."[2] These patients receive only ordinary medical measures and sufficient amounts of pain medication to assure comfort after their choice is made explicit. Fluid resuscitation is discontinued, they are admitted to a private room, and visiting hours become unlimited. An experienced nurse and, frequently, a chaplain are in constant attendance, using their expertise to comfort and sustain the patient and his family, chiefly by their continued presence and willingness to listen.

The patients who understand that survival is unprecedented in their case but, nevertheless, choose a maximal therapeutic effort are admitted to the burn intensive-care unit. Fluid resuscitation is continued, and full treatment measures are instituted, as with any other patient in the unit. As with those who choose only ordinary care, however, they may change their minds at any time; their decision is reviewed with them on a daily basis.

In general, when patients are mentally incompetent on admission because of head injury or inhalation injury or some other injury and may reasonably be expected to remain so indefinitely, the socially designated next of kin or other relatives are allowed to speak for the patient.[13] With children who are legally incompetent because of age, however, we have for the past five years been unwilling to declare any burn as being without precedent of survival, chiefly because mortality rates for very large burns in pediatric patients appear to be improving more rapidly than can be reported.

After interviewing the patient or his family, the physician is responsible for recording the salient points and decision in the patient's chart. Accurate

. . . those who interpret this diagnosis of a burn without precedent of survival as an indication to avoid heroic measures typically become quite peaceful.

documentation serves to clarify communication with other team members and avoids legal ambiguity.

"Postvention," described by Shneidman as "those activities which serve to reduce the aftereffects of a traumatic event in the lives of survivors,"[4] is now being evolved on our unit. Nurses are learning how to help survivors comfort each other and, together with the chaplain and social worker, are arranging for safe transportation of the bereaved to their homes, counseling families on the difficult matters of explaining death to children and explaining such points as legal necessity of an unwanted autopsy. Our hospital chaplain is available to conduct the funeral services if the family does not have its own pastor. He gets in touch with the families on the first anniversary of their loved one's death to answer any unfinished questions that may have been bothering them. The social worker also offers her continuing services to the bereaved.

Results

During 1975 and 1976 there were 748 dispositions from our burn center, excluding readmissions, transfers, and nonthermal injuries. Of these patients, 126 died—18 children and 108 adults. Of the adults who died, 24, or 22 percent, were diagnosed on admission as having injury without precedent of survival. Twenty-one of these patients or their families chose nonheroic, or ordinary, medical care. Only three chose full treatment measures, and their desires were fulfilled.

The following case histories illustrate our approach.

Cases 1 and 2. Two sisters, 68 and 70 years of age, and their husbands were searching for a schizophrenic daughter who had disappeared after her discharge from a psychiatric hospital. While their car waited for a stoplight, a nearby construction machine hit a gasoline line. The spraying gas exploded, leveling a city block and igniting the car.

The sisters arrived in our burn center two hours later. The younger sister had 91 percent full-thickness, 92 percent total-body burn, with moderate smoke inhalation; the older had 94.5 percent full-thickness, 95.5 percent total-body burn, with severe smoke inhalation. The burn team agreed that survival was unprecedented in both cases. Both women were alert and interviewed separately.

The younger sister asked about death directly, looking intently into the physician's eyes. When he answered, she replied matter-of-factly, "Well, I never dreamed that life would end like this, but since we all have to go sometime, I'd like to go quietly and comfortably. I don't know what to do about my daughter . . ."

After she was made comfortable, the nurse obtained a description of the missing daughter and possible whereabouts. The social worker alerted the police to look for her and telephoned relatives, informing them of the accident as gently as could be conveyed by telephone. The husbands were located at another burn unit. An attempt was made to arrange a final spousal conversation, but both husbands were intubated.

Meanwhile, the older sister doubted whether her injuries were as serious as reported. "I feel so good, wouldn't I be hurting horribly if I were going to die?" The effect of full-thickness burns on nerve endings was explained. The physician reiterated that we wished to do what she thought was best for her. She hedged, "What did my sister say? I'll go along with her decision." Since the patient seemed unsure of her decision, she was offered full therapy in the room with her sister. She then refused the therapy adamantly but denied that she was dying.

The sisters' beds were placed next to each other so that they could see and touch each other easily. They discussed funeral arrangements and then joked, in the next breath, about the damage done to their hair. The hospital chaplain prayed with them. By active listening, he was able to convey to the older that her husband was not to blame for the accident as she had thought. "It's good to go out not cursing him after all our years together," she said. The younger sister died several hours later after her sister lapsed into a coma; the older died the next day. The daughter was not located.

Case 3. A 58-year-old man was cleaning his kitchen with an aerosol when the fumes were ignited by the stove pilot. He arrived at the hospital one hour later with a 97 percent full-thickness burn, severe smoke inhalation, and corneal abrasions. The team consensus that survival was unprecedented was unanimous. When the physicians talked with him, the man replied that he preferred his wife and her mother-in-law to decide for him. His wife and her mother, stunned and horrified by the accident, refused. Further conversation with the patient revealed that he wished to live by any and all means "until God is ready for me." In the burn intensive-care unit he required a tracheostomy and respirator. He continued to communicate, although imperfectly, by "writing" letters in the air. Despite an armamentarium of intensive nursing care, a cardiac-output monitor, silver nitrate dressings, Swan-Ganz catheter, and intravenous dopamine, he died three days later in septic shock.

Discussion

Unlike diseases such as uncontrolled cancer, the prognosis of burns without precedent of survival is evident almost immediately at the time of admission, because the extent and severity of burn are easily recognized and rapidly quantifiable, and mortality statistics are more detailed and complete than for most other pathologic processes. Although such severe burns are rapid and even violent in onset, the patient is usually alert and mentally competent on admission and may remain so for hours to a day after the burn—longer if aggressive fluid resuscitation is given. There is no way to predict the length of this lucid interval for a particular patient, but certainly there is little time for the patient to gain a gradual awareness of his condition or for the burn team suddenly to acquire insight into the ethical issues involved.

The California Natural Death Act requires a 14-day waiting period after a "terminal" condition is diagnosed and the appropriate document is signed and witnessed before a person's wish for nonheroic measures is legally binding. It is not applicable to these patients because death almost always occurs before the waiting period has lapsed. The lack of specific legal guidelines, however, does not negate the desirability of a planned and efficient approach.

The approach described above evolved slowly and unevenly through experience, interdisciplinary conferences, and informal debate. Although

> . . . the patient is usually alert and mentally competent on admission and may remain so for hours to a day after the burn. . . .

When dealing with an alert, competent patient, we need not struggle against distractions and prejudice to imagine what the patient wants; we need only ask.

medical factors were always involved, the final issues invariably proved to be primarily ethical and could be stated approximately by the question, "Which is better for this patient, maximal therapy or ordinary care, and upon whose value system should the judgment be based?"

As pointed out by Kübler-Ross, when a patient is severely ill, he is often treated like a person with no right to an opinion.[4] Yet it is the patient's life and rights that are at stake. Statistics may describe past experience with a given type of injury receiving maximal therapy or ordinary care; physicians may cite such an experience and are experts in carrying out programs of maximal therapy or ordinary care, but only the patient may choose between them because only he has the right to consent to one or the other.

Just as Lincoln stated that "No man is good enough to govern another man without that other's consent,"[15] so no physician is so skilled that he may treat another without the other's consent.[16] If asked, the physician may offer his opinion about the choice, but it will be merely his personal, inexpert opinion about whether it is better to accept death or fight to make history as the first survivor in such an injury.

Bioethicists Joseph Fletcher and Paul Ramsey, as interpreted by Robb,[17] urge that *agape* or unselfish love for the patient and regard for his full stature as a person should be the criterion upon which we base our answers to bioethical questions such as those posed above. When dealing with an alert, competent patient, we need not struggle against distractions and prejudice to imagine what the patient wants; we need only ask. Who is more likely to be totally and lovingly concerned with the patient's best interest than the patient himself? Whenever in the past we as care-givers tried to decide these matters for the patient, issues such as what was best for the morale of the nursing service, or for the solvency of the hospital, constantly clouded our judgment. It is for this reason that we oppose decision making by select committees convened "[to] explore what the best interest of the patient and his relatives require" without necessarily asking or respecting the opinions of either.[5]

It took many months before we could shed a "we-know-best" defense and actually ask the patient what he wanted on admission when he was most competent to decide. Our approach seems obvious and right to us now; the first few times were agonizing. Our words seemed clumsy and awkward. If we had acted individually, without colleague support, the plan would probably have reverted rapidly to denial, or even worse, to a paternalistic decision making for the patient. Our patients and their families were able to see the human concern behind our first faltering phrases. Their warmth, gratitude, and peace confirmed what we later read: that what we say to the patient, the exact words, matters less than how we say it in an atmosphere of honesty, caring, and constant human presence.[18]

Weisman wrote, "The pervasive dread in dying seems not only to be the extinction of consciousness, but the fear that the death we die will not be our own. This is the singular distinction between death as a property of life and being put to death."[19] We believe that on our burn unit, death for these patients has become a property of life. It would be hypocritical to imply that all life-and-death decision making or all "decisions not to resuscitate" are now straightforward and anxiety-free on our burn service. Many patients admitted with head injuries or inhalation injuries are confused or unconscious on admission and never regain competency. Initially competent patients with small but measurable chances of survival still tend to have complications and to become incompetent before we learn what they would want us to do in the event that continued therapy became more a prolongation of death than a prolongation of life. Turning to the family for decision making when death seems imminent for an incompetent patient is rarely satisfactory; guilt-ridden families often find it very difficult to be objective and unselfish in their decision making. The more voiceless and vulnerable the patient, the more easily we have found ourselves slipping into a paternalistic role, using terms such as "hopeless," which we realize now are so obviously prejudicial (literally, judging before the fact). Yet our experience continues to convince us that "truth is the greatest kindness." It seems inevitable that more and earlier communication with the patient will prove to be the most honest and compassionate answer to many of the remaining problems of ethical decision making in the intensive care unit.

References

1. Jackson, D.M. The psychological effects of burns. *Burns* 1:70–74, 1974.
2. Muir, I.F.K., Barclay T.L. *Burns and their treatment*. Second edition. Chicago, Year Book Medical Publishers, 1974, p. 110.
3. Stone H.H. The composite burn solution. *Contemporary burn management*. Edited by H.C. Polk Jr., H.H. Stone. Boston, Little, Brown, 1971, p. 96.
4. Kübler-Ross, E. *On death and dying*. New York, Macmillan, 1969.
5. Critical Care Committee of the Massachusetts General Hospital. Optimum care for hopelessly ill patients. *N. Engl. J. Med.* 295:362–364, 1976.
6. Tagge G.F., Adler D., Bryan-Brown, C.W. et al. Relationship of therapy to prognosis in critically ill patients. *Crit. Care Med.* 2:61–63, 1974.
7. Skillman J.J. *Intensive care,* Boston, Little, Brown, 1975, p. 21.
8. Rabkin M.T., Gillerman G., Rice N.R. Orders not to resuscitate. *N. Engl. J. Med.* 295:364–366, 1976.
9. Cassem N.H. Confronting the decision to let death come. *Crit. Care Med.* 2:113–117, 1974.
10. Bull J.P. Revised analysis of mortality due to burns. *Lancet* 2:1133–1134, 1971.
11. Feller I., Archembeault C. *Nursing the burned patient*. Ann Arbor, Institute for Burn Medicine, 1973, p. 10.
12. Kavanaugh R.E. *Facing death*. Los Angeles, Nash, 1972, p. 67.
13. Brody H. *Ethical decisions in medicine*. Boston, Little, Brown, 1976 p. 98.
14. Shneidman E. *Death of man*. New York, N.Y. Times Book Company, 1973, p. 33.
15. Lincoln Abraham. In Peoria, Illinois during Lincoln-Douglas debate on Oct. 16, 1854. Quoted in Bartlett J. *Familiar quotations*. Boston, Little, Brown, 1968, p. 635a.
16. Ramsey P. *The patient as person*. New Haven, Yale University Press, 1970. p. 7.
17. Robb J.W. The Joseph Fletcher/Paul Ramsey debate in bioethics and the Christian ethical tradition. Religion in Life (in press).
18. Feifel H. Attitudes toward death in some normal and mentally ill populations. *The meaning of death*. Edited by H. Feifel. New York, McGraw-Hill, 1959, p. 124.
19. Weisman A.D. *On dying and denying: A psychiatric study of terminality*. New York, Behavioral Publications, 1972.

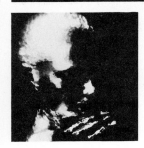

21

Practice

A re you a future-oriented person? Do you always work for something down the road? Perhaps a grade at the end of a course, a college diploma at the end of four years, or children and a career within the next ten years are your milestones. In this chapter, Orville Kelly suggests that we should shift our values in order to "make today count." Kelly, himself a cancer patient, has created an organization with 183 chapters to represent this value shift. The following Appendix exercises are particularly relevant to this chapter.

        E.   Confronting the Realization of Death

        K.   Planning for Living

        O.   Values Grid

Making Today Count

Orville E. Kelly

My exposure to illness and the prospects of dying are perhaps not untypical. What is emerging from my personal encounter with death, however, is unique. Although I had been ill at various times for over a year, and had to resign from my job as editor of a newspaper, I never thought anything was seriously wrong with me! I had several physical examinations during this time and pneumonia twice. I did think I had been working too hard while trying to hold my family together. So, after I left my newspaper job, I drove my wife, Wanda, and four children from our home in Illinois to Colorado. I felt the change of climate might be beneficial. I even felt as if I might be leaving my problems behind as we drove westward along Interstate 80. For a while, I was happy once again. But soon I was back in bed again, too ill to look for a job. When my condition grew worse, we returned to southeastern Iowa, where my wife and I grew up.

One April morning, in 1973, I was shaving when I noticed a swelling beneath my left arm. I was concerned enough to go to a doctor. I finally ended up in a surgeon's office who after examining me told me the swelling was a tumor, maybe two, and that he had found another one in my groin. He suspected lymphoma, a form of cancer.

The surgeon surgically removed one of the tumors from beneath my arm. The second tumor there was located too near the heart to remove. A biopsy was performed immediately. The surgeon's suspicions were confirmed. I had cancer.

When I heard the word "cancer" I thought I was going to die, very soon. My world fell apart. My only hope then was that possibly a mistake had been made and someone with authority would come into my room and tell me everything was going to be all right. I lived in a state of fear, dreading what each new test would reveal.

I felt they didn't understand my feelings and were deserting me at a time when I most needed their support.

After spending several days as a patient in the hospital in Burlington, Iowa, where I reside, the surgeon arranged for me to be transferred to the University of Iowa Hospitals and Clinics at Iowa City, Iowa.

By this time, I was depressed, and even contemplated suicide. I felt as if I had become a burden to my family. I still did not officially know what to anticipate as far as my future was concerned, but I suspected I would soon die of cancer. Yet, I still could not accept what was happening to me. I knew cancer touched the lives of many people, but I never thought it would affect me.

One bright summer afternoon, as white clouds drifted lazily through the sky outside my hospital room window, a physician came into my room, shutting the door behind him. Somehow I knew (perhaps because of the closing of the door) that he had some bad news for me.

"Has anyone talked with you about your prognosis and what you might expect?"

"No."

"You have a type of cancer known as 'lymphocytic lymphoma!' Tests we have conducted indicate is has metastasized. In other words, you can be treated, but not cured."

Now it was official. I was going to die of cancer. But the scene I had a part in seemed unreal. Such things were supposed to happen in movies and novels, but not in my life.

The doctor really didn't want to give me a time limit, but he quoted some statistics. (A general consensus seemed to be somewhat between a few months and six years.)

When I was able to travel, I was allowed to return home on weekends. It was then I discovered I had more to cope with than the physical problems of living with cancer. Many of my friends and relatives were obviously uncomfortable around me. Not only did they not know what to say to me, but I didn't know what to say to them. They viewed me as a "dying man" because of the diagnosis of cancer. I felt they didn't understand my feelings and were deserting me at a time when I most needed their support.

"If you ever need anything, just let me know," one well-meaning friend said over the telephone.

I needed *them,* and I needed them now!

"I've just been *dying* to meet you," a lady stated. Then she apologized for using "that word." It bothered her more than it did me.

One day while I was home on a weekend visit from the hospital, a family friend visited us. My wife and I met her at the door.

"How's he feeling?" the friend asked my wife, pointing at me.

Why didn't she ask me? I didn't know it then, but she didn't want to confront me directly. And I'm certain she didn't *really* want to know how I was feeling, since I felt terrible. The question, and the expected response, are supposed to go something like this:

"How are you feeling?"

"Just fine."

"Good. You're going to live another 20 years."

During this period of time I thought often of my past life, "when everything was all right." I remembered previously forgotten incidents, which had been lost somewhere during the course of my life prior to the diagnosis of cancer. I remembered a trip to a park near my home in Illinois, and how Wanda and I had sat beneath a large shade tree while the children played nearby. I remembered the plans we made for the future, and the dreams we had. For a while, I let myself become lost in reverie, and then I would suddenly remember the cancer and realize my dreams had become much shorter and my future was now associated with a group of statistics. I had lost control of my life.

I reported for tests when instructed to do so. My apparently limited future was dependent upon my response to drugs and many other intangibles. The actual prognosis ranged from "zero" onward. But the tragedy was that I died many deaths in my mind. Over and over again, I thought about my impending death. It really never occurred to me that the death rate for every generation is 100 percent and that we don't all live to be 70 years old or more. All I could think of was now. I had been cheated out of a normal life. I could not think about leaving my wife and children behind when I died. What would happen to them? Who would be a father to my little son, Britton? I thought that, God, if indeed there existed such an entity, must punish one needlessly. Some persons had told me that God punished sinners by inflicting cancer upon them. In my confused mind, therefore, I blamed God for my cancer.

At the hospital, my tests continued. I became reluctantly acquainted with bone marrow biopsies, lymphangiograms and berium dye tests. Such denying and impersonal statements as "it's only going to hurt for a little bit" and "bring in the lymphoma patient" became familiar to me.

Finally, I was released from the hospital. The oncologist treating me decided that chemotherapy would be the desired drug therapy for me. Prior to the first treatment, an oncologist briefed Wanda and me about the possible side effects associated with the toxic chemicals to be used, including nausea, a lowered white count resulting in a lowered resistance to infectious illnesses, and such complicated things as bone marrow depression.

I dreaded receiving the first treatment, but one September day, I drove to Iowa City and received the first injections of drugs. I was given a 5-day supply of a drug to be taken orally. Driving home, I had some time for contemplation and realized that fear itself is often more difficult to cope with than the thing you fear. I had endured the diagnosis; the weeks of testing at the hospital; the depression, rejection, isolation, increasing impotence, and anger; and my first chemotherapy treatment. And I was still alive.

My heart was still beating. I could still love, and be loved. I still had a lifetime left to live. It occurred to me that I had some choices about how I would live the rest of my life. I could continue wasting time, or I could make an attempt to live despite the cancer. I felt I should try living again.

A miracle didn't suddenly occur. But when I began talking openly about cancer, and told my children what was wrong with me, the quality of our family life commenced to improve.

It occurred to me that I had some choices about how I would live the rest of my life.

The Birth of an Organization

I discovered it helped *me* to know I was not alone and that other patients shared some of my emotional problems.

I had no desire initially to write after the diagnosis of cancer, but in December 1973 I decided to describe the life of a cancer patient in an article for the newspaper in Burlington. It appeared in January 1974. Two paragraphs of the article suggested that an organization for persons with life-threatening illnesses, their families, and other interested persons be formed. People began calling me. I discovered it helped *me* to know I was not alone and that other patients shared some of my emotional problems. I found doctors, nurses, ministers, and others were concerned about what was happening to me. They *did* care. I realized that people had difficulties expressing their concern, but if I met them halfway it was easier for them to tell me they did care. When they realized I needed to talk about my problems, they were willing to listen, and I soon realized they, too, needed someone who would listen to *them*.

We held our first meeting of seriously ill patients and other interested persons on January 24, 1974, in Burlington, Iowa. Eighteen persons attended. We all had so much to say the first night that I found it difficult to end the meeting. But before closing, we decided to call our new organization, "Make Today Count." After all, that is what we were trying to do.

Today, over four years since the first meeting, we have 183 chapters of Make Today Count in the United States, Canada, and Europe. We plan to have 500 chapters within the next year. Obviously, there is a need for our group, not only in America, but elsewhere.

What happens at a typical MTC meeting? Open discussion periods are the most popular part of a meeting. Sometimes family members and patients meet in separate groups, then come together for general discussions. Sometimes oncologists, chaplains, nurses, patients, family members, social workers, and others speak about topics of interest to our groups.

Because of the informal atmosphere of the gatherings, patients and family members can discuss their emotional problems openly with others who share their feelings or who want to understand. In addition, health care professionals can express their own problems encountered while treating seriously ill patients.

"I do care," a nurse might remark, "so I feel guilty when I think, 'I hope Mrs. Smith doesn't die during *my* shift.' "

"I was taught not to become emotionally involved with my patients," a doctor confesses, "but I'm a human being and I *do* get involved. I think the physician-patient relationship has improved as it applies to me, now that there is no barrier present. And it has not affected my professional standards. In fact, my patients have benefited, I feel, from our mutual candor."

Many pleas of help come from patients and family members around the world. These people generally are not members of an MTC chapter, but we try to help them. One letter reads:

"I am the daughter of a 70-year-old terminal patient. He has cancer and a heart problem. He has intense pain. The hospital has released him—

to die at home, I assume. He has no appetite; nothing tastes good to him. He complains all the time. I don't think he even knows he is dying. He has no will. How can we help him prepare for death when we don't even like to discuss this subject ourselves? How can we talk about legal matters without making it sound as if we are greedy? And is it fair for our children to be subjected to all this?''

Another letter reads: "My brother has cancer. They cannot operate and he has been given six months to live. How can we help him understand what is happening, when we don't know either? What is cancer?''

Or: "I, too, am a cancer patient. I don't know whether or not it's the same as yours. All I know is that I have lots of pain and I'm scared. I don't want to die. I'm only 27 and I have two children. Why did this have to happen to me? I read all about terrible things people do and I've tried to be a good Christian. What did I do wrong?''

There is no magic formula, but these people can be helped. Usually I listen to them, without offering any suggestions. Then, one day, after they have "talked themselves out", they will say, "Thank you, Mr. Kelly, for helping me. Now I can cope with my problems." But actually they have helped themselves. I have just listened!

Most doctors tell me they do not place a time limit on people's lives, since it accomplishes very little. In spite of this many patients appear to be living under a time limit. Communications typically are ineffective among members of the health care profession, patients, and their families. There are many patients and their families who feel that there is "nothing more that can be done." Perhaps nothing more can be done to effectively treat the disease, but the patient can be made as comfortable as possible. Death should not represent failure to the medical profession since nature will eventually have its own way no matter what we do.

Even though 80 percent of America's deaths occur in hospitals, only approximately two percent of these hospitals are prepared to care for dying patients. And only a very small number of the 122 medical schools in America effectively teach future physicians how to treat dying patients. The emphasis is on "curing" and "healing." With this orientation toward survival, our society has tended to disregard the quality of life of seriously ill persons and pay attention only to quantity of life. With two out of three cancer patients dying from their disease, or its complications, it makes more sense to make today count than to work toward a cure for tomorrow.

I have discovered considerable interest among the students at medical and nursing schools in hearing a view "from the other end of the stethoscope." Their professors, however, display little enthusiasm and consider this interest in "death and dying" in America only a fad. Yet, the same persons who wrap their emotions in a protective cloak sometimes become patients.

"It's terrible to suddenly become just a number," commented a physician-turned-cancer patient. "I wanted someone to call me by my name. I felt terribly alone.''

> . . . they will say, "Thank you, Mr. Kelly, for helping me. Now I can cope with my problems." But actually they have helped themselves. I have just listened!

We don't die! Instead, we "pass away," "expire," "cross the River Styx," or "go to the great beyond."

"The doctors treating me really couldn't help me with my emotional problems," stated a surgeon, after he became a cancer patient. "I needed to talk with someone who could understand what it's all about."

"I can tell you something about loneliness," said a physician who prior to a stroke had been the chief of staff of a hospital. "My colleagues haven't visited me. I'm lonely and I want to have friends. And I apologize for crying in front of you, but I'm angry."

But doctors *do* care. It's just that we're all taught, indirectly, that death is an enemy. It represents failure.

"If we can put a man on the moon, why can't we cure cancer?"

"After all the billions of dollars spent on research, why isn't there a cure for cancer somewhere on the horizon?"

Our fears of death seem to encourage a language of denial. We don't die! Instead, we "pass away," "expire," "cross the River Styx," or "go to the great beyond."

As a matter of fact, we generally don't die of cancer. We "pass away after a lingering illness," or a "lengthy" illness, or a "prolonged" illness.

Society is changing its attitudes toward life-threatening illnesses and death. But it is a slow process.

"We admire you because of what you are doing, Mr. Kelly . . ."

However, there often is an unspoken sentence lingering in the speaker's mind: ". . . but just don't involve us."

The prospects of facing our own personal death are always difficult. Several weeks ago I visited a lung cancer patient in his hospital room. He had completed the maximum chemotherapy and radiation therapy. He seemed to accept the fact that he was dying and even talked about his visits with other seriously ill cancer patients.

"It was obvious the majority of them hadn't accepted the possibility of death," he said.

Then he commented about his own prognosis:

"Now I feel I'm going to return home and live some more. I'm not ready to die yet. I've got some unfinished business to take care of before *I* die."

He died ten days later, without having left the hospital.

A Personal Update

Where am I today? Certainly I am pleased to have been a part of the growth of the organization I founded.

I have traveled over 400,000 miles and have made approximately 700 appearances, speaking about the MTC organization and how the quality of life can be improved for patients and their families. I have had a part in changing some attitudes. I don't think that ten years ago a cancer patient would have been asked to speak at major medical conferences attended by physicians, or at junior and senior high schools. But this has happened to me.

I still become depressed. Not a constant period of depression, but a realization on certain days that probably my time, statistically, is running out. It does not help for me to know that time is running out for all of us. I am thinking about my life, and my family. Yes, I am concerned about other persons, but I want to live. Actually, my desire to remain alive has increased in proportion to my new awareness of life and the intensity of my emotions. Each day of life, for me, represents a day I never thought I would live to enjoy—or to be depressed in. So if I am depressed, I no longer feel guilty about it. But I am not satisfied with my depression. I endure it, and make plans for tomorrow.

I have completed three and one-half years of chemotherapy. I have lived through the various side effects, some of which are still evident. I have lived through four years of impotence, intensified by anti-hypertension drugs. I estimate that I have consumed over 20,000 pills of various sizes and ingredients in addition to the injections of drugs and the liquid medicines.

Today, as I write these words, I pause to look outside, through my fifth floor office window in the downtown area of Burlington. I see the Mississippi River flowing by, bordered on one side by my city, and on the other side by the green forests of Illinois. There is life around me, and I am a part of it. But in my mind, as a part of my memories, are thoughts about the hundreds of cancer patients I have known who are now dead. I did not want them to die, but neither am I responsible for their deaths. Whether I like it or not, death is a part of our lives.

Gone from this earth, but not from my mind, are Steve's smile and Mrs. Owen's familiar "Good morning, Mr. Kelly." Gone are all the patients from the first MTC meeting in Burlington.

I don't know whether I feel fortunate because of my additional, unexpected longevity, or sad because the statistics are increasing against my future life span. I suppose I have a mixture of feelings.

Five days from this day is the fifth anniversary of my diagnosis of cancer. I will not celebrate it. But neither will I be dismayed. It will be another day.

What have I learned during the past five years?

I have learned the importance of caring, of listening, of touching. I have learned to appreciate life more and not take it for granted. My relationship with Wanda and our four children has taken on a new meaning for me. I have learned I should not waste time. Most important of all, I have learned to value love.

No matter what happens in the future, my life *has* been worthwhile. I am not happy because I have cancer, but it took the specter of death to make me aware of life.

And I still have my dreams—they're just shorter!

> **I have learned the importance of caring, of listening, of touching.**

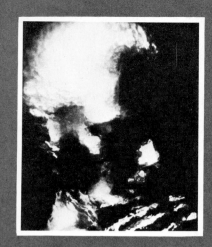

Part 3

Community and Societal Dynamics

Among the notable transitions of our ever-changing society is the trend toward advanced technology. With our increased wisdom and technological skills we have attempted to control all aspects of human existence for several centuries. Until recently, the crisis of death was considered a realm outside this province of control. "Can we control?" and "Why should we control?" questions have now been submerged by the more familiar question, "How?" Our technological capability to control heartbeat and respiration have resulted in a quandary relating to definitions of life and death. On top of these developments came the advent of heart and other organ transplantation, which posed additional ethical, legal, and social questions about the definition of death. The lowering of death rates through the control of infectious diseases has also left our society with the belief that longevity is the norm—to be expected. Quantity of years has emerged as a standard over quality.

Part 3 of this book now addresses the impact of micro-level transitions on the societal fabric within which we all live. Numerous issues will be explored. How has our care of the dying been affected by the passing of functionally meaningful extended families? What elements have characterized our societal shift from a moral to a technological order? If the modern hospital represents the successful strivings of medicine to conquer death, should we view the presence of nursing homes as our resignation to it? Is society failing to meet the obligation it has to its dying members? Are we confusing the dying role with the sick role? Should there be a constitutional right to die? What is euthanasia? How do we differ in our attitudes toward euthanasia? Do ethnic communities differ in the ways death is presented in their newspapers? Do stressful environmental events such as relocation and mandatory retirement contribute to premature death in the elderly? What cross-cultural differences exist in the treatment of cancer? What successful community innovations exist for patients and families facing life-threatening illness? How can death as the "ultimate indignity" be humanized through right-to-die legislation?

Part 3 begins with a chapter entitled "Dying in a Technological Society," by Eric Cassell, whose basic premise is that we as a society have moved from a moral order to a technological order. A moral order defines what is right; it is based on values, sentiment, and conscience. A technological order relies on the functional utility of things; it is based on practicalities and necessities. With death becoming a technological phenomenon, we no longer believe it is necessary to die. We believe instead that death is reversible through judicious use of mechanical and professional means.

Depersonalization of care is one consequence of this transition to a technological order. The dying person is viewed in terms of a beating heart—pulse and organ viability. Such a narrow view of the body falls far short of the goals of holistic health. Dying patients are persons with emotional, social, and spiritual needs too! We must not blame the physicians alone for this impersonalization, warns Cassell. We have seen how the whole society has shifted its public focus from moral to technical in many areas of life. We have constructed the modern medical center as a "temple to this technical order, revered both by medicine and the public." Our way out of this dilemma seems to lie in restoring a balance between moral and technological needs.

Russell Noyes and John Clancy believe that society is failing to meet obligations to dying persons. In their article "The Dying Role: Its Relevance to Improved Patient Care" Noyes and Clancy distinguish between the "sick role" and the "dying role." They believe society has confused the two roles, much to the detriment of total patient care. Dying persons have been assigned the "sick role," which implies expectations to get well, or at least to live as long as possible. Physicians too have confused the roles. Thus they use technological advances to achieve temporary treatment successes.

Noyes and Clancy identify the signs of role confusion and suggest how the confusion may be corrected. They show how reestablishment of the "dying role" can result in improved care of dying people. What we must realize, they suggest, is that while treatment is appropriate to acutely ill persons, it may "unnecessarily prolong the suffering and disability of the dying people."

We have seen that often advances in technology prolong life primarily by delaying death. The result is to make dying slower, more painful, and more undignified than ever before. Pamela Koza addresses the consequences of this dilemma in her paper "Euthanasia: Some Legal Considerations." Even in Canada, Koza recognizes, the Karen Quinlan court case in the United States has focused attention on euthanasia. Her paper is concerned with the definition of euthanasia and the legal sanctions that may be applied under Canadian law to someone who is involved in such a case. She identifies specific sections of the Canadian Criminal Code relevant to the issue of euthanasia. She also considers the value placed on the sanctity of life by the law, the failure to recognize motive in cases of euthanasia, and disparate legal and medical definitions of death. Koza concludes by asking whether innovative legislation is needed at all, or whether a more sensitive interpretation of existing laws would be preferable.

There are many opinions about euthanasia. Winget, Kapp, and Yeaworth's review "Attitudes toward Euthanasia" explores the variations among seven samples of people: college students, first-year nursing students, senior nursing students, registered nurses, first-year medical students, senior medical students, and physicians. All respondents completed a fifty-item questionnaire relating to euthanasia. Not surprisingly, attitudes appeared to be "harder" in proportion to how professionally established the respondents were and how much experience they had had dealing with patients. Thus, of the seven groups questioned, practicing physicians showed more positive attitudes to euthanasia. Their responses did not differ significantly from those of senior medical students. These and other findings of the report are interpreted in terms of interpersonal and intrapersonal role theory.

A fascinating and important three-year longitudinal investigation of comparative societal attitudes regarding death is reported by Reynolds and Kalish in their article "Death Rates, Attitudes, and the Ethnic Press." These authors studied the presentation of death in community newspapers, attitudes toward death, and its statistical presence among four different ethnic groups. The four ethnic groups and their respective newspapers were as follows: black Americans, *Los Angeles Sentinel;* Japanese Americans, *Rafu Shimpo;* Mexican Americans, *La Opinion;* and white Americans, *Los Angeles Times.* The study provided evidence supporting each of four hypotheses: (1) Different ethnic communities represent death in different ways. (2) Newspaper presentations of death are reflected in community attitudes and expectations regarding death. (3) Official death statistics are correlated to both community attitudes and newspaper presentations of death. (4) Violent death is overrepresented in newspapers. Results are also discussed in terms of location, age, sex, religion, occupation, and affective tone.

Even more significant, however, is that the environment or community events can affect people's *behavior.* In her review article entitled "Environmental Events Predicting Death for the Elderly," Kay Rowland describes evidence that stressful environmental events may be linked to a subsequent decline in health or even to death of an individual. The effects of three stressors are reviewed: death of significant other, relocation, and retirement.

Essentially, relocation and death of a significant other are found to be fairly accurate in predicting death, especially under certain circumstances. The relationship between retirement and premature death, however, appears less substantiated. Since these environmental events are common features of our society, it behooves us to understand why they have the impact they do and what can be done to temper the effects. Rowland reviews Caplan's crises theory, Eisdoyer's reinforcement model, and Seligman's learned helplessness model. She relates theories to each other as complementary and shows how they might lower death rates following the death of a loved one, relocation, or retirement.

The point is repeatedly made throughout this part that the medical establishment is overzealous in treating illness but underzealous about more holistic health concerns. Patrick McGrady focuses our attention on treatment and challenges us with the query: "A man has three weeks to live. Do you make him comfortable or do you work like hell?" His article "The American Cancer Society Means Well, but the Janker Clinic Means Better" compares cancer treatment in the United States and Bonn, Germany. He concludes that nowhere in the United States does a patient have access to the professional involvement or range of techniques available at the Janker Clinic in Germany. The National Cancer Institute and the Food and Drug Administration are seen as more conservative than the Janker Clinic. Specific beliefs that seem to differentiate these two societies include: (1) the notion that all radiation or drug treatment must be terminated if a person's white blood cell count dips below 1,500; (2) notion that all cancers should be managed by surgery, radiation, or drugs; and (3) the notion that postoperative drug therapy interferes with wound healing and therefore should not be used. McGrady's observations and criticisms are specific and accusatory, but they do help us question the structural rigidities of our health care delivery system.

Health care delivery at the community level can be accomplished in very innovative ways, as described by Charles Garfield and Rachel Clark in their article "The SHANTI Project: A Community Model of Psychosocial Support for Patients and Families Facing Life-Threatening Illness." The SHANTI project is a model of health care in the San Francisco Bay Area which addresses the psychological and social needs of patients, their families, and the professionals who serve them. Staffed by volunteers, the project responds to requests for information and services. The SHANTI project captures the best of a viable community psychology. Its efforts are primarily preventive, its staff predominantly paraprofessional, and its locus clearly community- based. Once a client-volunteer relationship is established, the volunteer continues to work with his or her client at home, during hospitalizations, or during relocations to extended-care facilities. This continuity of care is a distinguishing characteristic of the project and represents the kindness and compassion that should be the norm in our treatment of the terminally ill.

Recognition of the need for compassion and humanistic care for the terminally ill is best symbolized by passage of "right-to-die" legislation. In their article "Control, Quality of Life, and 'The Right to Die,' " Bugen, Tullos, and Bolton describe the emergence and passage of such legislation in

Texas. The Natural Death Act is a written document voluntarily executed by a patient to give a directive to an attending physician to withdraw life-sustaining procedures in the event of a terminal illness.

The bill is presented in its entirety following a discussion of control and quality of life. The Natural Death Act of Texas is one of the first of its kind in the United States and is viewed as increasing the freedom to control health care delivery while insuring respect for a patient's quality of life. In order to more fully represent the impact of this innovative legislation, the viewpoints of both a terminally ill consumer and a health care provider are also presented. The intent, as Tullos points out, is to help doctors, and society in general, to "stop seeing a patient's death as a personal defeat but rather as a biological process which the patient may choose to hasten by relinquishing life supports."

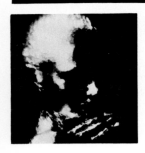

22

Theory

Have you ever felt overwhelmed by the impersonality of an unattended toll booth machine as you dropped your money in—particularly when you were lost and needed directions? Machines are becoming ever more prominent in our lives—and deaths as well, affecting when, where, and how we die, as we discover in this chapter by Eric Cassell. When you have completed the chapter, any of the following Appendix exercises will be helpful to your learning:

B.   Appropriate Death Fantasy

I.   Life and Death Attitudes: Dyadic Encounter

J.   Mortuary Form

P.   Warm-up Exercise

Dying in a Technological Society

Eric J. Cassell

The care of the terminally ill in the United States has changed as the business of dying has shifted from the moral to the technical order. The moral order has been used to describe those bonds between men based on sentiment, morality, or conscience that describe what is right. The technical order rests on the usefulness of things, based in necessity or expediency, and not founded in conceptions of the right.[1] The change of death from a moral to a technical matter has come about for many reasons based in social evolution and technical advance, and the effects on the dying have been profound.

One reason for the change has been the success of modern medicine in combating death. For most, in the United States, premature death is no longer imminent. The death of infants is unusual, the death of children rare, and the death of young adults so improbable that it must be removed from the realistic possibilities of young life. Further, the nature of death has also changed. The degenerative diseases and cancer have become predominant. Lingering sickness in the aged is a less common event because medicine is able to combat the complications of chronic disease that so often in the past kept the sick person from functioning. Accompanying these changes brought about by technical advances, there has been a change in the place where death occurs. Death has moved from the home into institutions—hospitals, medical centers, chronic care facilities and nursing homes.

This material was first published in *Death Inside Out—The Hastings Center Report*, pp. 43–48, edited by P. Steinfels and R. Veatch; New York: Harper & Row, 1974. Reprinted by permission.

1. Robert Redfield, *The Primitive World and Its Transformations* (Ithaca: Cornell University Press, 1953), pp. 20ff.

From the Moral to the Technical

Death is a . . . failure of technology. . . .

There are other reasons for the shift of death in the United States from the moral to the technical order. One is the widespread acceptance of technical success itself. Because life expectancy has increased, the dying are old now. But, life expectancy is not an individual term, it is a statistical term. For individuals, what has changed is their death expectancy; they do not expect to die. They may use fantasies of early death or fears of death for personal or psychological reasons, but the reality belief is that death need not occur in the foreseeable future, that death is a reversible event. That belief in the reversibility of death, rooted in the common American experience of modern medicine, begins to move death out of the moral order. Death is a technical matter, a failure of technology in rescuing the body from a threat to its functioning and integrity. For the moment, it does not matter that the death of a person cannot be removed from the moral order by the very nature of personhood; what matters is the mythology of the society. The widespread mythology that things essentially moral can be made technical is reinforced by the effect of technology in altering other events besides death; for example, birth, birth defects, or abortion.

The fact that technology can be seen so often as altering fate nurtures an illusion that is basic to the mythology of American society—that fate can be defeated.

From the Family to the Hospital

Another reason why death has moved away from the moral order lies in the changes in family structure that have occurred over the past decades in the United States. The family remains the basic unit of moral and personal life, but with the passing of functionally meaningful extended families have come changes directly related to the care of the dying. The old, both the repository of knowledge about what is right and the major recipients of moral obligation, have left the family group. For many reasons, not the least their desire for continued independence in the years when previously material dependency would have been their lot, the aged frequently live alone. In retirement they may live far from their roots or their children, associating largely with others of their own age. An age-graded way of life has emerged that depends again on technical success and public responsibility (such as old age benefits) to solve problems for the aged that previously would have been the primary concern of the family. There is the belief, reinforced by the advantages of the change in family structure and geographic mobility, that essentially moral problems—obligations to parents, for example—have become part of the technical order amenable to administrative or technical solutions.

On the other hand, in his search for continued independence and comfortable retirement, the old person has allowed his family to separate, allowed the young to achieve their independence. In previous times and in other cultures, the mantle passed to the next generation only with the death of the old. Here it is voluntary. But, a problem is created for the dying patient. The old person who is going to die is already out of the family. To die amidst his family he must return to them—reenter the structure in order to leave it. Reenter it in denial of all the reasons he gave himself and his children for separation, reasons equally important to them in their pursuit of privacy and individual striving and in their inherent denial of aging, death, and fate.

Thus, by reason of technological success and changes in family structure that are rooted in the basic mythology of America, death has moved from the moral order to the technical and from the family to the hospital.

The Context of Dying

It is interesting to examine some of the consequences and corollaries of the shift. In individual terms, moving the place of death from the home to the hospital, from familiar to strange surroundings, means changing the context of dying. The picture of the old person, independent and swinging free—promulgated as much by the old as by others—while part fact, is also a partial fiction dictated by the old person's love for, and nurturance of, the independence of the young. Becoming a burden is the great fear not only for what it may mean personally, but for the threat it poses to the fragile economic and personal structure of today's nuclear family. But part fiction or no, the hallmark of "golden age" is independence. With independence and its mobility, the belief arises that each person is the sole representative of his own beliefs, values, and desires. In health that may seem to be true, but the fact is as fragile as the body. In health a person can struggle for his rights, pronounce his values, and attempt their fulfillment. But the sick, bound to their bodies by their illness, are different. The values and desires dearly held during life give way in terminal illness. Pain and suffering erode meaning and deny dignity. The fiction of independence and the denial of fate give way to reality. In terminal illness, the individual must give over to others and to the context of his dying the defense of his dignity and the statement of his values. But the context of dying and the people at the bedside have changed. The aged no longer die surrounded by their loved ones. An essentially private matter takes place in the public sphere surrounded by symbols of individual sameness, not personal difference. The family and its needs are the intruders. The patient's values, spoken by others, compete with the values of the institution. There is a final, ironic independence as the person dies alone.

Thus, there are personal or value problems created for the individual when death moves from the moral to the technical order. Characteristically, our society seeks solutions to these problems not by reasserting the moral, but by attempting technical solutions for moral imperatives. We are seeing

In terminal illness, the individual must give over to others and to the context of his dying the defense of his dignity and the statement of his values.

There are two distinct things happening in the terminally ill, the death of the body and the passing of the person.

increasing attempts in the United States to find quasi-legal or legal means to reassert the rights of the dying—some technical means to give as much weight to the person who dies as the hospital gives to his body.

Mechanical Events in the Moral Sphere

In the process of the shift of death from the moral to the technical, a basic confusion arises that confounds the usefulness of technical solutions in what are essentially moral problems. The mechanical events involved in a body becoming dead, which occur in the technical sphere, are confused with the process of dying, which occurs in the moral sphere. It is a natural error but one that we do not frequently make in health. That is to say that while we are aware that the mechanical event that is a beating heart is essential to life, we do not confuse ourselves with our heartbeat. As a matter of fact, if someone becomes too conscious of his heartbeat, we consider it a symptom, or neurosis. But in the sick or the dying the confusion is rampant. There are two distinct things happening in the terminally ill, the death of the body and the passing of the person. The death of the body is a physical phenomenon, a series of measurable events that are the province of physicians. The passing of the individual is a nonphysical process, poorly defined, largely unmeasurable and closely connected to the nature of the dying person. It is the process by which he leaves the group and during which we take leave of him. Indeed, in the manner in which many act toward the newly dead body—as though it still contained some part of the person—the passing of the individual, at least for the onlooker, may not end with death. It is obvious that in sudden death a person may pass away who was never dying; or conversely, in the depressed, the person may be dying with no evidence of impending death.

The passing of the individual is also part of the work of physicians; but, of more importance, it is the province of family, friends, and clergymen—indeed the entire group. But in a technical era, the passing of the person, since it is unmeasurable and does not fit the technical schema, is not a legitimate subject for public discourse.

Those feelings within that relate to the dying person are difficult to organize, to deal with, or to speak about. The social rituals that previously enabled those confused meanings and feelings to spend themselves appropriately have diminished or disappeared along with the extended family. In the moral order, time slows down for those around the dying; but in the world of things, of necessity or expediency, time moves on relentlessly, making its case for those around the dying to return to that world. Furthermore, with decreasing practice in moral matters, even when social forms remain, the content becomes increasingly sterile. Men obscure the moral content of the passing of the person by using the facts and artifacts of the death of the body as the vehicle for their interchanges—much as talk about the weather or sports draws the sting on other occasions.

The confusion of the mechanical events of the death of the body with the personal and social nature of the passing of the person confounds attempts to solve the essentially moral problems of the dying—problems of sentiment, conscience, or the knowledge of what is right. Thus, in matters such as when the respirators should be turned off, and by whom—essentially moral questions—the mechanical events loom so large that attention is diverted away from the moral, back to the technical. And this is the corollary problem to that raised earlier: the context of death no longer gives weight to the values of the dying person and forces a resort to legal or administrative protection of his rights.

> **The confusion of mechanical events for moral processes creates**
>
> **· · ·**
>
> **depersonalization of care.**

Depersonalization of Care

The confusion of mechanical events for moral processes creates the further problem of depersonalization of care. And it is seen in the greater attention paid to diseases than to people by doctors and their institutions—a common complaint about physicians and particularly about physicians in their care of the dying. Frequently we explain this depersonalization by saying that it is the physician's psychological defense against the emotional burden imposed by the care of the dying. Though that may be true, it is only part of the truth. We have seen how the whole society has shifted its public focus from moral to technical in many areas of life: doctors are no exception to the trend. The problem cannot solely lie among physicians, or the society would not let them get away with it. Social forces would drive doctors back toward a more holistic view of their patients. Indeed, such a change is beginning to occur in response to the increasingly vocal dissatisfaction with medical care.

Because depersonalization is so much a part of the technical order, not only in medicine, and so antithetical to the values of personhood, let us further examine how depersonalization takes place. Each dying patient is not only a person, but also the container of the process or events by which his body is dying. By definition, since he is dying, these processes or events cannot be controlled by existing technology. Because of the inability of the technology to control such things—and cancer or heart failure are examples—they acquire independent meaning apart from the person containing them. From the viewpoint of caring for the terminally ill, such depersonalization may be justly deplored. But from the viewpoint of medical science, the pursuit of the meaning of the resistant body process, apart from the person containing it, is a legitimate end in itself. That is to say, the heart as an abstraction, as a pump, an electrical system, or what have you is a proper object of technical concern and quite distinct from the fact that human hearts are only found in humans. Further, it is the nature of any system of abstract or formal thought not to be content with mystery but to continue operating on any problem until understanding results. Mystery is a threat to the adequacy of the system of thought itself. Consequently, the disease process must be probed and probed, not only because of its relevance to the care of the sick and dying, but also because lack of a solution poses a threat to the entire logical construct of which the body process is thought to be a part. Thus, the depersonalization and abstraction of body mechanics is both necessary and legitimate within the framework of science, and understanding of the body-as-machine is impeded by consideration of human values.

The problem of depersonalization depends in part on the degree to which the dying person's disease process is understood. For example, in the care of the patient with bacterial pneumonia, easily treated with antibiotics, depersonalization poses little difficulty. The abstractions necessary for understanding microbes, antibiotics, and so forth are so much a part of the physician's thinking that he or she is able to integrate them back into a total concept of man, patients, etc. Withdrawal and depersonalization are not frequent, I think, when experienced doctors and nurses care for the dying, if the cause of death is something acceptably inevitable, such as pneumonia in the very old, or stroke. If it is correct that persons dying of a poorly understood process are more likely to be depersonalized by their physicians, we can better understand why the accusation of depersonalization is most often brought against young physicians. To the inexperienced doctor almost everything about the dying person is unfamiliar or poorly understood, thus requiring the abstraction that leads to depersonalization. Effective integration of the learned technical material with human needs, values, and desires comes only at a later stage of learning.

Temples of the Technical Order

In the United States the modern medical center is the very temple of the technical order, revered both by medicine and the public. As medical science, in its effort toward understanding, has taken the body apart system by system, it has departmentalized the intellectual structure of the hospital. By that I mean not only the well known division of medicine into specialties, but the further subdivisions that represent specific body functions. The corridors of any American medical center reveal rooms whose doors bear titles such as pulmonary function laboratory, cardiographics laboratory, nuclear medicine, sonography, and so forth. Each of these specialized functions has contributed immeasurably to the diagnostic and therapeutic power of the modern physician, and no doctor who has grown accustomed to their use will feel wholly comfortable in their absence. They are unlike the traditional clinical or research laboratory which, when examining a function of the patient's body, takes the whole patient along; it is not his blood or urine that goes to the laboratory, it is the patient. But it is not the person who holds the interest for the specialized laboratory; instead the interest centers on the person's lungs, or heart, or whatever. A good coronary arteriogram is not necessarily a good patient or even good for the patient, it is merely a technically good example of coronary arteriograms. Patients are usually not aware of or interested in those distinctions, and all too frequently, but in an opposite sense, neither is the physician who performed the test. One can see the hospital, thus compartmentalized, as the concrete expression of the depersonalization resulting from the abstract analytic thought of medical science. Thus, the dying patient in the modern hospital is in an environment ideally suited for the pursuit of knowledge and cure, but representing in its technology and idealized representative—the young doctor—technical values virtually antithetical to the holistic concept of person. This does not imply that the most personal and humane care cannot be and is not given in such hospitals, but rather that those who do give such care must struggle against their technical, depersonalized thinking about the body and against the structure of the hospital that such thought has produced.

No discussion of the care of the terminally ill in the United States can avoid the problem of the nursing home. Whereas the modern hospital represents the positive strivings of medical science and the technical order— the belief that nature, disease, and fate can be conquered—the nursing home represents the tattered edges of that philosophy. Medicine and medical care are seen primarily as the application of medical science to disease: if science fails the body, medicine fails the person. Nursing homes contain the failures and frustrations of medicine as well as the homeless or unwanted sick. They are a place to linger and to die. Walking their halls is deeply depressing because hopelessness is overwhelming. It is the hopelessness one experiences whenever one sees the sick completely over-taken by their sickness, forever apart from the comfort of group. None of the many reasons for their proliferation and crowding explains why they are the hopeless places that they usually are. We know they can be better because of the success of the occasional institution given over to the care of the terminally ill in a positive sense. Such successful nursing homes are often run by religious orders or by others whose belief in their mission is deeply moral. Thus, what we see in the usual American nursing home is by no means inevitable in the way that death is inevitable, but rather a vacuum of care. The promise of science and technology has failed here. The old family solutions to the problems posed by the care of the terminally ill have been altered past utility by social change. No new solution has come forward to fill the void.

We have seen how the care of the terminally ill has changed in the United States. They are older now and die more frequently in institutions. But that bare frame of facts conceals increasing distress within the society over the quality of their dying. When death occurs in the modern hospital, there seems to be more concern for the disease than for the dying person, more concern for life as a succession of heartbeats than life as meaning. When death occurs in nursing homes, it is as if life just dribbled out— custodial care seemingly inconvenienced by individual difference or tenacity for life.

When death occurs in nursing homes, it is as if life just dribbled out. . . .

A Balance of the Moral and Technical

We have seen that the problem is larger than widespread insensitivity which might be corrected by new educational programs. Rather, there has been a shift of death from within the moral order to the technical order. The technical, the expedient, the utilitarian that has worked so well in so many material ways seemed to promise easier solutions to the problems previously seen as matters of conscience, sentiment, or obligations between men. But the promise has not been fulfilled; not in the United States nor elsewhere where the technical order spreads its dominance.

Even if it were possible, the solution is not a return of American society to technical innocence. I do not believe that men were inherently more moral in the past when the moral order predominated over the technical. The path seems to lie in the direction of a more systematic understanding of the moral order to restore its balance with the technical. Understanding the body has not made it less wonderful, and the systematic exploration of the moral nature of man will not destroy that nature but rather increase its influence. In the care of the dying, it may give back to the living the meaning of death.

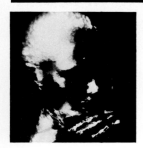

23

Theory

Think back to the last time you were ill. What kind of expectations of people around you were you aware of? Were you encouraged to get well as soon as possible because you were such an inconvenience at the time? Noyes and Clancy believe that there is a definite social role that our society expects of the "sick" and that this should be distinguished from the "dying" role. When you have read the chapter and understand this distinction, the following Appendix exercises are recommended:

     I.   Life and Death Attitudes: Dyadic Encounter

    L.   Privacy Circles

    O.   Values Grid

The Dying Role: Its Relevance to Improved Patient Care

Russell Noyes, Jr.

John Clancy

Sick Role

The social role accompanying illness was first described by Parsons (1951). Like other roles it is a constellation of expectations involving both rights and duties. In the case of the sick role there are two of each. Within this role a patient is, first of all, exempt from the responsibilities of his usual social role. Important business or social obligations may be broken without fear of censure. The second right is that of being cared for. The sick person is not responsible for becoming ill, and, consequently, members of society become obligated to him. This obligation falls primarily upon the family, and, of course, the physician.

The duties of the sick person are twofold, as well. Because society regards illness as an undesirable state, the patient must wish to get well. A person lacking this desire is not favorably regarded by his fellows and may be denied the rights of the sick role. Secondly, the sick person is obligated to obtain competent help in an effort to regain his health and is expected to cooperate with the treatment prescribed. A person who does not seek professional help is regarded as a drag on society.

Like other social roles, the sick role determines how a person perceives his situation. When sick he adopts a new set of expectations relative to his behavior, his obligations toward others, and their duties toward him. At the same time family members, physicians, and others in the social system are made to see their role in caring for the sick person. Both sick and well perceive a set of reciprocal obligations.

This material was first published in *Psychiatry,* vol. 40, pp. 41–47, February 1977. Copyright © 1977 by The William Alanson White Psychiatric Foundation, Inc. Reprinted by special permission of The William Alanson White Psychiatric Foundation, Inc.

Dying Role

As a person enters the dying role, it is important for him to desire to remain alive. . . . The obligation appears to continue, in some degree, as long as family and friends maintain meaningful attachments to the dying person.

The social role of the fatally ill person is, like that of the sick person, time limited. However, while the one terminates in the restoration of health, the other ends in death. Both are conferred by medical authority via the diagnosis, which for the dying person carries an unfavorable prognosis. The expected duration of life is important in assigning this role, and the physician therefore has an obligation to the parties concerned to estimate this in terms that reflect the limitations of his knowledge.

As a person enters the dying role, it is important for him to desire to remain alive. By so doing he assures his family and community that he is without responsibility for his approaching death. If he too readily accepted his fate he might appear to "give up" and reject loved ones or social obligations. The obligation appears to continue, in some degree, as long as family and friends maintain meaningful attachments to the dying person. He may relinquish unrealistic hope of recovery but must retain the "will to live," a motivational set commonly attributed to dying persons. Later appreciation and acceptance of death's reality do not mean that the final parting is willful. Only suffering or disability justifies a wish to die.

When an individual becomes ill he temporarily vacates healthy social roles. For a period of time they are held open in anticipation of his return. The dying person is obliged to transfer them to others on a more permanent basis. It is, therefore, a second duty of a person in the dying role to exercise the prerogatives he may have and arrange for an orderly transfer of property and authority. The person who fails to execute a will or participate in decisions regarding the future of his business or family may become an object of disapproval. The social disruption consequent to his death can be great. On the other hand, timely decisions and transfer of responsibility make a smooth transition possible.

The dying person has an obligation to avail himself of the necessary supports to life and to cooperate in their administration. If he fails to do so, he may impose a burden upon his family and overload those on whom he has grown dependent. He is not expected to remain dependent upon the physician, who has already, in the process of diagnosing a fatal illness, transferred him from the sick to the dying role. Having done so, the doctor no longer holds a position of primary importance in the person's care although he may oversee supportive and palliative treatments. Society reserves the physician's role for the more important restorative function and, in so doing, jealously guards against inroads upon the physician's time and energy.

Another of the important aspects of the dying person's cooperation is his acceptance of the curtailment of freedom and loss of privileges imposed by caregivers. If institutional care is required he is expected to abide by the rules and routines which enable the facility to deliver that care efficiently. Such routines are, in large measure, supportive and permit a higher level of functioning within a limited range.

Lastly, dependency is encouraged in the sick role, whereas independence, within the limits of an individual's declining resources, is encouraged in the dying role (Twaddle, 1972). In this regard it appears to resemble the impaired role described by Gordon (1966). The dying person is expected to limit his claim on others for attention and rely upon himself to a greater degree. Cooperation with caretakers especially calls for independence. The dying person who appears capable but unwilling to feed himself is often viewed with irritation by those looking after him. He is regarded as imposing an unnecessary burden upon the caretaking system. Attendant to this expectation of greater independence, dying persons are encouraged to keep certain complaints to themselves, use a minimum of medication, remain active, and care for themselves to the extent possible.

The dying person has a right to exemption from social role responsibilities and commitments. As he undergoes physiologic decline, he is free to withdraw from active engagement in the social system of which he has been a part (Cumming and Henry, 1961). Ultimately the dying person may be freed from every expectation save that of cooperation in the maintenance of physiologic functions—e.g., eating and eliminating. As an individual dies, his attachment to and interest in the world around him diminishes, and his need, or even ability, to respond to the attachments of those about him is reduced. The emotional demand upon his family declines as he moves toward final disengagement.

A second right of the dying person is to be taken care of. Because his plight is not of his own making, society feels obligated toward him. Again, the duty falls primarily on his family or on whatever nursing care the family secures to assist it. And the family's obligation usually extends beyond the provision of physical care to decisions regarding that care and the general welfare and well-being of its dying member. No family is obligated to respond to its detriment, however, or beyond the limits of its physical, emotional, or economic resources.

Finally, the dying person is entitled to continuing respect and status despite his loss of health and function. His dignity is maintained by those caring for him so long as he meets the obligations of the dying role. The dying man makes room in the social order for others. In the process he is expected to do what he can to make a smooth transition and to impose as little burden as possible. If he does so he is entitled to the continuing care and concern of his family and community.

To summarize, both the sick and dying roles are time limited and defined by physician authority. In addition, both maintain for the individuals occupying them the continued respect and status of their community. Beyond this point there appear to be important differences. The duty of the sick person is to desire to get well; that of the dying person is to desire to live as long as he can. The sick person is obliged to cooperate with a physician for the purpose of getting well. The dying person must cooperate with nonphysician caretakers in the hope of functioning at a high level, with minimal distress, for as long as possible. Important differences also appear to exist

The sick person is obliged to cooperate with a physician for the purpose of getting well. The dying person must cooperate with nonphysician caretakers in the hope of functioning at a high level, with minimal distress, for as long as possible.

In recent years dying persons have been assigned to the sick role. . . . The trend toward more vigorous and active treatment of terminal patients by physicians is one manifestation.

as far as rights are concerned. The sick person has the right to be cared for and is encouraged to become dependent. The dying person is also entitled to care but is encouraged to become independent within limits. While both sick and dying persons are exempt from social responsibilities, the dying person is permanently freed from them and allowed to disengage from family and community.

Role Confusion

In recent years dying persons have been assigned to the sick role. Signs of this confusion of roles are not difficult to identify. The trend toward more vigorous and active treatment of terminal patients by physicians is one manifestation. Technological advances have given the physician increased control over physiologic aberrations, which he has naturally exercised with enthusiasm. In so doing he has often lost sight of the fact that he has done little to alter the fatal course of an illness. And, caught up in temporary treatment successes, both doctor and patient have tended to indulge in false hopes. It is, of course, natural for the physician to be energetic in his treatment. Within his professional role the life-saving cure of disease has first priority. Confronted, in an emotionally charged atmosphere, with a patient having high expectations and a family wishing "everything to be done," the doctor responds in an active manner. What we have begun to realize is that such treatment is often more appropriate to actuely ill persons and may unnecessarily prolong the suffering and disability of dying people.

Dying persons are treated as acutely sick ones with respect to the information they are given about their disease and prognosis. In fact a "conspiracy of silence" often surrounds the dying person, maintained by the family, community, and patient himself. Early denial is supported by those who judge the person too frail or vulnerable to cope with the anticipation of his death. It is common practice to withhold bad news from actuely ill persons lest their weakened system be overloaded and their condition aggravated. Our approach to chronically impaired persons is quite different, however. We strive to provide information which, for them, is a source of independence and a foundation for adjustment to physical limitations. Clearly a person needs knowledge of his illness and prognosis if he is to fulfill the obligations of the dying role. The behavior of a dying patient who clings to the sick role, long after the diagnosis of a fatal illness, places inordinate demands upon his family and care-givers. His false hopes, insistence upon restorative treatment, and dependent behavior often lead to a deterioration of relationships with family and physician.

Another sign of confusion between the dying and the sick roles is the increasing tendency to care for dying persons in hospitals. These institutions are primarily oriented toward diagnosis and treatment. Chronic support of function and rehabilitation are, in fact, looked upon by personnel as a drain on the hospital care-giving system. Persons in need of such services are viewed with annoyance as occupying beds needed for the acutely ill. It is hardly surprising that dying patients are neglected on acute medical and surgical floors. Which of their needs competes with falling blood pressures, rising temperatures, and other matters of life or death consequence. Yet, are they truly neglected? Or, do the observers who make this accusation— including some patients—harbor the mistaken notion that dying persons should receive the same kind of attention that sick persons receive? The hospital is a relatively authoritarian community where privacy and autonomy are limited. Such a setting is optimal for the diagnosis and treatment of acute illness but may encourage dependency among the chronically ill or dying.

Open communication with persons suffering from fatal disease appears essential to reestablishment of the dying role.

Reestablishment of the Dying Role

Open communication with persons suffering from fatal disease appears essential to reestablishment of the dying role. The notion that dying persons may be overwhelmed by learning about their prognosis remains unsupported, and unilateral decisions to withhold information ignore a person's right to it and the likelihood that he is already aware of it. Significant tasks may be completed by the dying person providing he knows what lies ahead of him. A will insures that property shall be distributed according to his wishes and in a giftlike manner. Timely decisions regarding business or household affairs allow a smooth transfer of authority. Participation in decisions regarding treatment increases the dying person's sense of mastery and reduces the possibility of his becoming a burden to his family. Awareness of a fatal illness may be spiritually meaningful to a religious person. And, finally, a dying person may draw together a variety of loose ends as he seeks a sense of completion.

Open communication does not imply insensitivity on the part of the physician who must share his understanding of a fatal illness. It does imply a common or shared awareness between the dying person and significant others such that family members or friends may aid that person in carrying out the aforementioned tasks. As a part of the growing consumerism, dying persons can be expected to insist upon a larger say in how they are cared for. And many, as a part of this movement, are already making arrangements for funerals and medical care well in advance of a final illness. The attitude reflected in such actions will, no doubt, contribute to greater independent cooperation on the part of dying persons.

The doctor has an important part to play in reestablishing the dying role. It must be clear to him that once he has made the diagnosis of a fatal illness and exhausted possible curative treatments, his obligation to the dying person changes. He must follow the course of his patient's illness, respond in the event of complications, see to the patient's comfort, and counsel the family and patient regarding his care. Though his role continues to be one of importance it is no longer primary. Other professionals, in

Persons with fatal illnesses should be cared for in an appropriate setting by personnel who regard their needs as having high priority.

charge of supporting function and controlling symptoms, must assume major responsibility when care is needed.

The physician should begin to modify the relationship he has with his dying patient. While assuring him of his continuing availability, he should encourage the patient to assume more responsibility for his care, e.g., medications, diet, and exercise. In contrast to the parent-child mode of interaction that may have characterized the relationship during the acute or undiagnosed phase of the patient's illness, the doctor should strive for one of mutual cooperation (Szasz and Hollender, 1956). While in acute illness he may order analgesic medication according to the need he observes, in chronic illness the physician should rely to a greater extent on the patient's observations and opinions, sharing with him responsibility for safe administration of the drug. When he does so, the dying person may gain a greater sense of control and experience less anxiety.

Persons with fatal illnesses should be cared for in an appropriate setting by personnel who regard their needs as having high priority. As has been pointed out, in most hospitals the needs of dying persons are overshadowed by more urgent affairs unless special programs or units are set up to meet them. Home care is ideal in many ways but the community at large must be prepared to support families and furnish institutional placement when the burden exceeds their resources. The requirements of the chronically ill, whether convalescing of deteriorating, appear sufficiently similar to the needs of dying persons that they may be cared for together, thereby avoiding the stigma of the "death house."

Those who care for the dying must be mindful of three important privileges or rights granted to persons meeting the obligations of the dying role. The first of these is the right of disengagement. As the dying person's energy declines, he withdraws his investment in the world around him and shifts his remaining interest to his body and its disordered function. The process is, of course, stimulated by his anticipated separation. Such disengagement is complicated by a family or community that resists it and clings to him. Inordinate demands are then placed upon the dying person. Too often his emotional needs are assessed by healthy persons, who judge them to be like their own. Sentimentalism is an impediment to solving the problems of dying persons; what is needed are practical answers to difficult questions.

The dying role carries with it the right of unchanging status or valuation within the community. The fact that dying persons have not been held in high esteem by our society may be another reason why the role has been avoided in favor of the sick role. If these persons are to assume the role described, attitudes must begin to change. Of course, appropriate behavior by persons occupying the dying role should result in increased respect for them from families and community.

Finally, the dying role confers the right of protection from abuse. Too many dying persons are exposed to inadequate or neglectful care. Consequently their care must become a matter of higher priority. Unfortunately, it, like the care of chronically ill persons in general, will probably remain a matter of lesser importance regardless of changing attitudes. Still, the vocal concern currently focused on another issue—the rights and status of aged persons—may bring with it constructive change in the approach to dying people.

Implementation

The dying role, if properly established, should clarify the expectations a dying person and his community might reasonably have of one another. But if community leaders and administrators become more aware of an obligation to their dying members, how should they act? What type of programs should they develop? There is, of course, no final solution and simply shifting dying people from one setting to another is not the answer. The plight of chronic mental patients is an example of how a variety of relocations have, in the end, only recreated the poor conditions they were designed to correct (Siegler and Osmond, 1974). Most recently such patients have been moved from crowded and poorly staffed hospitals to the community. Now, however, it has become clear that programs to care for them there are inadequate and they are neglected in the community as they were in the hospital.

Any new programs to improve the care of the dying should be undertaken with caution lest they make matters worse instead of better. At this time, guiding principles are more to be relied upon than uncertain, action-oriented objectives. Foremost is a need to clarify the confusion surrounding the sick and dying roles through public education. Much of the current emphasis on death and dying is backed by emotionalism and based on individual experience. Such a thrust makes the public aware and ready for change but does not point to the direction that change should take. Improved care for dying persons can begin within the existing health system through the application of proven practices of care and delivery.

Continuity of care is a high priority. It allows persons to move about in the care system without major disruptions or abrupt transitions in the services delivered. The needs of the dying are not static and the provision of adequate care may require a high degree of professional expertise. Flexibility in a program goes hand in hand with continuity and helps to individualize the services required. Essential to coordination of activities within the system is communication. In many instances, particularly in smaller communities, communication among a dying person, family, and health personnel may be an easy matter. In larger communities, public hospitals, multiple clinics, rotating personnel, and geographical isolation from families all combine to fragment communication. Special services and personnel may be required to prevent this from occurring.

In a time of increasing consumer awareness health professions are being called upon to account for the quality of care delivered. Utilization reviews, medical audits, and federal standards are all designed to improve

> **Any new programs to improve the care of the dying should be undertaken with caution lest they make matters worse instead of better.**

care and provide for consumer satisfaction. It may also be appropriate for institutions to set standards for and examine the care given dying persons in a manner similar to their monitoring of care provided the sick. Ultimately, high quality care rests upon continuing public awareness and support of the needs of dying people.

Conclusion

The dying role appears to be a distinct and useful concept. It helps clarify what dying persons and those caring for them can reasonably expect of one another. If these expectations can be met, the care of dying persons will be improved and their status in the community enhanced. And, because they occupy an important, life-affirming role, their improved position can only serve the betterment of their communities. The care given dying persons reflects the value placed on life and, in turn, has an influence upon it.

References

Blauner, R. Death and social structure. *Psychiatry* (1966) 29:378–394.

Cumming, E., and Henry, W. *Growing Old: The Process of Disengagement.* Basic Books, 1961.

Gordon, G. *Role Theory and Illness: A Sociological Perspective.* New Haven: College and University Press, 1966.

Kübler-Ross, E. *On Death and Dying.* Macmillan, 1969.

Parsons, T. *The Social System.* Free Press, 1951.

Reynolds, D. K., and Kalish, R. A. The social ecology of dying: Observations of wards for the terminally ill. *Hosp. and Community Psychiatry* (1974) 25:147–152.

Siegler, M. and Osmond, H. *Models of Madness, Models of Medicine.* Macmillan, 1974.

Sudnow, D. *Passing On: The Social Organization of Dying.* Prentice-Hall, 1967.

Szasz, T. S. and Hollender, M. H. A contribution to the philosophy of medicine, the basic models of the doctor-patient relationship. *Arch. Int. Med.* (1956) 97:585–592.

Twaddle, A. C. The concepts of the sick role and illness behavior. *Adv. Psychosom. Med.* (1972) 8:162–179.

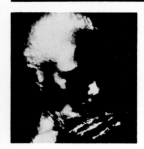

24

Theory

I magine that you have been comatose for seven months with no apparent brain waves. Your family is incurring sizable hospital bills and also getting pressure to find an alternate institutional setting. You are being kept alive by machines. If you were able to make a decision which would influence your care what would it be? Pamela Koza's chapter may help you make this decision, as will the following Appendix exercises:

    A.   Announcing One's Own Death

    B.   Appropriate Death Fantasy

    F.   Euthanasia Exercise

    L.   Privacy Circles

Euthanasia: Some Legal Considerations

Pamela Ennis Koza

The long-awaited decision in one of the most complex court cases to come to public attention was not totally unexpected: New Jersey Supreme Court Judge Robert Muir ruled that Karen Quinlan, who lapsed into a coma on April 15, 1975, must be kept alive with a mechanical life-support system because "there is no constitutional right to die." What is surprising in Judge Muir's ruling, however, is his statement that "the nature, extent and duration of care is the responsibility of the physician. What justification is there to remove it from the control of the medical profession and place it in the hands of the court?"[1] The justification for such action resides in Judge Muir's very words. They exemplify the reluctance on the part of the law, medicine, religion, and philosophy to deal decisively with the issue of euthanasia. Had the Quinlan parents intentionally disconnected the respirator in order to allow their daughter to die, they would have likely been prosecuted for homicide. However, precedent indicates that convictions in such cases are rare, or else that penalties are greatly reduced. The cynic might speculate that it may have been wiser for the Quinlans to follow this course of action rather than to request prior court approval to remove life-support systems. The fact that one may even consider such alternatives is surely a sad commentary on society's failure to take a stand on the euthanasia issue.

Etymologically, the term "euthanasia" is derived from the Greek *eu,* meaning good, and *thanatos,* meaning death. Yet this apparently benign notion of a good or peaceful death now has come to evoke value-laden associations with suicide, murder, and genocide. Today the term is used to refer to any death, or means of death, which from one or more perspectives may be viewed as being of a good or better kind. According to Marya Man-

This material was first published in *Essence, Issues in the Study of Ageing, Dying, and Death,* vol. 1, pp. 79–89, 1977. Copyright 1977 by Atkinson College Press and reproduced by permission.

> **Clearly what is needed is a more objective framework within which to categorize the various ways in which the term "euthanasia" has been employed.**

nes (1974, p. 61) euthanasia "is simply to be able to die with dignity at a moment when life is devoid of it. It is a purely voluntary choice, both on the part of the owner of this life, and on the part of the doctor who knows that this is no longer a life." For Kohl (1974, p. 95) euthanasia is "the painless inducement of a quick death." Gould and Craigmyle (1971, p. 16) use the term to refer to "those techniques and procedures deliberately intended to interrupt the patient's ability to sustain life, to legalize which an act of Parliament would be necessary."

These definitions reflect the lack of consensus about the meaning of euthanasia, and are probably more representative of the particular moral viewpoints of the writers. While moral questions strike at the very heart of the euthanasia controversy, they tend to confuse the issue for definitional purposes. Clearly what is needed is a more objective framework within which to categorize the various ways in which the term "euthanasia" has been employed. Fletcher (1973) has outlined a fourfold typology of elective death that is based on the concepts of voluntariness and directness. While it is unlikely that any specific case could ever be so neatly classified along these two orthogonal dimensions (as demonstrated by the Quinlan case), this schema does have utility in terms of clarity. Euthanasia may be:

1. Voluntary and direct: Death is chosen and carried out by the patient and is a matter of simple request and personal liberty. Suicide falls into this category.
2. Voluntary but indirect: The patient gives to others, such as his physician, lawyer, family, and friends, the discretion to end it all as and when the situation requires, if the patient becomes comatose or too dysfunctional to make the decision pro forma. The "Living Will" has been designed for this purpose.
3. Direct but involuntary: A "mercy killing" is performed on a patient's behalf without his present or past consent. This form of euthanasia is also called active euthanasia. To disconnect the respirator that is keeping Karen Quinlan alive would be an act of direct but involuntary euthanasia.
4. Indirect and involuntary: The patient is "let go." Nothing is done positively to release him from his condition, and what is done negatively is decided *for* him rather than in response to his request. "Passive euthanasia" is another term which has been used to describe such an act. If a patient is beyond recovery and on the verge of death, it is far more natural to speak of the cessation of life-support systems as "permitting" rather than "causing" death. There are sufficient causal factors present for the harm to eventually occur without the physician's contribution.

It must be emphasized that there is an infinitely graduated spectrum from the clear cases to the cases that are far from clear. However, these "typical" categories are useful for understanding the legal sanctions which may be applied in cases of euthanasia.

Within the last few decades the emergence of two factors has demanded a profound change in our whole attitude toward death. This new awareness has made euthanasia a salient focus of attention. Coupled with the mounting longevity of man, advances in the technical skill of the medical profession have allowed doctors to prolong life beyond its long-accepted limits. Yet while medicine can now often delay death, in the process it sometimes makes dying slower, more painful, and more undignified than it has ever been before. In earlier times, by contrast, nature itself made many of man's life and death decisions. According to Slater (1969, p. 51), "Death performs for us the inestimable office of clearing up a mess too big to mend; if we are going to intervene, then we must have at least some hope of doing this ourselves." Medicine is suddenly forced to deal with value-laden questions: where the physician was once concerned only with the morality of doing something to put people mercifully out of hopeless misery, the new question is now whether he may morally omit to do any of the ingenious things that he *could* do to prolong people's suffering.

A second important consideration which has made euthanasia a topical issue involves our growing respect for individual integrity. This respect is based on two humane and significant concerns. First is the compassion that almost all of us feel for those who are painfully and terminally ill. It is inhumane to keep the dying alive when they are in great pain or when they have lost almost all of their usual functions. What is important is the quality as opposed to the quantity of life. Fletcher (1973) argues that in any code of ethics where humanness and personal integrity are put above biological life and function, it is harder morally to justify letting somebody die a slow and ugly death, dehumanized, than it is to justify helping him to escape from such misery.

A second related aspect is the recognition of the freedom of the individual to maintain and exercise his rights over matters affecting his life and death, his mind and body. In the practice of medicine, this respect requires that a patient be permitted to determine the course of the treatment that he will receive; a patient should not be subjected to medical treatment to which he does not consent. Those who are in favor of voluntary euthanasia extend this notion by arguing that the choice to withhold techniques that would prolong life is a choice to shorten life. Therefore, if one can choose to shorten one's life, why can't one ask a physician to put an end to one's life by a simple and direct act of intervention?

Yet, in spite of our heightened sensitivity to these issues, the euthanasia controversy has not been resolved. Perhaps the major obstacle in this debate is the fact that euthanasia is inextricably bound up with the law. Abstract considerations about the ethics and morality of euthanasia are not as salient as the concrete legal sanctions which may be applied to one who is involved in such a case.

> . . . while medicine can now often delay death, in the process it sometimes makes dying slower, more painful, and more undignified than it has ever been before.

The Treatment of Euthanasia Under Canadian Law

In Canada there are no laws dealing specifically with euthanasia, although there are a number of sections in the Criminal Code (R.S.C. 1970, chapter c.-34) which are potentially applicable in such cases. Should a doctor inject a fatal dose of a drug into the veins of his patient, this act can be construed as culpable homicide under s. 205(1):

A person commits homicide when, directly or indirectly, by any means, he causes the death of a human being. Where a doctor causes the death of his patient by discontinuing a life-saving device like a respirator, this act could be construed as noncapital murder (s. 212), for a doctor has a duty to preserve life and is expected to exercise it. Even if the physician does this act with the permission of the patient, as through instructions in a Living Will, he has aided his patient to commit suicide and could be charged under s. 224:

> Every one who (b) aids or abets a person to commit suicide, whether suicide ensues or not, is guilty of an indictable offense and is liable to imprisonment for fourteen years.

Similarly, a physician may be liable under the preceding section if he leaves fatal tablets within reach of the patient, knowing that he will take them for the purpose of committing suicide. These two examples are rather paradoxical, given the fact that suicide itself is no longer a crime in Canada.

Where a doctor is responsible for the death of his patient by omitting to give him the benefit of life-saving devices which are available, he is potentially liable under two different sections of the Criminal Code. S. 198 states:

> Every one who undertakes to administer surgical or medical treatment to another person or to do any other lawful act that may endanger the life of another person is, except in cases of necessity, under a legal duty to have and to use reasonable knowledge, skill and care in so doing.

By s. 202:

> (1) Every one is criminally negligent who
>   (a) in doing anything, or
>   (b) in omitting to do anything that it is his duty to do, shows wanton or reckless disregard for the lives or safety of other persons.
> (2) For the purpose of this section, "duty" means a duty imposed by law.

What about the case where doses of morphine are increased to relieve pain? As the body becomes resistent to the effects of this drug, the next dose might be the fatal one. This is a grey area in legality because every patient suffering from continuous pain is entitled to be relieved of his suffering, even to the extent of being kept in an unconscious state on a constant basis. If it could be determined that the final and fatal dose of morphine was unavoidable, no criminal charges could be laid against the doctor.

Finally, there is the peculiarly legal notion of acceleration of death, contrary to s. 209:

> Where a person causes bodily injury to a human being that results in death, he causes the death of that human being notwithstanding that the effect of the bodily injury is only to accelerate his death from a disease or disorder arising from some other cause.

If there is only the slightest spark of life in a person and this is extinguished, such an act is as much a homicide as the killing of a healthy and vital person. In a legal sense, euthanasia may be viewed as the acceleration of death that is already in progress. One can see possible difficulties with such a legal concept in transplant cases.

. . . since mercy is not differentiated from malice, there is no legal basis for distinguishing euthanasia from murder.

The Rationale Behind the Law

A fundamental value underscored by the legal system is the sanctity of life. According to the present law, every life is to be preserved for as long as possible, no matter what its quantity or quality.

Homicide is a generic term that denotes the killing of a human being. As a legal concept, it refers to any act that causes or contributes materially to a person's death. The only exceptions which are legally acceptable are cases of self-defense, the defense of family or property, or the performance of a legal duty. In connection with the practice of medicine, homicide applies to any act or omission that precipitates a patient's death, even though he may be fatally ill or on the verge of dying. There is no legal equivalent to the moral distinction between causing and permitting a patient to die which will allow a doctor to bring about death by withholding or terminating life-preserving measures. The criminal law is only concerned with the fundamental distinction between acts and omissions.

Maguire (1974, p. 22) has argued that the law "plods along encumbered by faded and inadequate categories that do no justice to the moral and medical facts of life." This certainly appears to be true with respect to the legal status of euthanasia. The present categories of the law are incapable of encompassing the realities involved in death by choice cases where, by omission or commission, one's own death or the death of another is opted for in preference to continued living. A prime example is the failure of the criminal law to appreciate the essential difference that motive makes in euthanasia cases.

From a moral point of view, motive is usually one of the most important considerations in the evaluation of human behavior. From a legal viewpoint, motive has far less significance and is not regarded as a necessary component of any crime, except to demonstrate self-defense. Therefore, since mercy is not differentiated from malice, there is no legal basis for distinguishing euthanasia from murder. Where euthanasia is planned and deliberate, premeditation, the basic element in murder, is present. The fact that the person to be killed is already dying is no justification. The end of both actions is the same under the law: an individual's life has been shortened. However, Maguire (1974) notes several ways in which the motives of the mercy killer and the murderer may vary. One major difference is that the mercy killer is not motivated by a disrespect for law, but by a respect for life. Yet such distinctions are meaningless under a law which does not recognize an individual's right to die. For this reason, a patient's consent is not regarded as a legitimate defense in criminal homicide cases.

In addition to the failure to recognize motive in euthanasia cases, there is no legal definition of death based on twentieth century facts.

Legal and Medical Definitions of Death

The legal concept of death is quite general and does not take into account the changes that have occurred in the practice of medicine. The law makes the assumption that the medical criteria for determining death are settled and not in doubt among physicians. The law further assumes that the physicians' traditional method for the determination of death is to ascertain the absence of all vital signs. According to Black's Law Dictionary (4th ed., 1951), death is defined as, "The cessation of life, the ceasing to exist, defined by physicians as a total stoppage of the circulation of blood, and a cessation of the animal and vital functions consequent thereupon, such as respiration, pulsation, etc." The courts usually interpret death simply as the antithesis of life, and as an event which takes place at a specific point in time when vital functions cease and can no longer be revived. Therefore a patient is considered to be alive as long as any heartbeat and respiration can be perceived with or without instruments, regardless of how these signs of life are maintained.

In contrast to the legal view, medicine views death as a dynamic process rather than as a single event. It is now possible to prolong the signs of life long after the loss of vital functions is permanent. Modern resuscitation and supportive measures can now restore "life" as judged by the ancient standards of persistent respiration and continuing heartbeat, even when there is not the remotest possibility that consciousness will be recovered after massive brain damage. The Ad Hoc Committee of the Harvard Medical School (1968) has developed new criteria for a definition of death. It has defined irreversible coma as the criterion of death, with a permanently nonfunctioning brain exhibiting the following characteristics: (1) unreceptivity and unresponsivity to external stimuli; (2) no movements or spontaneous breathing for one hour; (3) absence of elicitable reflexes. Although these three criteria are the most important, a flat EEG repeated at 24 hours has confirmatory value. However, its utility depends on the exclusion of two conditions: hypothermia, or central nervous system depressants like barbiturates.

The Ad Hoc Committee has urged physicians to universally adopt irreversible coma as the criterion of death, as this could form the basis of a change in the current legal concept. No statutory change in the law should be necessary, since the law treats the question essentially as one of fact to be determined by the physician in each case. Yet, until this definition is agreed upon, disparate concepts of the moment of death in law and medicine may have crucial implications for the parties in the final illness. The legal concept, which overrides the medical when the two do not agree, may determine civil or criminal liability in such areas as initiation of resuscitation, interruption of sustaining devices, or other acts or omissions relating to the deceased.

The Law in Practice

That the legal norm is severe and uncompromising does not necessarily mean that the people who administer the legal system are also severe and uncompromising. The law in practice does not always correspond to the law in theory. Kamisar (1969) has provided a thorough discussion of particular cases reported in the press and in law reports, and it is evident that there is a high incidence of acquittals, suspended sentences, and even failure to indict mercy killers. Convictions are rare [or] . . . typically . . . carry lenient sentences and probation. As Fletcher (1973, p. 121) argues, "there is something obviously evasive when we rule motive out in charging people with the crime of mercy killing, but bring it back in again for purposes of determining punishment." Acquittals are usually based on an acceptable defense such as temporary insanity. There appears to be a flight to psychiatry when there is no help from the law; the court offers a diagnosis in place of a verdict.

There is no case in Anglo-American tradition in which a doctor has been convicted of murder or manslaughter for having killed to end the suffering of his patient. In 1950 U.S. doctor Herman Sander was tried and acquitted after he confessed to injecting air into the veins of a terminal cancer patient.[2] In a more recent American case, Dr. Vincent Montemarano was accused of the "wilful murder" of a cancer patient into whose veins he allegedly injected a lethal dose of potassium chloride. His defense lawyer told the jury that, "It's not a case of mercy killing, it's a case of murder—pure and simple."[3] To have admitted euthanasia would be tantamount to a guilty plea of murder, and would have relieved the state of the burden of proof. Dr. Montemarano was found "Not Guilty" by the jury after only fifty-five minutes of deliberation.

Until there are legal justifications and procedures to allow doctors to practice euthanasia, those who do act out of mercy must, in turn, rely on the mercy of others who judge their actions. The law in theory is a product of medical ethics and social norms that take seriously the role of the physician as the preserver of life. It therefore underscores the expectation that

There is no case in Anglo-American tradition in which a doctor has been convicted of murder or manslaughter for having killed to end the suffering of his patient.

Today more and more individuals are arguing for the establishment of a legal right for euthanasia. . . .

life be preserved as a legal responsibility, yet it does not reflect the ambiguities and conflicts that arise when other medical and social values are incompatible with this requirement.

Do We Need a Law Dealing Specifically With Euthanasia?

In 1974 the following question was asked by a Gallup Poll in Toronto: "When a person has an incurable disease that causes great suffering, do you or do you not think that competent doctors should be allowed by law to end the patient's life through mercy killing if the patient has made a formal request in writing?" Fifty-five per cent of the respondents approved, while 35 per cent disapproved. In 1968 when this same question was asked, approval just marginally outweighed disapproval.[4] While society's attitudes toward euthanasia appear to be changing, this trend is not reflected in our present laws where inconsistencies among medical, social, and legal values are expressed by the law in practice. Trubo (1973) points out that foreign countries such as Uruguay and Switzerland, by contrast, have made great strides in the legal treatment of euthanasia. They have gone to the extent of recognizing motive, the victim's consent, and even, in some cases, the legalization of passive euthanasia.

Today more and more individuals are arguing for the establishment of a legal right for euthanasia, without the patient, family, or those who provide or administer the means of death incurring any legal penalty or stigma. What many advocates are seeking is legal recognition of the Euthanasia Educational Council's Living Will. This is a short testament addressed to the patient's family, physician, clergyman, and lawyer. It says, in part, "If there is no reasonable expectation of my recovery from physical or mental disability, I request that I be allowed to die and not be kept alive by artificial means or heroic measures . . . I do not fear death as much as I fear the indignity of deterioration, dependence, and hopeless pain. I ask that medication be mercifully administered to me for terminal suffering even if it hastens the moment of death." In Florida, legislation called the Death with Dignity Bill, permitting people to decide when medical treatment should be withheld from close relatives who are incurably incapacitated, has been passed in the Legislature's lower house.[5]

Some supporters of euthanasia believe that such actions do not go far enough in that they only sanction passive forms of euthanasia which have been occurring all along. What is desired is the enactment of legislation permitting active or voluntary euthanasia, within strict and clearly defined limits and conditions. Yet such attempts have been struck down in Great Britain successively in Parliamentary debates in 1936, 1950, and 1969. The first debate took place in the House of Lords on December 1, 1936 when the second reading of the Voluntary Euthanasia (Legislation) Bill was moved by Lord Ponsonby. "Briefly, our desire is to obtain legal recognition for the principle that in cases of advanced and inevitably fatal disease, attended by agony which reaches or oversteps the boundaries of human endurance, the sufferers after legal enquiry and after due observance of all safeguards, shall have the right to demand and be entitled to receive release."[6] By this Bill, euthanasia could be effected only if a patient was over twenty-one years of age, was suffering from an incurable and fatal illness, and had signed a form in the presence of two witnesses asking to be put to death. A special court would then consider the case and, if satisfied, would issue two certificates: one to the applicant and another to the practitioner deputed to administer euthanasia. At the end of this 1936 debate, 14 voted in favor of the Bill, with 35 against.

The next debate in the House of Lords was on November 28, 1950. This was not a debate on a Bill but on a Motion in the name of Lord Chorley, "To call attention to the need for legalizing voluntary euthanasia, and to move for papers."[7] The motion was withdrawn. In 1968 a draft bill was prepared by the Euthanasia Society with the aim of eliminating many of the death-bed formalities that were inherent in the 1936 Bill. Under this proposed Bill, anyone might make a declaration in advance stating that he or she wished in certain circumstances to be put painlessly to death. Anyone making such a declaration became a "qualified patient" once two physicians had certified in writing that the patient appeared to them to be suffering from what was termed an "irremedial condition." This was defined as a serious physical illness or impairment reasonably thought, in the patient's case, to be incurable and expected to cause him severe distress or render him incapable of rational existence. If such a condition was satisfied, a physician might lawfully "administer euthanasia" to a qualified patient. A declaration would not come into effect until one month had elapsed, but then, unless revoked, was to remain in force during the lifetime of the declarant. However, a declaration could be revoked at any time by actual destruction or notice of cancellation, either by the declarant or by his order. Finally, no physician or nurse would be required to administer euthanasia if he or she were opposed to the practice.

Lord Raglan introduced this same Bill with minor modifications in the House of Lords for debate on March 25, 1969. However, he was defeated by a vote of 61 to 40.[8] One criticism against the Bill was that there was no requirement that a person making a declaration be of sound mind. In addition, many opponents argued that the provisions for revocation of the declaration appeared to be defective. What if, for example, a declarant changed his mind but could not locate his declaration? The definition of irremedial condition was also considered to be far too wide: an individual with an amputation could be said to be suffering from an irremedial condition. Finally, there were no provisions in the Bill to prohibit discrimination against doctors or nurses who were conscientiously opposed to euthanasia.

An even more subtle problem, however, is whether the adult patient is really in a position to consent to death.

While these technical difficulties could theoretically be solved by revising and rewording the Bill, the strong opposition against such legislation in general stems from much more deep-seated issues. Kamisar (1969), who has been a most vocal opponent of voluntary euthanasia legislation, argues that there is too great a risk of abuse and mistake to warrant a change in the existing law. He feels that any effort to legalize euthanasia, however guarded, will form the "thin edge of the wedge." Gould and Craigmyle (1971, p. 88) agree: "Once the principle of the sanctity of human life is abandoned, or the propaganda accepted that to uphold it is old-fashioned, prejudiced, or superstitious, the way is open to the raising of—and the satisfaction of—a demand for so-called euthanasia for the severely crippled, the aged, and ultimately for all those who are a burden on community services and the public purse."

An even more subtle problem, however, is whether the adult patient is really in a position to consent to death. When does he make this decision—while heavily drugged, or during a period when narcotic relief is withdrawn for the decision? Mental side-effects of narcotics, pain, and toxic effects of disease or the violent reactions to certain surgical procedures may change our capacity for rational and courageous thought. How does one distinguish lucidity? The likelihood of confusion, distortion, and vacillation in such circumstances would appear to be a serious drawback to any voluntary plan. Is the suggested alternative of consent in advance a satisfactory solution? Can such a consent truly be deemed an informed one? "Is this the kind of choice, assuming that it can be made in a fixed and rational manner, that we want to offer a gravely ill person? Will we not sweep up, in the process, some who are not really tired of life but think others are tired of them; some who do not really want to die, but who feel they should not live on, because to do so when there looms the legal alternative of euthanasia is to do a selfish or a cowardly act? Will not some feel an obligation to have themselves "eliminated" in order that funds allocated for their terminal care might be better used by their families or, financial worries aside, in order to relieve their families of the emotional strain involved?" (Kamisar 1969, pp. 95–96).

Another argument deals with the fatal mistakes that would inevitably occur should these proposals receive legislative implementation. Diseases go into unaccountable remission, and the power of life is unpredictable. What if a cure is found? This objection is not as valid as the preceding one, for it tenders a vague hope of medical miracles as an argument against death by choice. At most, continuing medical advances suggest that we may never despair of finding a cure *some* day. However in the meantime, some cases may become too advanced for a cure to offer any hope of benefit. A related argument is that diagnosis and prognosis are fallible. Yet it is an inescapable feature of the human condition that no one is infallible about anything; mistakes occur in every sphere of life. We cannot avoid making a decision to act or abstain even in matters of life or death.

Perhaps the most critical problem is the psychological effects that legalized euthanasia would have—on the patient, his family, and on medical personnel. Should the patient to be killed be segregated from the members of his family, or should he be attended by them to be supported by their affection? Should they be present at the fatal ministration, or only before and after? Should the patient or his family members know at which precise moment the ministry of death is to be applied, or should all be in ignorance? And if all are in ignorance, what will be the effect on the patient and his relatives every time a doctor or nurse enters the room? What are the effects on other patients? Could their sense of security in doctors and nurses be undermined by watching events in the wards and noticing that others have died? Are ward patients to be told which patients have died naturally and which have been legally euthanatized? How would other chronically ill patients care to be attended by these same doctors and nurses who administer euthanasia? Doctors and nurses could be put in a self-contradictory situation, expecting themselves to observe one set of values with some of their patients and a contradictory set of values with others. What are the attitudes of doctors and nurses who are being made the ministers of death? Is there not an implicit understanding on the part of a doctor who knowingly accepts the care of a "qualified patient" to kill him either at the patient's request or if a condition supervenes which might cause further deterioration? Should the administration of euthanasia even be a part of a doctor's role, or should there be a cadre of professional euthanatizers? Would they charge for this service? All of the above presupposes a patient who has been informed of his condition. Yet, even in this area, there is ample evidence that physicians are often far from candid with their patients (Mount, Jones, and Patterson 1974).

Such questions spiral on and on, but they all serve to illustrate the point that the problem of euthanasia cannot be considered in terms of the dying person alone. The relatives and friends of each dying person are intimately associated with the death. Also, the care and treatment of the dying is ultimately the concern of the whole of society.

Perhaps the most critical problem is the psychological effects that legalized euthanasia would have—on the patient, his family, and on medical personnel.

Conclusions

In the light of the foregoing discussion, one must ask whether or not specific legislation about euthanasia would be an overly rigid solution to a problem that changes dimensions with each individual case. Perhaps we should invoke a more sensitive interpretation of the law as it now stands, a simple negative proposal involving the removal of euthanasia from the ban of the criminal law. Williams (1958) suggests that the most hopeful line of advance would be to bring forward a measure that does no more than give legislative blessing to the practice that is approved of by the great weight of medical opinion. Such a move would give the medical practitioner a wide discretion and would require that we place our trust in his good sense. Williams (1958, p. 303) states that it should merely be provided that "no

Coming to grips with the issue of euthanasia will probably be one of the biggest problems which the law will confront in our lifetime.

medical practitioner should be guilty of an offense in respect of an act done intentionally to accelerate the death of a patient who is seriously ill, unless it is proved that the act was not done in good faith with the consent of the patient and for the purpose of saving him from severe pain in an illness believed to be of an incurable and fatal character.'' Under this formula, it would be for the physician, if charged, to show that the patient was seriously ill, but for the prosecution to prove that the physician acted from some motive other than the humanitarian one allowed to him by law. Under such a formula, the moral question would no longer be whether euthanasia is right or wrong, but whether the doctor should be punished. If the law were to remove its ban on euthanasia, the effect would be to leave this subject to the individual conscience.

No one would say that Williams's proposal is an ideal solution, although it does merit serious consideration. There is an absence of safeguards, a risk of abuse, and the possibility of mistakes. Furthermore, there is the important question of whether the physician would even want to accept this responsibility. According to Maguire (1974), doctors should never be involved in decisions of this nature, as the choice for death is a moral one involving personal, nonmedical factors and values over which the doctor has no special competence.

Coming to grips with the issue of euthanasia will probably be one of the biggest problems which the law will confront in our lifetime. Whether the controversy is to be resolved by positive legislation or by reinterpretation of existing laws is itself a question that will undoubtedly generate much debate. A discussion of euthanasia should certainly be given high priority by the federal Law Reform Commission. However, a strong argument can be made against any law which defines or impinges upon the manner in which men and women choose to live—or die.

Notes

1. Dad ''numb'' as judge rules girl in coma must live. *The Toronto Star,* Nov. 11, 1975, p. 1.
2. *Time Magazine,* March 6, 1950, p. 20.
3. U.S. doctor's mercy killing trial begins today in New York. *The Toronto Star,* Jan. 14, 1974, p. 1.
4. Qualified mercy killing approved by 55 per cent. *The Toronto Star,* May 15, 1974, p. B5.
5. To depart at choice? *The Globe and Mail,* Feb. 8, 1975, p. 6.
6. *Hansard,* House of Lords, Vol. 103, Cols. 465-506.
7. *Hansard,* House of Lords, Vol. 169, Cols. 552-598.
8. *Hansard,* House of Lords, Vol. 300, Cols. 1143-1254.

References

A definition of irreversible coma. Report of the Ad Hoc Committee of the Harvard Medical School to examine the definition of brain death; Henry Beecher, Chairman. *Journal of the American Medical Association* 205(6)(1968):85-88.

Fletcher, Joseph. Ethics and euthanasia. In R. Williams (ed.), *To Live and to Die.* New York: Springer-Verlag, 1973.

Gould, J. and Lord Craigmyle (eds). *Your Death Warrant? The Implications of Euthanasia.* London: Geoffrey Chapman, 1971.

Kamisar, Y. Euthanasia legislation: Some non-religious objections. In A. B. Downing (ed.), *Euthanasia and the Right to Death*. London: Peter Owen, 1969.

Kohl, Marvin. *The Morality of Killing*. London: Peter Owen, 1974.

Maguire, D. *Death by Choice*. Garden City, N.Y.: Doubleday & Co., Inc., 1974.

Mannes, M. *Last Rights*. New York: William Morrow and Company, 1974.

Mount, B. F.; A. Jones; and A. Patterson. Death and dying: Attitudes in a teaching hospital. *Urology* IV(6)(1974):741–747.

Slater, E. Death: The biological aspect. In A. B. Downing (ed.), *Euthanasia and the Right to Death*. London: Peter Owen, 1969.

Trubo, R. *An Act of Mercy: Euthanasia Today*. Los Angeles: Nash Publishing, 1973.

Williams, G. *The Sanctity of Life and the Criminal Law*. London: Faber and Faber, Ltd., 1958.

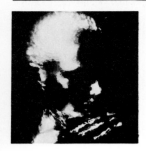

25

Research

Do you think that your views about euthanasia are more favorable than those of most of your friends? How do you think senior medical students, physicians, registered nurses, first-year medical students, senior nursing students, first-year nursing students, and college students compare in their attitudes toward euthanasia? This chapter by Winget, Kapp, and Yeaworth sheds some light on these questions as well as others. The following Appendix exercises are suggested follow-ups to the chapter.

B.   Appropriate Death Fantasy

F.   Euthanasia Exercise

L.   Privacy Circles

Attitudes toward Euthanasia

Carolyn Winget

Frederic T. Kapp

Rosalee C. Yeaworth

This study is a report on attitudes toward euthanasia as reflected in a survey of medical, nursing and college students, and practicing physicians and nurses. These attitudes are of crucial significance in the decision-making process when issues of fighting for life or maintaining existence are posed.

The word "euthanasia" arouses a mixture of feelings and images in most people. On the basis of its Greek derivation, the word comes from *eu,* meaning well, and *thanatos,* meaning death. Thus, euthanasia is defined as "good" or easy, painless death. It is more fully defined in Webster's Dictionary (1961) as the "act or practice of painlessly putting to death persons suffering from incurable and distressing disease." As medical technology has advanced, the subject of euthanasia has been the topic of debate not only by physicians and other health professionals, but also by lawyers, theologians, politicians, and the lay public.

The philosophical question may become a clinical dilemma for physicians and nurses or for patients and their families when the question of fighting for or maintaining life is posed and a decision cannot be avoided. This decision making may be an active or a passive process. Just as failure of those in authority to exercise control does not mean absence of control, but rather control exercised by other forces, so, making a decision not to discontinue treatment may imply making a decision to prolong marginal existence (Skinner, 1971).

Parsons and his colleagues (1973) have recently focused our attention on the importance of greater societal knowledge and participation in decision making in medical ethics. However, most of the literature stresses that the onus of making a decision ultimately falls on the physician. This is a heavy burden for the physician, but once the decision is made, the nurse, the patient and the family may live more closely with it than the doctor (Braverman 1969; Gustafson 1973).

This material was first published in the *Journal of Medical Ethics,* vol. 3, pp. 18–25, 1977. Copyright 1977 by the Society for the Study of Medical Ethics. It is printed here in slightly modified form by permission.

Areas of Conflict in Attitudes to Euthanasia

A recent survey of the American public (Harris 1974) indicated that 62 per cent of those polled believed that a patient with a terminal disease ought to be able to tell his doctor to let him die rather than to extend his life when no cure is in sight.

There are a number of areas in which attitudes toward euthanasia may give rise to conflict. One way to conceptualize such problems is to classify them as primarily interpersonal in nature in contradistinction to those that are intrapersonal. In the latter area, one starts with the premises that persons strive for cognitive balance or consistency in their attitudes and beliefs (Brown 1965) and that the process of socialization into a professional role involves learning attitudes and beliefs as well as skills (Vollmer and Mills 1966; *Society today,* 1973). Hence, the intrapersonal problem is exemplified by the individual in whom there exists inconsistent attitudes relating to a particular subject, i.e., the physician who believes individual freedom includes the freedom of choice to live or to die, but who also believes that every effort should be made to keep patients alive as long as possible. There is the further possibility that a professional may hold certain personal beliefs, attitudes, and values that are incongruent with what he perceives as the prescriptions or proscriptions for his professional role. Thus, a physician or nurse might believe that persons should ultimately have freedom of choice regarding matters of life and death, but believe that his or her professional role requires doing everything possible to preserve or prolong life for any patient in his care. The longer the socialization process for a role the more likely that the attitudes and beliefs associated with that role will become internalized and integrated into the individual's overall belief system.

Interpersonal attitudinal problems focused on euthanasia exist when the attitudes and beliefs of physicians or nurses are in conflict with each other or with those of the larger society, the patient, or the family. Such interpersonal issues are confounded and made more difficult to elucidate by the very lack of congruence and consistency which may characterize the intrapersonal area. In addition, very subtle nuances of definition become magnified and of marked significance, as is true in the specialized literature on euthanasia.

A recent survey of the American public (Harris 1974) indicated that 62 per cent of those polled believed that a patient with a terminal disease ought to be able to tell his doctor to let him die rather than to extend his life when no cure is in sight. However, only 37 per cent believed that the patient who was terminally ill should be allowed to tell his doctor to put him out of his misery. The American Medical Association's stand reflects this wider societal perspective. The statement adopted by the House of Delegates of the American Medical Association on 4 December 1973 was:

> The intentional termination of the life of one human being by another—mercy killing—is contrary to that for which the medical profession stands and is contrary to the policy of the American Medical Association.

The cessation of the employment of extraordinary means to prolong the life of the body when there is irrefutable evidence that biological death is imminent is the decision of the patient and/or his immediate family. The advice and judgment of the physician should be freely available to the patient and/or his immediate family.

The second part of the AMA statement above would put the onus of making the decision on the patient and his immediate family. But it is still the physician who must make the decision that biological death is imminent. The statement does not attempt to deal with situations where biological death might not be imminent, but the judgment to be made centers around the possibility of the person's life ever being "meaningful" or "useful." McCormick (1974) tries to resolve this dilemma by suggesting that "life is a value to be preserved only insofar as it contains some potentiality for human relationships."

Rachels (1975) has argued against the AMA stand on active euthanasia or so-called "mercy killing," pointing out that "the process of being allowed to die" can be relatively slow and painful, whereas being given a lethal injection is relatively quick and painless. He argues that there is no moral difference between active and passive euthanasia. The differentiation hinges on making the decision that, for a given patient, death is less an evil than that patient's continued existence.

Fletcher (1968) has defined four types of euthanasia: (1) direct voluntary; (2) indirect voluntary; (3) indirect involuntary; (4) direct involuntary. "Indirect" implies discontinuing a treatment, while "direct" involves initiating an action. The patient participates in the direct voluntary type of euthanasia by collaborating in an act to bring about his own death, and in the indirect voluntary type by asking that life-sustaining measures be omitted or discontinued. In the two involuntary types of euthanasia, a conscious decision by the patient is not involved. For example, in the case of a comatose patient decisions are usually made by the family.

Shils and Schweitzer (Kohl 1972), proponents of the "sanctity-of-life principle," hold that life is the most primordial experience of man and therefore that it ought always to be inviolable. They contend that man cannot either create or destroy life for life is sacred and must be so treated. To them, to take life no matter how it is done or for what reason, is to punish and any violation of the sacredness of life must inevitably lead to undesirable consequences. Data relating to both the interpersonal issues and to the problem of intrapersonal conflict are presented below.

Shils and Schweitzer . . . hold that life is the most primordial experience of man and therefore that it ought always to be inviolable.

Method: The Questionnaire

An interdisciplinary research group at the University of Cincinnati Medical Center, as part of a larger study, developed a "Questionnaire for understanding the dying patient and his family." The construction of the questionnaire has been described elsewhere (Yeaworth, Kapp, and Winget 1974). Embedded in the 50 items of part I of the questionnaire are five items that relate to euthanasia. These are:

Item 1. Regardless of his age, disabilities, and personal preference, a person should be kept alive as long as possible.
Item 13. Those who support the principle of "death with dignity" endorse active as well as passive euthanasia.
Item 14. No matter what my personal belief, in my role as a medical or nursing professional I would fight to keep the patient alive.
Item 16. Individual freedom of choice ultimately should mean freedom of choice to live or die within a context of responsibility for self and others.
Item 33. Some patients should be allowed to die without making heroic efforts to prolong their lives.

Each item could be responded to on a five-point scale ranging from "strongly agree" to "strongly disagree." Weights were assigned to statements so that responses indicative of a favorable attitude toward

Table 1 Characteristics of groups studied

	Type of group						
	College students	First-year nursing students	Senior nursing students	Registered nurses	First-year medical students	Senior medical students	Physicians
No. in group	75	108	69	75	110	90	30
Setting of data collection[1]	Classroom	Classroom	Classroom	Hospital	Take home	Mailed	Mailed
Sex							
Male	17 (23)[2]	2 (2)	0	0	92 (84)	82 (91)	30 (100)
Female	52 (69)	106 (98)	69 (100)	75 (100)	11 (10)	5 (6)	0
Not answered	6 (8)	0	0	0	7 (6)	3 (3)	0
Age (yr)							
20	38 (51)	99 (92)	0	0	0	0	0
20-25	26 (35)	2 (2)	56 (81)	17(22)	97 (88)	28 (31)	4 (13)
26-35	5 (7)	2 (2)	11 (16)	29 (39)	6 (6)	59 (66)	9 (30)
35	0	0	0	29 (39)	0	0	17 (57)
Not answered	6 (7)	5 (4)	2 (3)	0	7 (6)	3 (3)	0
Religion							
Catholic	23 (31)	38 (35)	23 (33)	22 (29)	22 (20)	24 (27)	1 (3)
Protestant	33 (44)	52 (48)	37 (54)	51 (68)	41 (37)	30 (33)	2 (7)
Jewish	4 (5)	4 (4)	2 (3)	0	15 (14)	14 (16)	24 (80)
None/other	8 (11)	0	0	0	17 (15)	10 (11)	0
Not answered	7 (9)	14 (13)	7 (10)	2 (3)	15 (14)	11 (13)	3 (10)

[1] Protocols were administered anonymously and subjects were recruited after approval by appropriate committees monitoring research on human subjects in the various colleges.
[2] Numbers in parentheses are percentages, numbers rounded to equal 100 per cent.

euthanasia were assigned a low score, i.e., a weighting of 1 or 2, while attitudes favorable to the "sanctity-of-life principle" were assigned a score of 4 or 5. Responses indicative of indecision or uncertainty were weighted 3.

The responses to the five euthanasia items were abstracted from the completed questionnaires of a variety of subjects: college students, first-year and senior nursing students, first-year and senior medical students, practicing registered nurses and practicing physicians. Table 1 provides information on the composition of these samples.

Results

Table 2 indicates the percentage responses to the five euthanasia items for each of the seven groups. Most individuals in all the groups disagree with Item 1. This disagreement with keeping a patient alive regardless of age, disability, and personal preference is most marked in the senior medical student group and is least marked in the first-year nursing students and the college students. Both nursing students and medical students show a decided difference in the proportion of those who are undecided when first-year men are compared to seniors.

Item 13 asks for attitudes regarding the issue of equating active with passive euthanasia within the overall rubric of "death with dignity." This item contains ambiguous cognitive and attitudinal components which apparently evoke ambivalence and uncertainty. The variance in weighted responses is great and the proportion of those answering "undecided" in each group is very high compared to responses to the other four items about euthanasia. Physicians and nurses in practice show proportionately the fewest "undecided" and "agree" responses and, thus, the highest percentage of responses presumably distinguishing active from passive euthanasia.

Responses to the statement about fighting to keep a patient alive (Item 14) again reveal marked differences among the seven sampled groups. Practicing physicians, nurses, and senior medical students are the three groups that indicate the most disagreement with the notion of fighting to keep a patient alive at any cost. Indecision in this area is greater for senior than for first-year nursing students but is considerably less for senior than for first-year medical students.

Issues of autonomy for the terminally ill patient are raised in Item 16. While the majority of all seven of our subject groups agree on the abstract notion of freedom of choice, the two groups of practicing professionals show greater disagreement proportionately than any of the student groups. First-year medical and senior nursing groups are, again, the two with the highest proportion of "undecided" responses.

There is overwhelming agreement with Item 33, "some patients should be allowed to die without making heroic efforts to prolong their lives." For both the nursing and medical students there are markedly fewer "undecided" responses in senior students as compared with those of first-year students.

There is overwhelming agreement with Item 33, "some patients should be allowed to die without making heroic efforts to prolong their lives."

Table 2 Percentage response to five euthanasia items by seven groups of respondents

No. Group	Strongly agree (%)	Agree (%)	Undecided (%)	Disagree (%)	Strongly disagree (%)
Item 1 Regardless of his age, disabilities, and personal preference, a person should be kept alive as long as possible					
75 College students	8	19	19	37	17
108 First-year nursing students	4	13	30	41	12
69 Senior nursing students	3	11	13	28	45
75 Registered nurses	4	11	23	34	28
110 First-year medical students	2	6	21	36	35
90 Senior medical students	0	0	9	38	53
30 Physicians	10	7	10	33	40
Item 13 Those who support the principle of "death with dignity" endorse active as well as passive euthanasia					
75 College students	0	21	59	17	3
108 First-year nursing students	1	19	46	25	6
69 Senior nursing students	0	14	54	22	10
75 Registered nurses	0	19	32	33	16
110 First-year medical students	4	21	45	23	8
90 Senior medical students	0	9	35	40	16
30 Physicians	3	10	13	50	23
Item 14 No matter what my personal beliefs, in my role as a medical professional I would fight to keep the patient alive[1]					
75 College students	25	35	24	12	4
108 First-year nursing students	24	45	22	6	1
69 Senior nursing students	13	28	32	19	9
75 Registered nurses	11	36	24	25	4
110 First-year medical students	7	25	41	23	5
90 Senior medical students	0	24	23	43	10
30 Physicians	13	20	17	40	10
Item 16 Individual freedom of choice ultimately should mean freedom of choice to live or die within a context of responsibility for self and others					
75 College students	17	48	19	15	1
108 First-year nursing students	18	45	18	14	4
69 Senior nursing students	17	42	25	16	0
75 Registered nurses	13	46	21	15	5
110 First-year medical students	19	47	24	7	4
90 Senior medical students	23	51	16	9	1
30 Physicians	3	67	10	20	0
Item 33 Some patients should be allowed to die without making heroic efforts to prolong their lives					
75 College students	20	41	16	13	9
108 First-year nursing students	19	47	19	11	5
69 Senior nursing students	29	59	7	1	3
75 Registered nurses	50	44	5	1	0
110 First-year medical students	27	50	19	3	1
90 Senior medical students	62	34	3	1	0
30 Physicians	40	53	0	7	0

[1] Nonmedical personnel answering this question were asked to respond as they might *if* they were a doctor or a nurse.

For each subject within the seven groups, a score was derived for the five euthanasia items by summing the weights. A low score (14 or less) indicated a tendency toward a favorable attitude toward "death with dignity." A high score (15 or more) was indicative of a positive attitude toward the "sanctity-of-life principle." Table 3 shows the average scores for the seven groups for the euthanasia subscale as well as the average for other attitudes toward death and dying. The correlation (Pearson r) of these two scores is also shown. The least accepting attitudes on issues of euthanasia are held by college students, although first-year nursing students are quite similar. The most accepting attitudes are held by senior medical students and by practicing nurses and physicians.

Using Duncan's multiple range test and a confidence level of 0.01 (Edwards 1964), each mean was tested against every other mean. Table 4 displays the differences among the means for our seven groups and allows ready comparison. Thus, senior medical students do not differ significantly from physicians on euthanasia as measured by our five items, but are significantly lower than the five other groups. Physicians, registered nurses, first-year medical students, and senior nursing students are significantly lower than first-year nursing students and college students, while the latter do not differ significantly from each other.

If one looks at general issues of relating to the dying patient and his family, as indicated in the responses to the total questionnaire, the most understanding and emphatic responses, on the average, are those of senior nursing students. Table 3 shows that nurses and physicians who have been working at their professions yield the highest mean scores. This difference in the rating of the euthanasia subscale and the 28 weighted items of the other areas of care of the dying patient is revealed in the wide fluctuations in the correlation coefficients for the seven groups. For the three nursing groups, attitudes toward euthanasia appear to have no relationship to other attitudes toward the dying person and

The least accepting attitudes on issues of euthanasia are held by college students. . . . The most accepting attitudes are held by senior medical students and by practicing nurses and physicians.

Table 3 Means and standard deviations on euthanasia and other attitudes toward death and dying

Group	No.	Five euthanasia items Mean	S D	Other attitudes toward death & dying Mean	S D	Pearson r	P
College students	75	14.27	3.56	65.36	8.03	0.248	< 0.05
First-year nursing students	108	14.09	2.92	64.67	7.63	0.126	ns
Senior nursing students	69	12.32	2.81	55.49	6.83	0.038	ns
Registered nurses	75	12.17	2.49	66.65	17.70	0.134	ns
First-year medical students	110	12.29	2.81	63.94	7.62	0.338	< 0.01
Senior medical students	90	10.01	2.15	61.72	8.36	0.382	< 0.01
Physicians	30	11.40	3.76	67.10	8.04	0.743	< 0.001

his family. For college students, the two measures of attitudes are somewhat correlated (P<0.05) while for medical students both near the beginning and near the completion of the medical school experience there is a high correlation (P<0.01). For the sample of 30 practicing physicians, the correlation is extremely high (P<0.001).

Not only are there significant differences among these seven groups of subjects on attitudes toward euthanasia and other issues relating to the dying patient, there are also marked differences in the apparently inconsistent responses as indicated by within-person variation. A person was identified as having "discrepant" responses if his five weighted responses contained weightings indicative of both positive and negative attitudes toward euthanasia. Thus, persons whose weightings on the five items were 1–2–1–2–3 or 4–5–3–4–5 were not labeled discrepant, but persons with scores of 1–5–3–2–4 or 2–2–2–3–5 were so identified. Table 5 shows the number and percentage of individuals with "discrepant" responses for each group. Student nurses, whether first-year or senior,

Table 4 Differences between the means on euthanasia items for seven groups of subjects[1]

Group	$\overline{X}$	A (1) Senior medical students 10.01	B (2) Physicians 11.40	C (3) Registered nurses 12.17	D (4) First-year medical students 12.29	E (5) Senior nursing students 12.32	F (6) First-year nursing students 14.09	G (7) College students 14.27	Shortest significant ranges
Senior medical nursing students[A]	10.01		1.39	2.16	2.28	2.31	4.08	4.26	$R_2 = 1.33$
Physicians[B]	11.40			0.77	0.89	0.92	2.69	2.87	$R_3 = 1.39$
Registered nurses[C]	12.17				0.12	0.15	1.92	2.10	$R_4 = 1.42$
First-year medical students[D]	12.29					0.03	1.80	1.98	$R_3 = 1.45$
Senior nursing students[E]	12.32						1.77	1.95	$R_3 = 1.47$
First-year nursing students[F]	14.09							0.18	$R_4 = 1.49$
College students[G]	14.27								

[1] Any two means *not* underscored by the same line are significantly different at < 0.01, while any two means underscored by the same line do not differ significantly.

and practicing nurses, were all higher in percentage of discrepant responses than beginning or senior medical students or practicing physicians. First-year nursing students with 73 per cent discrepant responses showed the greatest inconsistency within the five euthanasia items.

Discussion

If one considers the five statements on euthanasia, three of them (Items 1, 14, and 33) deal directly with attitudes toward dying patients. Of these three, the statement which evokes the most agreement with the concept of euthanasia is Item 33, "Some patients should be allowed to die without making heroic efforts to prolong their lives." Ninety-six per cent of the senior medical students and 93 per cent of the practicing physicians agree. The practicing registered nurses and the senior nursing students indicate, respectively, 94 per cent and 88 per cent agreement. It appears that only the naïve, college students and first-year nursing and medical students, have much ambivalence or disagreement. One wonders what cultural factors have created the expectation in these three groups of young subjects that heroic efforts should be made to prolong the lives of everyone, no matter what the circumstances.

Item 1 introduces individual variables to influence the decision: "Regardless of his age, disabilities, and personal preference, a person should be kept alive as long as possible." This evokes an increase in indecisiveness in comparison to Item 33 and a decrease in the amount of agreement with the idea of euthanasia. Item 14 evokes role expectations: "no matter what my personal beliefs, in my role as a medical professional I would fight to keep the patient alive." Once such expectations are considered, the agreement with the idea of euthanasia decreases for all groups. Aside from the practicing registered nurses, there is a marked increase in indecisiveness. Generalizing the reactions to these three statements, indecision increases as modifying variables are introduced. A complex choice lends itself less well to a strong position.

Table 5 Number and percentage of discrepant responses by groups

Group	No.	No. of individuals with discrepant response
College students	75	46 (61.3%)
First-year nursing students	108	79 (73.1%)
Senior nursing students	69	41 (59.4%)
Registered nurses	75	52 (69.3%)
First-year medical students	110	54 (49.1%)
Senior medical students	90	33 (36.7%)
Physicians	30	12 (40.0%)

The senior medical students have the most positive attitudes toward euthanasia, followed by practicing physicians and first-year medical students. There is less consistency among practicing nurses and nursing students.

Item 13, "Those who support the principle of 'death with dignity' endorse active as well as passive euthanasia," introduces a primary cognitive component. All student groups showed much more indecision in their responses to this statement. This finding suggests lack of knowledge of the "death with dignity" concept and a poor understanding of the meanings of "active" and "passive" euthanasia.

Item 16, "Individual freedom of choice ultimately should mean freedom of choice to live or die within a context of responsibility for self and others," moves away from professional role expectations and specific variables. It taps a broad philosophical approach to individual rights and responsibilities. Registered nurses and senior student nurses both have 59 percent agreement with this statement, less than the other five groups.

If one discounts the responses to Item 13, which depend more on cognitive than affective components of attitudes to euthanasia, there is a consistency among first-year medical students, senior medical students, and practicing physicians. The senior medical students have the most positive attitudes toward euthanasia, followed by practicing physicians and first-year medical students. There is less consistency among practicing nurses and nursing students. The data also indicate that nurses' attitudes toward euthanasia are not correlated with their overall attitudes toward death and dying. A greater proportion of nurses, whether students or practicing professionals, have discrepant responses to statements about euthanasia.

These findings pique our curiosity and stimulate speculation on a post hoc basis. Such a state of indecision could be favorably viewed as an openness to shift to one position or another on the basis of additional information. Attitudinal research indicates that a strongly held attitude is usually resistant to change. Krech et al. (1962) indicate that the ability to alter our concepts and beliefs is determined by our ability to deal with ambiguities and inconsistencies. Studies of the nursing role have shown that it is especially fraught with inconsistencies and conflicting expectations, not only because of the nature of the job itself, but also because 95 per cent of nurses are female and women's role in our society is changing and has poorly defined expectations. This suggests that women, especially nurses, have learned to tolerate more indecision and inconsistencies in their attitudes than men, who are more likely to have a clearer professional identity. An alternative explanation could be that women have not thought through their attitudes to the point of an integrated perspective. This would leave them more vulnerable to emotional indecision. As more men enter the nursing profession and more women become physicians it will be easier to delineate the extent to which professional identity rather than gender is the crucial factor.

Another possible explanation of the differences between the disciplines in consistency of personal attitudes may be attributed to differences in socialization to roles (Kramer 1968). Sociological theory indicates that the longer the socialization process, the more likely the attitudes, values, and beliefs associated with a role will be internalized. Medical students have a longer period of professional training and so are more likely to internalize the attitudes, values, and beliefs that are associated with the physician's role. If this assumption is valid, practicing physicians and physician teachers therefore have a more consistent set of attitudes, values, and beliefs to convey to students. Nurses not only have shorter periods of professional training, but with the multiplicity of programs, there are marked differences in the length of nursing education. Because of this variation, nurses are less likely than physicians to have a consistent set of attitudes, values, and beliefs to transmit to nursing students.

Conclusion

In a survey of medical, nursing, and college students and practicing physicians and nurses, there were significant attitudinal differences in responses to statements about euthanasia. Senior medical students and practicing physicians did not differ significantly from each other but were more positively oriented toward euthanasia than registered nurses, first-year medical students, senior and first-year nursing students, and other college students. Attitudes toward euthanasia were positively correlated with other attitudes toward the dying patient and his family for all groups but the two groups of nursing students and the practicing nurses. These three nursing groups and the college students also showed proportionately the greatest within-person inconsistency in responses to the euthanasia items.

References

Braverman, S.J. (1969). Death of a monster. *American Journal of Nursing* 69:1682–1683.

Brown, R. (1965). *Social psychology*. Pp 549–609. New York: The Free Press.

Edwards, A.L. (1964). *Experimental Design in Psychological Research*. New York: Holt, Rinehart and Winston.

Fletcher, J. (1968). Elective death. In *Ethical Issues in Medicine*. Ed. E. F. Torrey. Pp 139–158. Boston. Little Brown and Co.

Gustafson, J.M. (1973). Mongolism, parental desires and the right to life. *Perspectives in Biology and Medicine* 16:529–559.

The Harris Survey (23 April 1974). Chicago: *Chicago Tribune*.

Kohl, M. (1972). The sanctity-of-life principle. In *Humanistic Perspectives in Medical Ethics*. Ed. M. B. Visscher. Pp 39–61. Buffalo: Prometheus.

Kramer, M. (1968). Role models, role conceptions and role deprivation. *Nursing Research* 17:115–120.

Krech, D.; Crutchfield, R.S.; and Ballachey, E.L. (1962). *Individual in Society*. New York: McGraw-Hill.

McCormick, R.A. (1974). To save or let die. The dilemma of modern medicine. *Journal of the American Medical Association* 229:172–176.

Parson, T.; Fox, R.C.; and Lidz, V.M. (1973). The "gift of life" and its reciprocation. In *Death in American Experience*. Ed. A. Mack. Pp 1–49. New York: Schocken.

Rachels, J. (1975). Active and passive euthanasia. *New England Journal of Medicine* 292: 78–80.

Skinner, B.F. (1971). *Beyond Freedom and Dignity*. New York: Knopf.

Society today (1973, 2nd edition). Pp 161–173. Del Mar, California: CRM Books.

Vollmer, H.M. and Mills, D.L., eds (1966). *Professionalization*. Englewood Cliffs, New Jersey: Prentice-Hall.

Webster's New Collegiate Dictionary (1961). Springfield, Massachusetts: G & C Merriam Company.

Yeaworth, R.C.; Kapp, F.T.; and Winget, C. (1974). Attitudes of nursing students toward the dying patient. *Nursing Research* 23:20–24.

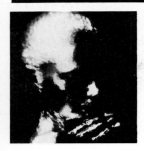

26

Research

Do you believe everything you read in the newspapers? Do you believe that you may unknowingly be influenced by what you read in the press? More specifically, to what extent do you believe that your attitudes and expectations regarding death are correlated with the newspaper in your community? Reynolds and Kalish raise these issues in discussing their research project which showed that different ethnic communities represent death differently in their press. The following two Appendix exercises may be helpful at the completion of this chapter:

      I.   Life and Death Attitudes: Dyadic Encounter

      O.   Values Grid

Death Rates, Attitudes, and the Ethnic Press

David K. Reynolds

Richard A. Kalish

The violence of death on television has often been noted, both in the academic literature and—even more—in the popular press. A great deal of heat and a sporadic glimmer of light accompany most such discussions. Although newspapers are not reluctant to provide ample airing of the sins of television, they have done little if anything to comtemplate the ways in which they themselves express death and violence.

The present study examines a small piece of this large puzzle. Due to an extensive three-year investigation of the meaning of death in a cross-ethnic context, we were able to interrelate attitudes toward death held by four ethnic groups, the image of death as presented in relevant ethnic community newspapers, and the statistical nature of death for ethnic groups reported through official enumerations. (See Kalish and Reynolds 1976).

Our hypotheses are very general. First, we would hypothesize that those newspapers serving specific ethnic communities differ among each other as to the ways in which death is presented. Second, we would hypothesize that newspaper presentations of deaths would be reflected in community attitudes and expectations regarding death. Third, we would hypothesize that official death statistics would be reflected both in community attitudes and expectations and in newspaper presentations. Fourth, we would assume that all forms of violent death would be overrepresented in the newspapers.

Methods of Procedure

Instruments
Three sets of measures were utilized for this study: content analyses of newspapers, survey of community attitudes through interviews, and official statistics indicating death by cause.

This material was first published in *Ethnicity,* vol. 3, pp. 305–316, 1976. Copyright © 1976 by Academic Press, Inc. It is printed here in slightly modified form by permission.

. . . to determine
the image of
death projected to
each ethnic
community by its
newspapers. . . .

Content Analysis

In order to determine the image of death projected to each ethnic community by its newspapers, we selected those newspapers with the largest circulations among each of three Los Angeles ethnic communities, plus the largest general circulation paper in the area. The publications and their approximate daily circulations were the *Los Angeles Sentinel* (Black Americans: 47,000), the *Rafu Shimpo* (Japanese Americans: 18,500), *La Opinion* (Mexican Americans: 20,000), and the *Los Angeles Times* (White Americans, general circulation: 1,200,000). We subscribed to each of these newspapers for one year.

We randomly selected sequences of issues (daily issues Monday through Saturday, except for the *Sentinel,* which is a weekly), representing all four seasons equally. In each newspaper selected in this fashion, we marked every article in which death was reported (ranging from war stories to obituaries). The total number of death-related articles examined was 320 for the Black Americans, 320 for the Japanese Americans, 166 for the Mexican Americans, and 354 for the White Americans. We had established 300 as the minimum number of articles for each group, but fell short of this number for *La Opinion*. Only the English-language section of the Japanese American newspaper was coded. Although each newspaper selected was perused in full for any death-related article, each article was tabulated as one unit, regardless of how many deaths were reported or discussed.

The articles were coded for: (1) type of death, (2) place of death, (3) age of deceased, (4) sex of deceased, (5) religion of deceased, (6) occupation of deceased, (7) survivors of deceased, (8) underlying affective component of the article, and (9) philosophic theme of the article. A single judge coded the articles in three of the newspapers and helped train the Spanish-speaking coder of *La Opinion*. Both raters were carefully trained for this task; they had been previously closely associated with the research project and were familiar with its purpose and progress. Close supervision was maintained. Although no reliability check was performed, we felt that, with the exceptions of (8) and (9), categorization was not a difficult task and did not require a second rater. Variable (9) was dropped from later analysis since it eventually became obvious that reliable ratings could not readily be made.

Interviews

As part of a three-year study of death and bereavement in a cross-ethnic context, 434 persons in the Los Angeles area responded to a one-hour, individually-administered interview. Interviews were conducted by highly trained, bilingual (when appropriate) interviewers of the same ethnicity as the interviewee. Interviews were translated into Japanese and Spanish. Although the sampling procedures are described in detail in Kalish and Reynolds (1976), a few matters should be explicated: First, the sampling design oversampled persons over age 60 and undersampled persons in the middle and upper income groups; second, this led to a disproportionate number of persons with viewpoints that appeared traditional in terms of the indicated ethnic groups; third, interviews were conducted in the autumn of 1970; fourth, telephone call-backs of a 15 percent sample 6 months later obtained an extremely high reliability for the 12 questions included.

For this paper, only two sets of questions are relevant. First, near the beginning of the interview, we asked each person, "How many persons that you knew personally (knew them by name, talked with them informally) died by accident?" Subsequent questions asked about natural causes, war, suicide, and homicide. Then, toward the end of the interview, we asked, "Try to put yourself into the future for the next few questions. If you had to predict . . . how do you suppose you will die?" And two questions later, "If you could choose, how would you like to die?" Both of these latter questions were given in open-ended fashion, with the interviewer normally coding them during the interview. (See Table 1.)

Death Rate Statistics
Since official Department of Public Health statistics do not differentiate between Mexican American and "Anglo" American, we utilized death rates based upon data from the Los Angeles County Coroner's Office.

Statistical Analysis
Given the nature of this study and of the data collected, we wished to learn the extent to which reading a given newspaper would bring the reader into contact with a particular kind of content. We therefore applied the Lambda technique, as described in Freeman (1965), to examine the relationships between (1) the ethnic community served by the newspaper and the types of death reported most frequently and (2) the ethnic community served and the location at which the deaths occurred. We utilized the Kolmogorov—Smirnov test of statistical significance, based upon chi square, between each pair of newspapers in analyzing differences in the age of the deceased. For religious affiliation, sex, occupation, and affective tone, we decided against using any statistical analysis beyond that of tabulating percentages, largely because the number of categories and the relatively small numbers in many categories made the use of available techniques questionable. Also, we felt that the tabulated statistics were—for the most part—quite adequate in and of themselves, without the addition of significance tests.

Results

In reporting results, we will take each variable separately, attempting to integrate the findings from the content analysis, the community survey, and the death rates as each pertain to that variable.

Type of Death
Each newspaper has a different emphasis in the kinds of deaths it reports most frequently. The *Rafu Shimpo* articles primarily discuss persons who died natural deaths (or at least, the newspaper reports them as natural

> Each newspaper has a different emphasis in the kinds of deaths it reports most frequently.

Table 1 Responses of 434 Los Angeles Residents to Selected Interview Questions

	Black Americans %	Japanese Americans %	Mexican Americans %	White Americans %
1. How many persons whom you have known personally died during the past two years?				
0	10	17	19	26
1–2	34	44	34	39
3–7	31	24	38	27
8 plus	25	15	9	8
2. Those knowing one or more who died in an accident.	37	19	28	22
3. Those knowing one or more who died in war.	13	5	8	8
4. Those knowing one or more who died by suicide.	2	3	5	2
5. Those knowing one or more who died by homicide.	10	0	3	0
6. Those knowing one or more who died by natural causes.	82	75	77	64
7. How do you suppose you will die?				
Natural	88	94	88	90
Accident	3	5	11	9
Suicide	—	—	—	—
Homicide	1	—	1	—
Other	7	1	—	1
(DK/NA)	(37)	(9)	(34)	(21)
8. How would you *like* to die?				
Natural	98	98	93	94
Accident	—	2	7	2
Suicide	2	—	—	3
Homicide	—	—	—	—
Other	—	—	—	—
(DK/NA)	(6)	(4)	(5)	(12)

deaths, since 20 percent of the Japanese respondents in the community survey—versus 5–7 percent of the others—stated that they knew of a suicide that had been reported as a natural death), while the *Sentinel* reports vastly larger numbers of homicidal deaths, and *La Opinion* pages tend to describe deaths from accidents. *The Los Angeles Times,* because its obituaries do not mention cause of death, does not carry this information for most persons, but nearly half of those that are reported refer to deaths by accident. (See Table 2).

Consistent with the practice of *La Opinion* to report extensively on accidental deaths, more Mexican American respondents in our community survey expect to die through an accident (11 versus 3–9 percent) and more would like to die by an accident (7 versus 0–2 percent). Mexican Americans were also more likely than Japanese or White Americans (but not more than Black Americans) to know at least one person who had died of an accident during the two previous years.

Also consistent was the reaction of the Black Americans toward homicide as a cause for death. Over half the death-related articles in the *Sentinel* referred to homicide, and more Black Americans than others interviewed had known a homicide victim (10 versus 0–3 percent). Similarly, of the four persons interviewed who expected to be a homicide victim, three were Black Americans. Only among Black Americans and White Americans did anyone state that he preferred suicide as a way to die, and it was the *Sentinel* and the *Los Angeles Times* that had the highest proportion of articles on suicidal deaths. Death articles in the *Rafu Shimpo* were almost all about persons who died of natural causes, and the Japanese Americans were most likely to expect to die of natural causes and to want to die of natural causes, although differences among ethnic groups for both these questions were very slight.

Even the death rates themselves were moderately consistent. Thus, the Black Americans, followed by the Mexican Americans, had the highest reported rates of deaths by homicide, while the White Americans had the highest suicide rates (and the highest proportion of persons wanting to die from suicide).

Not all findings were as consistent as those reported above, and some differences were negligible. However, there were no gross inconsistencies among these three sources of data. Moreover, the Lambda of 0.41 indicated that the ability to predict cause of death as a function of newspaper being read was substantial, i.e., by knowing which newspaper was read, we can eliminate 41 percent of the errors that would have accrued by guessing.

Location

In those deaths that mentioned some kind of location, more occurred outdoors than anywhere else. Only among the Black Americans was a substantial proportion of deaths reported to have occurred in the home, although fewer Blacks (44 versus 54–72 percent) than any other ethnic group inter-

> **. . . the ability to predict cause of death as a function of newspaper being read was substantial. . . .**

Table 2 Death-related articles in selected newspapers as categorized by type of death, location of occurrence, religious affiliation and occupation of deceased, and affective tone of article

	Percentage of responses			
	The Sentinel (N = 320)	Rafu Shimpo (N = 320)	La Opinion (N = 166)	L.A. Times (N = 354)
Type of death				
Natural	19.8	81.3	9.8	20.4
Accident	19.8	10.9	61.3	45.5
Suicide	3.4	1.5	1.4	3.6
Homicide	54.6	3.8	26.1	15.0
War-related	2.3	2.2	1.4	15.0
(Unknown)	(10.0)	(17.5)	(14.5)	(83.3)
Totals	99.9	99.7	100.0	99.5
Location				
Home	28.4	6.5	12.8	8.9
Hospital	18.0	18.7	15.3	11.9
Outdoors	40.8	64.2	44.3	62.1
Battlefield	3.1	9.9	1.6	5.3
Nursing home	6.0	—	1.6	—
Building	3.5	—	24.2	11.8
(Unknown)	(20.3)	(81.8)	(25.3)	(83.1)
Totals	99.8	99.3	99.8	99.9
Religion				
Catholic	15.2	4.9	93.4	68.8
Buddhist	—	57.7	—	3.1
Baptist	25.4	6.4	—	3.1
Methodist	20.5	9.0	6.6	6.3
Episcopal	4.9	3.3	—	12.5
Lutheran	1.2	0.4	—	6.3
Presbyterian	—	4.5	—	—
Protestant (other)	32.0	14.4	—	—
[Protestant (all)]	[84.0]	[38.0]	[6.6]	[28.2]
(Unknown)	(75.6)	(24.3)	(81.9)	(90.4)
Totals	99.2	100.6	100.0	100.1
Occupation				
Entertainer	8.5	—	8.2	8.8
Student	13.8	24.8	30.2	2.2
White-collar	21.5	16.8	15.0	28.7
Professional	30.0	27.2	13.6	17.6
Blue-collar	10.2	14.4	28.9	6.6
Service	7.7	9.6	—	6.6
Armed Forces	7.7	7.2	4.1	28.7
(Unknown)	(63.7)	(87.5)	(56.0)	(86.4)
Totals	99.4	100.0	100.0	99.2

Table 2 *continued*

	Percentage of responses			
	The Sentinel (N = 320)	*Rafu Shimpo* (N = 320)	*La Opinion* (N = 166)	*L.A. Times* (N = 354)
Affective tone				
Peaceful	1.8	5.2	5.1	12.6
Tragic	37.3	57.0	0.8	2.5
Violent	60.2	26.7	69.2	54.6
Heroic	0.4	10.3	25.1	30.3
(None)	(32.1)	(88.4)	(29.0)	(88.1)
Totals	99.7	99.2	100.2	100.0

Each of the newspapers appears to consider different age groups as particularly newsworthy in terms of their deaths.

viewed stated a preference for dying at home. We might assume that most of the deaths at unreported locations actually occurred in hospitals, while outdoor deaths would often be accidents. Differences among newspapers were not nearly so substantial in reporting location, and all papers had "outdoors" as the modal category. The Lambda of 0.00 confirms the impossibility of making a differential prediction regarding location of death from knowledge of which newspaper is being read.

Age, Sex, and Survivors
Each of the newspapers appears to consider different age groups as particularly newsworthy in terms of their deaths. The *Sentinel, La Opinion,* and the *Times* all give primary coverage to the deaths of persons in their early adult years, while the *Rafu Shimpo* shows increased concern as a function of age. Had the *Los Angeles Times* reported the age of persons with formal obituaries, their reports would be more similar to the Japanese-language newspaper, but this was not done. These numbers undoubtedly reflect the kinds of death that are reported (see above). In the Los Angeles area, deaths from suicide of younger persons have been increasing rapidly for both Black and White Americans; deaths from homicide and accidents are also high for these age groups. The *Sentinel,* however, reports relatively more deaths for persons in their teens and 30s, while the Spanish-language newspaper describes more deaths of children and teenagers.

As specified previously, we did not compute Lambda for the distribution of ages reported, but—partly to satisfy our own curiosity—did compute chi squares based upon a Kolmogorov—Smirnov test of goodness of fit between distributions. By matching each newspaper with each other newspaper, six such tests were required. All three tests involving the *Rafu Shimpo* were significant well beyond the .001 level; the *Times* and the *Sentinel* were differentiated beyond the .05 level of confidence, and the *Times* and the *La Opinion* at the .06 level of confidence; no difference was found between the *Sentinel* and *La Opinion*. (See Table 3.)

Interestingly, over two-thirds of all death-related articles are about men, although we would assume that actual deaths are very close to 50–50. Although a portion of this undoubtedly arises from the larger number of male suicide, homicide, and accident victims, some certainly reflect judgments that men are more newsworthy. The newspapers differed relatively little in proportion of male-based articles—from 63 percent of the *Rafu Shimpo* articles to 77 percent in *La Opinion*.

Survivors were mentioned in nearly half of the *Rafu Shimpo* articles (48 percent) and in over one-third of the *Times* articles (35 percent), but relatively few of the *Sentinel* or *La Opinion* articles (18 percent in each) made such references. This reflects the relative frequency of obituaries.

Religion

Specific religious background was mentioned in less than 10 percent of the articles in the *Times,* and most of these indicated the deceased as Catholic. Conversely, over three-fourths of the *Rafu Shimpo* articles stipulated the religion of the dead person, with over half being Buddhist and the rest being distributed over numerous Protestant denominations (and 4 percent Catholic). The 18 percent of *La Opinion* articles on death were almost all Catholic, and the *Sentinel* articles, like the *Times,* normally did not mention religious affiliation. (See Table 2)

Table 3 Death-related articles in selected newspapers as categorized by age of deceased

| | Percentages of responses and cumulative percentage | | | | | | | |
| | The Sentinel | | Rafu Shimpo | | La Opinion | | L.A. Times | |
Age	%	C%	%	C%	%	C%	%	C%
0–10	7.8	—	2.2	—	17.7	—	—	—
11–20	15.6	23.4	5.2	7.4	11.7	29.4	12.8	12.8
21–30	31.2	54.5	6.4	13.8	31.9	61.3	32.3	45.1
31–40	14.7	69.2	2.9	16.7	8.4	69.7	5.5	50.6
41–50	8.2	77.4	8.7	25.4	7.5	77.2	7.3	57.9
51–60	4.5	81.9	9.9	35.3	5.8	83.0	12.8	70.7
61–70	5.3	87.2	13.3	48.6	5.8	88.8	7.3	78.0
71–80	7.4	94.6	21.3	69.9	5.0	93.8	19.5	97.5
81–90	2.4	97.0	26.5	96.4	3.3	97.1	1.8	99.3
91 plus	2.4	99.4	3.2	99.6	2.6	99.7	—	99.3
(Unknown)	(24.0)		(3.4)		(28.2)		(83.6)	

Occupation

That each of the newspapers reported more deaths of persons from professional and white-collar groups than would be expected by chance is not surprising. Although between one-half and seven-eighths of the reported deaths did not refer to occupation, each newspaper does appear to have its own biases. Thus students are much more frequently mentioned by *Rafu Shimpo* and *La Opinion,* while the *Sentinel* and *Rafu Shimpo* were most likely to report the deaths of professional persons, and *La Opinion* described more blue-collar deaths. The *Los Angeles Times* was the only paper in which war-related deaths were mentioned relatively often (more the result of their *not* reporting as many accidents, homicides, and suicides, rather than of having numerous war stories), and their fairly extensive obituary columns meant the reporting of deaths that went unmarked in the other newspapers. (See Table 2.)

Affective Tone

The coders for the *Rafu Shimpo* and the *Times* felt that very few death-related articles had a discernible affective tone. However, of those that did, the former were categorized as primarily *tragic* and the latter, as primarily *violent*. Both the *Sentinel* and *La Opinion* reported substantially more violent deaths, although the Black American newspaper did have many more articles focused upon the tragic aspects of sudden death, while *La Opinion's* articles focused secondarily upon the heroic aspects.

Violent deaths of all sorts, accidents, homicide, suicide, and war-incurred, were reported far out of proportion to their actual occurrence in the population.

Discussion

There is little doubt that our first hypothesis was confirmed. Major differences in methods of reporting deaths were observed in the four newspapers selected. Had we selected other newspapers in Los Angeles, the results might have been different, but we still doubt whether this hypothesis would have been refuted. A comparison of death-related articles in the *Rafu Shimpo* and another local Japanese-American paper, the *Kashu Mainichi,* revealed few significant differences.

We also feel that our second hypothesis was basically substantiated. The expectations, experiences, and preferences of the individual ethnic groups resembled the kinds of death-related materials published in the relevant newspapers. Similarly, the third hypothesis seemed essentially supported. Official death statistics were reflected by the community attitudes and expectations of the ethnic groups toward death and by the newspaper content analysis.

And there is little doubt that the fourth hypothesis was confirmed. Violent deaths of all sorts, accidents, homicide, suicide, and war-incurred, were reported far out of proportion to their actual occurrence in the population.

. . . the newspaper turns a mirror upon its readers, and the policy makers may decide to be selective in this image to be reflected back.

An interview with Mr. William Thomas, City Editor of the *Los Angeles Times,* in September, 1970, helped to explicate the role of newspaper policy in determining which deaths would be reported. Most obvious are deaths that are considered newsworthy, which implied having readership appeal. Newsworthy deaths are very frequently violent, although sometimes it is the reputation of the dead person (or a relative of the dead person) rather than the method of death that makes the event newsworthy. However, it is not the violence per se that leads to the publication of the article, but because the circumstances surrounding violent deaths are relatively more likely to be unusual or otherwise interesting to the public. For example, the common occurrence of a husband shooting his wife because he found her with another man is not news and would rarely make the *Los Angeles Times.* However, if a bullet struck a passer-by or if someone in the triangle were well known, the story might be newsworthy.

A second factor determining which events are printed is the availability of information. Traffic accidents often have witnesses, and traffic deaths can be written about fairly readily, while suicidal deaths often occur without enough available information to provide a readable article.

Although Mr. Thomas stated that the publication of articles about violent death "does not sell newspapers" (and anyone familiar with his publication can attest to an underplaying of the violence of urban life in its pages), not all major newspapers follow such a pattern. The ethnic newspapers have a different problem. Since their audiences form much more cohesive groupings than the readers of the *Times,* and since their readers usually turn to general circulation newspapers or the radio or television for more general news, their task is to fill pages with what the ethnic community wishes to read so that they can maintain circulation and advertisers. One obvious source of such stories is events of violence in general and violent deaths in particular.

However, two other factors come into consideration. First, in order to report on violent deaths, there have to be violent deaths. Therefore, if the suicide, homicide, accidental, or war-related death rates are very low or nonexistent, the article cannot be legitimately written. Second, the newspaper turns a mirror upon its readers, and the policy makers may decide to be selective in this image to be reflected back. Obviously, there is no such thing as a standard regarding the proportion of violent deaths that should be reported in the newspaper. This decision evolves out of the actual extent of violent deaths in interaction with the decisions of the editors and publishers and with significant cooperation or resistance of the writers, the police, and various other involved persons.

We would, thus, surmise that the desire of the decision makers at the *Rafu Shimpo* and the *Times* is to present an image to their readers, and indirectly to nonreaders, of living in a relatively nonviolent community. They may well consider it an obligation to avoid arousing tensions and antagonisms that extensive reporting of violence could possibly encourage. On the other hand—and again we must emphasize that we are speculating—the policies of the *Sentinel* and *La Opinion* may reflect the beliefs that readers do wish to learn about violence in the communities. Moreover, deaths from homicide and accidents (but not from suicide) are more relatively common in the Black and Mexican American communities, and their editors may feel that exposure, rather than underplaying, of this violence may have the most salutary effect upon the communities.

Two questions arise from this study, neither finding an answer in our data. First, to what extent do newspaper policy makers make their decisions with an eye to circulation and to what extent do they think in terms of the welfare of their readers? Second, to what extent does the newspaper reporting reflect what is going on in the community and to what extent does it *shape* what is going on in the community?

The latter question appears far more important. Although it is true that relatively more Black and Mexican Americans die from homicide and accident, the actual figures are very low, while the ethnic self-image reflected back to the readers by the newspaper is that of a community filled with deaths from violence. Does such reporting increase the expectations of readers that they will, indeed, die violent deaths? If so, is there any element of self-fulfilling prophecy in these expectations?

We are obviously raising questions that we are unable to answer. We are also somewhat skeptical that these issues can be satisfactorily investigated through laboratory studies on persuasion, although we do not deny the usefulness of such research. It is our hope that studies might be conducted on these matters that combine quantitative and qualitative procedures and that combine the insights of journalists, political scientists, and behavioral scientists.

. . . to what extent does the newspaper reporting reflect what is going on in the community and to what extent does it *shape* what is going on in the community?

Summary

A content analysis was conducted of articles involving one or more deaths in four newspapers in Los Angeles. Three of these newspapers were directed primarily at local ethnic communities (Black, Japanese American, and Mexican American), and the fourth was a general circulation newspaper. The *Sentinel,* serving the Los Angeles Black community, reported a much larger proportion of deaths by homicide; *Rafu Shimpo,* a bilingual English and Japanese paper, contained primarily descriptions of natural deaths; *La Opinion,* a Spanish-language paper, and the *Los Angeles Times* both reported relatively more deaths by accident. Other meaningful differences were found in the age of the deceased persons and the affective tone of the articles.

References

Freeman, L. C. (1965). *Elementary Applied Statistics.* New York: Wiley.
Kalish, R. A., and Reynolds, D. K. (1976). *Death and Ethnicity: A Psychocultural Study.* Los Angeles: Andrus Gerontology Center.

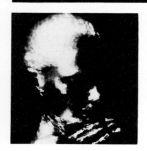

27

Research

Think back to the last time you moved, either from one house (or apartment building) to another or from one city to another. Was that relocation a stressful event at the time? Do you think that the stressful effects of moving would weigh more heavily on the elderly? Kay Rowland reviews research into how such events as relocation, the death of significant others, and retirement may contribute to premature death for the elderly. The conventional wisdom about the effect retirement has on how long a person lives may or may not be true. This chapter teaches us that we have much to learn about coping with major transitions. The following Appendix exercises are appropriate when you have completed your reading.

    C.   Awareness of Grief Process

    D.   Awareness of Losses

    H.   Fantasizing Grief Reaction of Significant Others

Environmental Events Predicting Death for the Elderly

Kay F. Rowland

In the field of psychosomatic medicine, in which one of the basic tenets is that psychological stress has a harmful effect on the physiology of the organism, attention has been directed to the importance of environmental factors to an individual's health. Indeed, there are many theorists who have linked environmental events to the subsequent death of an individual. Engel (1971), for example, documented 170 cases of sudden death during psychological stress, such as after the death of a close person. His finding that each death involved events impossible for the victims to ignore and to which their response was overwhelming excitation, or giving up, or both, led him to propose that death may be induced through the interaction of many factors. Similarly, Casler (1970),[1] in discussing death as a psychosomatic condition, hypothesized that death itself may stem from nonorganic causes. Giving as examples changes in residence, loss of a loved one, and retirement, Seligman argued that life changes that produce the psychological state of helplessness increase the risk of death (1975, pp. 166–188). Noting that there are cases that indicate that psychosocial factors seem to precipitate a fatal outcome, Weisman (1972) coined the term "psychosocial death" to signify that not only organic factors can be lethal.

Each of these theorists reasoned that environmental events have some relation to the health and subsequent chances of death in an individual. Birren (1965) believed that events involving environmental loss (e.g., death of friends and relatives, reduced contacts upon retirement, and change in residence) have both psychological and physiological consequences. These events, although difficult to handle at any age, are particularly significant in later life, according to Birren. Not only are losses more frequent in old age, but the elderly person must often adapt to these events with decreased physiological and psychological capacities.

This material was first printed in the *Psychological Bulletin,* vol. 84, no. 2, pp. 349–372, 1977. Copyright 1977 by the American Psychological Association. Reprinted by permission.

In the present article, the idea that environmental events may be related to death, particularly for the elderly, will be evaluated in terms of existing research. More specifically, research will be reviewed in which death of a significant other, relocation, and retirement as predictors of death for the elderly are investigated, as each of these events has been described as a stressful occurrence signaling death for many old people.

Although these events may have destructive effects short of death on the health of an elderly person, only research in which death is the criterion variable will be included in the present review. Declines in health are much more difficult to define and are more often open to dispute. For example, ill health must be considered in terms of severity (e.g., does a cold constitute a disease?) and duration (e.g., should a 24-hour virus be considered, or only a chronic condition?) and current discomfort (e.g., should arthritis be included when it is not subjectively aggravating to the person?). The many problems of definition are avoided when death, instead of illness, is used as the criterion variable. Unlike disease, death's existence is, at least after a period of time, subject to fewer disputes and is presumably a permanent condition. Because the idea in focus is that environmental events might predict an individual's death through physiological means, attention will be directed to research that has investigated natural deaths, rather than deaths that were accidental, homicidal, or suicidal.

With very few exceptions, the studies that have examined death of a significant other, relocation, and retirement as predictors of death have employed naturalistic designs. Usually, subjects for whom the event has occurred form the experimental group, and other subjects who have not experienced the event compose the control group. In the epidemiological study that is common in this body of research, mortality rates (defined as the number of deaths that occur during a given period of time per unit of the population) of the two groups are compared for differences. An obvious shortcoming in this type of research stems from the fact that subjects cannot be randomly assigned to experimental and control groups. There is always the possibility that the two groups may differ on characteristics other than whether they have been subject to the particular environmental event in question. These selection factors would then also be associated with the difference in mortality rates between the two groups, thus obscuring the effect of the environmental event. For instance, in many of the studies there are no controls for initial health and age of the subjects. The experimental subjects may begin the study older or less healthy than the control subjects, in which case they would, of course, be more likely to die.

Another method used in assessing environmental events as predictors of death employs the dichotomous variable, living or dead. At some arbitrary cutoff point, the predictor event is tested to see whether it discriminates between the survivors and the nonsurvivors. In other words, the event, death of a significant other, might be tested by first classifying each subject according to whether he had lost a spouse, and after some period of time, classifying him again as a survivor or a nonsurvivor. The extent to which the first ratings predicted the later status as living or dead would be the test of how well the environmental event could predict death. Palmore (1971a) pointed out that one difficulty with this method is that a relatively large number of cases is required for stable results. Another problem frequently encountered in studies of this type occurs when the research is carried out a considerable period of time after the event has taken place. When subjects are not solicited immediately after the event, it is possible that the elderly who are most susceptible to death after the event will have already died, with only those elderly not affected by the event remaining to be subjects. Thus, the timing of the study is a very important variable in research predicting death from environmental events.

Each event—death of a significant other, relocation, and retirement—is considered separately as a predictor of death in the elderly. Then, in a final conclusion the three events are related to current theories that explain how they might operate to predict death. Problems with existing research and suggestions for future research will also be discussed.

Loss of a Significant Other as a Predictor of Death

The first environmental event to be examined as a predictor of death in the elderly is the loss of a significant person. Probably the most likely significant other to be lost by an elderly person is his spouse. In the United States, 5.9 percent of all males and 20.5 percent of all females between the ages of 50 and 59 are widowed. These rates increase until, among those 75 and over, 38.5 percent of the males and 71.2 percent of the females have experienced the loss of a spouse (Shurtleff 1955).

When the mortality rates of widowed people have been compared with those of married people, it has been found that in all age groups the widowed have death rates approximately 1.4 times higher than those still married (Shurtleff). This discovery has led to the common speculation that the loss of a spouse may directly affect the remaining partner's life span. Offered in support of this claim are findings such as those of Rose (1964), which show that the longevous are frequently married. In his examination of 149 octogenarian veterans of the Spanish-American War, Rose found that 92 percent of the group had married and 61 percent were, in their advanced years, still living with a spouse. Although he showed that many long-lived veterans were still married, Rose provided no data on how many veterans dying at younger ages had also still been married. Without a control group of short-lived veterans, it is thus impossible to draw from these data any conclusions about the relationship between mortality and marital status.

There have been a number of studies of the claim that widowed people die earlier than married people. Powers and Bultena (1972), for example, interviewed a total of 611 persons over age 60 who were selected as being representative of the economic and rural-urban distribution of the state of Iowa. In a follow-up 11 years later, 32 percent were dead. Marital status was found to be a significant predictor of survival, with a higher incidence of widowhood occurring in those who died during the 11-year period. Similarly, after interviewing a total of 260 community volunteers, Pfeiffer (1970) compared a group of 39 who continued to be interviewed for the next 10 years (the long-lived group) with the 39 who had been the earliest to die after the first interview (the short-lived group). He found that among the short-lived women the proportion of those not married was significantly greater than in the long-lived group. For men the trend was in the same direction but did not attain statistical significance. Still another study (Butler 1967) produced comparable results when 47 healthy men over age 65 were followed for 5 years. Widowerhood was found to be associated with mortality.

Others (Goldfarb, Fisch, and Gerber 1966; Palmore and Stone, 1973) have obtained results that do not support the hypothesis that the widowed die before the married. Palmore and Stone found no difference in longevity between the married and widowed, whereas Goldfarb et al. found that in their institutionalized group followed for a year, married men had a higher mortality rate than did the widowed. Goldfarb and his colleagues also found that variables such as severity of brain syndrome, severity of physical dependence, and incontinence, all of which reflect physical health, were the best predictors of mortality. With these results in consideration, the authors speculated that the higher mortality rates of the married men may be attributed to the fact that their wives had cared for them until their illness had reached a more critical stage that demanded institutionalization.

The confounding of health and marital status may be found in many of the previously cited studies. In the Powers and Bultena (1972) study, for example, in which it was found that widowhood was a significant predictor of death, the subjects' age and health were also found to be highly significant predictors. It is thus possible that all of the differences between the group of subjects who died and those who lived throughout the 11-year period of the study were simply reflections of age-related changes. Perhaps the older subjects, those who were most likely to die, were also by virtue of their age more likely to be widowed and in poor physical health. Similar problems of interpretation arise in the Butler (1967), Pfeiffer (1970), and Palmore and Stone (1973) studies as well. Although the latter two groups of experimenters did control for age, there was no attempt to look at the independent prediction strength of marital status apart from health. In all three of these studies, health factors proved to be significant predictors of death. With only the information that both health and marital status can predict death, several interpretations are possible: (a) that of all widows, the healthiest tend to remarry and be classified as married and that those in poor health tend not to remarry and remain classified as widowed, (b) that loss of a spouse somehow produces a loss in physical health and resultant death, or (c) that some other factor, such as lack of medical care, makes it more likely that a subject's spouse will have died and also more likely that the subject himself will be unhealthy.

The first of the above listed explanations of the increased death rate of the widowed over the married—the selective remarriage of the healthiest widowed—can be evaluated in another type of study. Unlike the previously cited studies, which did not take into account how long subjects had been widowed, there have been several other studies in which death rates of subjects were examined immediately after the death of the subjects' spouses. In these studies the possibility of higher death rates because of selective remarriage was eliminated by looking at the immediate effects of widowhood.

Young, Benjamin, and Wallis (1963) followed for 5 years the death rates of all men 55 years of age and older who were widowed in England and Wales during January and July of 1957. These rates were compared to married men's death rates in the general population for the same age groups. The experimenters found that during the first 6 months of widowhood, the mortality rate was 40 percent greater than it was for married men of the same age. This increase was followed by a decline back to the level for married men in general.

A similar study was published in Sweden during the same year (Ekblom 1963). Again, the widowed (351 widows and 283 widowers) were followed from the day their partners died, for a period of 3 years, to measure the effect of loss of spouse. The subjects' mortality rates were compared with death risk figures given by Sweden's Central Bureau of Statistics for married people of the same age. The author reported, as did Young et al., that a relatively high risk of death was observed during the first 6 months of widowhood. In Ekblom's study, mortality rates for the widowed were 36 percent greater than for the married, figures very close to those of the British experimenters (Young et al. 1963).

Another more recent study, based on data from a small town in Wales, yielded similar results. Rees and Lutkins (1967) examined the death rates of 903 close relatives (spouse, parent, child, or sibling) of people who died during a 6-year period. These were compared with the death rates of a control group who were also known to have relatives living in the area. The relatives of the control group were matched with the dead by age, sex, and marital status. Of the recently widowed people, 12.2 percent died during the first year of bereavement, as compared with only 1.2 percent of the control group of spouses. As in the Young et al. and Ekblom studies, the death rates for the widowed were highest during the first 6 months of bereavement, after which they began to decline gradually.

In contrast to the Young et al., Ekblom, and Rees and Lutkins studies, Clayton (1974) has recently reported that one-year mortality rates for the bereaved and those for age- and sex-matched controls did not significantly differ. According to an earlier report in which the procedures for selecting the widowed were described (Clayton, Halikas, and Maurice 1971), the subjects were randomly chosen from obituaries and death certificates of St. Louis City and County. It is surprising that the 109 "randomly chosen" subjects all turned out to be white, since the population of the city of St.

Louis is over 40 percent black, according to the 1970 U. S. Census. Furthermore, the 109 who became subjects were those who agreed to be interviewed. Clayton stated that the acceptance rate was 58 percent, revealing that the subjects may have been a highly select group of people. With selection procedures that required that subjects agree to be interviewed within a month after the death of their spouse, a task that may not be considered very pleasurable by the recently widowed, doubts about the generalizability of the results from this sample to the general public become apparent. Clayton did report that the original refusers were contacted one year later and "none were found to be dead" (Clayton 1974, p. 747). It remains unclear, however, how many were found to be alive, or how many of those originally chosen from the death certificates and obituaries were neither accepters or refusers, but simply could not be located, perhaps because of death. It is impossible to tell from the report whether death rates were deflated, because the subjects consisted of the most cooperative and most easily located of the widowed. The studies of Young et al. (1963) and Rees and Lutkins (1967) have the advantage of looking at the entire population (England and Wales in the Young et al. study and an entire semirural community in Wales for the Rees and Lutkins study). In addition, status of subjects is more easily traced in England and Wales, since the National Health Service maintains a central register of all citizens.

Only the 1967 study of the 903 people whose close relatives died has examined the effect of loss of parent, child, or sibling on mortality (Rees and Lutkins). Apart from the widowed, there were 747 close relatives in the bereaved group and 712 in the control group. During the first year of bereavement, significantly more bereaved relatives died, as compared with the controls. There was an increase in mortality for each type of relative, but it was significant only when a parent or sibling was lost.

Paralleling the reports that death of a spouse or other close relative may increase the risk of death is an experiment that tested the extent to which environmental loss could predict death (Butler 1967; Libow 1974; Youmans and Yarrow 1971). A total of 47 healthy men were assessed in 1956 with regard to personal-social deficits, which were defined to include death of persons close to them, mentally or physically incapacitating illnesses of spouses, and departures of children or friends. After a 5-year period, with 8 of the 47 dead, Butler (1967) reported that the losses were not predictive of mortality. However, when the group was followed for an additional 6 years, bringing the total dead to 23, environmental losses were found to have been significantly more severe among the nonsurvivors than among the survivors (Libow 1974; Youmans and Yarrow 1971). Again, however, health was confounded with degree of loss, which led to problems in interpreting the results.

It was stated earlier that the association of widowhood with increased death rate could be interpreted in a number of possible ways. The first explanation, selective remarriage of the healthiest, proposed that the healthiest of the widowed remarried, whereas those in poor health remained widows. It followed that those left classified as widowed would experience a higher death rate simply because of their poorer health. This interpretation, although it perhaps accounted for part of the higher death rate of the widowed, could not explain why, in studies comparing mortality rates, the widowed died more often in the first year of bereavement than did married controls (Ekblom 1963; Rees and Lutkins 1967; Young et al. 1963).

Another interpretation, that some third factor may be responsible for both the death of the subject's spouse and that of the subject himself, has been discussed (Young et al. 1963; Parkes, Benjamin, and Fitzgerald 1969). Young and his colleagues suggested several possible outside influences that could effect a sudden short-run increase in death rate: *homogamy,* or the tendency of the fit to marry the fit and the unfit to marry the unfit, *mutual infection,* or the possibility that the husband and wife will die of the same infectious disease, and finally, *joint unfavorable environment,* or that fact that both spouses share a pathogenic environment.

Parkes et al. (1969), using the same 4,486 widowers as did Young et al. (1963), did a more extensive analysis of the physical cause of death during the first 6 months of bereavement to determine which of these influences could be operating to increase the death rate. A total of 213 widowers died within 6 months of their wives; the number attributed to each of the causes of death of these 213 was compared with the number that would have been expected, had these widowers had the same mortality rate as did married men of the same age in England and Wales. Significantly more of the widowers were diagnosed as dying of coronary thrombosis and other arteriosclerotic and degenerative heart diseases than would have been expected, whereas the percentage of widowers dying from infectious diseases did not differ significantly from the expected. These findings suggest that mutual infection of both spouses probably can not account for the increase in death rate following the loss of a spouse.

A comparison of the causes of death of the wives with the causes of death of the 213 who died in the 6-month period reveals that there was a tendency in all disease groups for the spouses to die from the same or a similar disease. This finding lends support to the contribution of homogamy or joint unfavorable environment to the increased mortality rate. The authors argued, however, that if either of these factors were the main cause of increased mortality following bereavement,

> one would expect to find the greatest concordance in diagnosis in those diagnostic groups that account for the increased mortality rate. This is not the case, and in fact the number of husbands and wives who died from arteriosclerotic and other degenerative heart diseases was only three greater than expectation. (Parkes et al. 1969, p. 743).

Thus, although the increased mortality following death of a spouse seems to be largely accounted for by diseases of the vascular system, the widowers

... the widowed died more often in the first year of bereavement. ...

who died from this cause frequently had wives who died of other causes. It remains unresolved from these findings what part of the increased mortality is contributed by homogamy or joint unfavorable environment.

Still another way of interpreting the increased mortality rate of the widowed is to describe the state of living without one's spouse as one that could be detrimental to both psychological and physical health. Among the suggested harmful effects of widowhood are loss of care, loss of social interaction with others, and grief, with accompanying changes in the function of the endocrine and central nervous systems.

There have been attempts to show that social interaction, both in amount and quality, may be predictive of death. In other words, elderly people with few social contacts or whose social interactions are unrewarding would be expected to die sooner than those who are able to maintain many meaningful relationships. However, most of the investigators who have attempted to demonstrate this relation between social interaction and death have not been successful (Lieberman 1971; Palmore 1969, 1971b; Powers and Bultena 1972; Youmans and Yarrow 1971). In general, these researchers have asked a group of elderly volunteers about their contacts with friends and family or about their participation in organizations. The subjects were then followed for 2–11 years to see if the degree or quality of social contact predicted death during the follow-up years. One problem with this approach is that there is no objective measure of amount or quality of social interaction; it is obtained merely by the self-report of the subject. One method of overcoming this shortcoming involves studying institutionalized groups in which direct observation of the subjects' interactions can be made. Brody, Kleban, Lawton, Levy, and Waldow (1972) obtained behavior ratings from the nursing staff and from a psychiatrist on each of their 64 female institutionalized subjects. Although the behavior rating by the nursing staff was not a significant predictor, interpersonal responsiveness as measured by the staff psychiatrist did predict death during the one-year follow-up. It is quite possible that much of the psychiatrist's rating of interpersonal responsiveness was influenced by his knowledge of the subject's physical status, since there was no attempt to ensure that he was blind to the hypotheses of the study or to measure the reliability of his ratings.

A behavioral predictor of survival was found in another study of hospitalized patients, in this case, 48 patients entering the coronary care unit of a large teaching hospital (Garrity and Klein 1971). Observations of the patient's behavior were made by members of the patient care staff during the first 5 days following hospitalization for a heart attack. At the end of two work shifts, two independent observers rated each patient on a 21-item check list, consisting of items such as "seeks reassurance from personnel," "unfriendly to others," "complains," and "withdrawn." These ratings were used to form a measure of positive behavior and a measure of behavior disturbance for each patient. Based on their scores over a 5-day period, the patients were divided into adaptors, those with higher positive behavior scores and lower behavior disturbance scores, and nonadaptors, those who exhibited behavior patterns with few positive behaviors and more behavior disturbance. The investigators found that significantly more of the nonadaptors (41 percent as compared with 8 percent of the adaptors) died within 6 months after discharge. It was also reported that the behavioral pattern was significantly related to mortality, independent of the severity of attack leading to hospitalization and of prior heart trouble, although the behavior pattern was related to the presence or absence of prior heart trouble. Because prior heart trouble and behavior pattern accounted for much of the same variance, the authors suggested that previous heart trouble may be a determinant of behavioral response and behavioral response may be a determinant of death. However, it is also possible that the behavior pattern could predict recurring heart trouble, as has been suggested in research on the Type A "coronary-prone" behavior pattern (Jenkins, Zyzanski, Rosenman, and Cleveland 1971).

. . . social interactions may somehow be related to life span.

If a patient's social interactions or behavior pattern can predict whether he will die following hospitalization for a heart attack, perhaps a similar relation exists between whether a widowed person's death will follow shortly after the death of his spouse. A study by Casler (1967), though designed to investigate the effects of suggestive therapy, revealed that some type of social interaction may prolong life. Casler's 30 institutionalized volunteers were divided into two groups equated for age, duration of institutionalization, sex ratio, and physical and mental health. The experimental group received weekly 1/2-hour visits from Casler, in which he attempted to suggest to them that they would live for many more happy years. Noting that his subjects often talked more than he, Casler admitted that a weekly talk with an attentive, relatively younger person may have been all that was necessary to produce the different mortality rates between the two groups. Although this study was only a pilot study and although its lack of controls obscures the determination of which variables affected mortality, it does illustrate the possibility that social interactions may somehow be related to life span.

In addition to the possibility that the social interactions of the widowed may predict whether death will soon follow, there is also some indication that there may be a sex difference in the mortality rates following death of a significant other, with males being more strongly affected by the death. In the United States population as a whole, the difference in mortality rates between the married and the widowed is greater for men than for women (Shurtleff 1955). These increased death rates for widowers could be accounted for by the fact that men tend to remarry proportionately more often than do women. Particularly among the older age groups, in which the available women considerably outnumber the men (Riley and Foner 1968), it is more likely that the widowers, as compared with the widows, will be able to find an eligible spouse. Prospective studies of the recently widowed would have to be examined in order to rule out the possibility of selective remarriage accounting for the higher rates. Unfortunately, Young and his colleagues (1963) used only male subjects. Neither Ekblom (1963) nor Clayton (1974) found any difference in mortality rates between widows and widowers. However, Rees and Lutkins (1967) reported the same sex dif-

The risk of death is highest during the first year of bereavement; once people are past this period the risk gradually returns to normal.

ference in their British population as Shurtleff (1955) reported in the United States, that is, during the first year of bereavement the mortality rate for widowers was significantly higher than the mortality rate for widows. Likewise, the risk for male relatives in general was significantly higher than for female relatives. Although there is not enough information to reach any conclusions about why widowers might be more likely than widows to die within a year following the death of their spouse, there are at least two plausible hypotheses. First, perhaps women are hardier than men to begin with and are thus better able to withstand the stress of losing a spouse. An alternative view could suggest that the single life, particularly in old age, is less stressful for a female than for a male. Bock and Webber (1972) discussed the social factors that might produce this sex differential in the stressfulness of a single life: (a) Domestic roles present a problem area for the male but are quite familiar to the female who continues to perform them, (b) the aged female is more likely to be closely supported by relatives, since the maintenance of kin networks has depended more heavily on females than on males, and (c) the aged male tends to be more isolated because he has been removed from his chief sources of self-identity, his occupational role and his relationships with co-workers.

Summary

In looking at loss of significant others as a predictor of death, the most convincing evidence comes from prospective studies of the recently bereaved, which compare their mortality rates with those of controls. Unfortunately, only four studies (Clayton 1974; Ekblom 1963; Rees and Lutkins 1967; Young et al. 1963) have been conducted using this design. Of these, the reports of Rees and Lutkin, Ekblom, and Young et al. have presented persuasive evidence of an increased mortality rate during the first 6–12 months following bereavement, followed by a decline to the level of married people. Although Clayton found no difference in death rates between the recently widowed and the married controls, his failure to find differences may have been influenced by his selection procedures. Most of the research examining loss of a significant other as a predictor of death has used the spouse as the significant other. However, there is some indication that loss of his parent or sibling may also predict death for the elderly person.

Thus, it appears that for some people, especially males, the loss of a significant other may be detrimental. The risk of death is highest during the first year of bereavement; once people are past this period the risk gradually returns to normal. Available evidence does not clarify whether these increased rates are due to the fact that the relatives shared the same harmful environment, to the tendency of the unfit to marry the unfit, or to some damaging aspect of widowhood itself. Widowhood has been described as involving a number of stressful changes—loss of emotional support and loss of social interaction—that might somehow alter physiological functioning and increase the risk of death. This explanation, however, remains speculation until further research is conducted.

Relocation as a Predictor of Death

A number of investigators have reported high death rates for old people during the first few months following their admission to institutions.

Just as death of a significant other may be viewed as representing environmental loss, another type of event affecting many elderly— relocation—may be viewed similarly. Changes in residence may involve loss of familiar surroundings and social ties. In this paper, relocation includes moves the elderly person makes from his private dwelling to some type of home for the aged, such as a mental institution or nursing home, from one institution to another, and from one building to another. Other relocations do of course take place—for example, from hospital to home or from one private dwelling to another. However, these moves probably do not involve the same losses; when a hospital patient moves home, he is returning to many of his old social ties, and when an older person moves from one private dwelling to another he is not necessarily losing as many of his familiar surroundings as is the elderly person entering a mental institution. At any rate, data are not available on the effects of these other types of relocation.

A number of investigators have reported high death rates for old people during the first few months following their admission to institutions (Camargo and Preston 1945; Josephy 1949; Whittier and Williams 1956). These rates, ranging from 16 percent to 25 percent dead during the first month after admission, are much higher than the expected mortality rates for elderly people of the same age in the general population. These high mortality rates have led to the widespread notion that the first type of relocation, entrance into an institution, may hasten death. Such a conclusion, based on the comparison of mortality rates of elderly who have just been admitted to an institution with mortality rates of the elderly in general, is questionable, since selection may influence the rates. In other words, those elderly who are admitted to institutions are likely to differ in health status from the beginning, when compared with the elderly in general. Since those who require institutional care are likely to be unhealthy, it is not surprising that they should die at a higher rate.

Another method of assessing whether the move into an institution increases the chances of death compares the mortality rate of a control group comprised of elderly on the waiting list with the mortality rates of a group that has just been admitted. Since the waiting-list group has been accepted into the institution, but not yet admitted, it is assumed to be in the same state of health as the recently admitted group. In a study using this design, Lieberman (1961) found that when comparing the mortality rate for the first year after admission with that of subjects on the waiting list there is a "considerably lower death rate on the waiting list" (p. 519). However, Lieberman's figures are misleading, as Kasl (1972) pointed out. Lieberman cited that 10.5 percent of his subjects died while on the waiting list, as compared with 24.7 percent who died during the first year of hospitalization. He did not compare equal time periods, however, since the average waiting-list period was only 6.4 months. Thus, according to Kasl, when the adjusted (annual) death rate for the waiting group is calculated, there is not an appreciable difference between the mortality rates for the two groups.

A similar design using a waiting-list control group was employed by Costello and Tanaka (1961). They reported a mortality rate of 38 percent in the first 6 months after admission, compared with an 11 percent death rate during a one-month waiting-list period. Again, when the rates are adjusted to compare equal intervals, the results do not support the hypothesis that entrance into an institution may effect death. Indeed, in the research of Costello and Tanaka, death was found to occur more often during the waiting-list period than it did after admission.

Although using elderly people who are awaiting admission to institutions as controls for those recently admitted helps to equalize health status between groups, this design is not without flaws. First, it is possible that the most severely incapacitated applicants to an institution are accepted without delay, while the healthier are allowed to wait. Thus, for institutions that accept patients on the basis of need, those admitted to the institution may still be less healthy than controls on the waiting list. On the other hand, for institutions that are regularly filled to capacity and all of whose patients routinely spend several months on the waiting list before admission, the less healthy may die during the waiting-list period, leaving the fittest to be admitted. In either case, selection of the admitted group is not random and results are likely to be biased. Still another problem with the comparison of waiting-list and postadmission mortality rates is that it is difficult to determine how much of the stress associated with relocation is due to the anticipation of moving and how much to the actual move itself. It is possible that the decision to enter an institution may be more predictive of death than is the admission itself.

In her 1967 discussion of the effects of environmental change, Blenkner reported data from two of her previous studies, which suggested that for older persons there may be a negative association between placement in an institution and survival, even when their physical condition is held constant. Her experimental design had the advantage of random assignment of the community elderly to experimental groups that varied in the amount of social work and public health services made available to them. Surprisingly, Blenkner found that in both studies the death rate for those subjects receiving the maximal, intensive service was higher than for those on the minimal, or control, program. She attributed the higher death rate to the fact that persons in the maximal service program were more often placed in institutions. She explained that social workers have a tendency to move people into protective settings when they become involved with them in an intensive, individualized fashion, although in her two studies the apparent result of such a move was to hasten death. Caution is necessary against relying fully on these results, since in both studies the difference in mortality rates did not reach statistical significance and the number of subjects was small. Nevertheless, the association between death and entrance to an institution was suggested, even when the selection factors that biased other studies of relocation into institutions were controlled by the random placement of subjects in experimental conditions.

By examining the effects of the other types of relocation, transfer from one institution to another, or from one building to another, two of the problems of the home-to-institution experiments can be minimized. In the relocation studies with home-to-institution moves, there is always the possibility that the higher mortality rates of those recently admitted to institutions are due to the selective application and acceptance of the less healthy, rather than to the relocation itself. This possibility is difficult to dismiss, except when subjects are randomly assigned to conditions, as in the Blenkner (1967) study. When the relocation is from institution to institution or from building to building, however, the subjects can be assumed to differ little in health status, since they are all already institutional residents. Thus, the problem of initial differences in health status is eliminated. A second problem in the home-to-institution studies is that the higher mortality rates could be produced not so much by the environmental change as by the exposure to some aspect of the institutional environment. For example, poor diet, infection, poor medical care, and sensory deprivation could raise the mortality rates (Kasl 1972). Again, the relocation studies involving between- and within-institution moves are more easily interpreted, since all subjects are assumed to be exposed to similar institutional environments.

Several of the studies examining relocation between and within institutions have used a design in which mortality rates of relocated patients were compared with mortality rates of patients who were not moved (Goldfarb, Shahinian, and Burr 1972; Killian 1970; Markson and Cumming 1974). These studies have produced different findings on the effects of relocation. For example, Killian matched patients who were transferred to other institutions with other patients on the basis of sex, race, organic or functional diagnosis, age, ambulatory or not at the time of transfer, and length of hospitalization and followed both groups for a 4-month period. His results revealed that the geriatric patients who were transferred had a significantly higher mortality rate than did the matched control patients who were not transferred. These death rates were especially higher for the older nonambulatory patients. In contrast, another study (Markson and Cumming 1974) produced no difference in mortality rates between transferred and non-transferred patients. When budget cuts necessitated the transfer of 494 elderly patients in New York State, these researchers took the opportunity to compare the patients' mortality rates for 11 months after relocation with those of another group of geriatric inpatients and a small group of old people living in the community and attending a psychogeriatric day-care center. Since the patients who relocated were healthier than were all chronic geriatric patients in general, both control groups were selected because they were relatively healthy physically. Acknowledging that they were studying a select patient population, the authors concluded that relocation may hasten an already impending death, but does not necessarily speed mortality among the relatively well.

> . . . relocation may hasten an already impending death, but does not necessarily speed mortality among the relatively well.

For those who were functioning relatively well physically, relocation may have actually been beneficial, the authors asserted.

Unlike Killian (1970), who found that transfer to another institution is associated with an increase in mortality, Goldfarb et al. (1972) discovered no significant differences in mortality for the year after relocation between relocated patients and groups of other nursing home residents. On closer inspection of patient characteristics, however, the authors found that relocation may differentially affect patients, based on the presence and severity of brain syndrome. Persons with severe brain syndrome and persons with considerable physical functional impairment were those at risk when relocated. For those who were functioning relatively well physically, relocation may have actually been beneficial, the authors asserted.

In each of these three studies (Goldfarb et al. 1972; Killian 1970; Markson and Cumming 1974), the relocated subjects were compared with patients who resided uninterruptedly in their original institutions. One possible problem with this approach is that, because the patients to be transferred are probably not randomly chosen, the likelihood that they are initially comparable to the remaining group is lessened. For example, in the Markson and Cumming study, patients to be relocated were chosen because of their good physical health, but the researchers made no attempt to match controls for physical disability, age, sex, or any other variable that might have contributed to the subjects' chances of dying. Only Killian selected his controls so that they would be matched with the relocated patients on six relevant variables. This stronger research design produced the most convincing data on the association between death and relocation.

Another method for examining whether relocation is predictive of death compares mortality rates before and after the move. Computing the mortality rate of a group residing in an institution or building is no clear-cut process, however. If the prerelocation period is considered as simply a number of months before the move (usually 3–12 months), the resulting mortality rate may simply reflect chance fluctuations. This possibility becomes evident from the finding of Markus, Blenkner, Bloom, and Downs (1971) that there was considerable fluctuation in mortality rates over a 15-year period. In an earlier study (1970), these same authors also found a cyclical trend in deaths over the quarters of the calendar. Such a trend may also confound the results of studies comparing pre- and postmove mortality rates for short periods of time. In an attempt to avert this biasing effect, several researchers (Aldrich and Mendkoff 1963; Markus et al. 1970, 1971; Zweig and Csank 1975) have employed different techniques for computing a prerelocation mortality rate. Zweig and Csank compared their postrelocation mortality rate with the rates for each of 3 years before the move; Aldrich and Mendkoff calculated an anticipated death rate based on the death rates for 10 years prior to the relocation date and then compared the observed mortality rate after relocation with this anticipated rate. The comparison used by Markus et al. was somewhat different. The mortality rates for 15 years before the relocation and that of the year following relocation were rank ordered. For the postrelocation mortality rate to be considered significantly different it had to rank either first or second—that is, it had to be either greater or smaller than the rate for 14 of the 15 control years. Using these longer comparison periods may have the effect of obscuring secular changes in death rates, thus creating stricter standards for comparison than are necessary. For example, it is possible that, because of improved medications or changes in staffing and practices, the mortality rates in a particular institution could be decreasing. The mortality rate after relocation may be significantly higher than that of the year before, but may not be different from the death rate 10 years before. Another possibility is that the patient population has changed due to altered admissions policies. If this were the case, it would be more legitimate to compare the relocated patients, not with patients of 15 years earlier, who may have had much different life expectancies, but with a more recent group. These possibly confounding variables should be subjected to further investigation to determine if they do in fact affect mortality rates. Also, in attempting to avoid many of the problems associated with these pre- and postrelocation comparisons, future researchers could use a time series analysis (Campbell and Stanley 1963). With this type of design, the change in mortality rate after relocation would be compared with the rate of change in previous years to determine whether relocation produces departure from the trend over time.

Several of the studies comparing pre- and postrelocation mortality rates have supported the notion that relocating an elderly person results in an increased chance of death (Aldrich and Mendkoff 1963; Aleksandrowicz 1961; Jasnau 1967). In Jasnau's study the death rates for the last 6 months of 1965, when the hospital was being reorganized and the majority of the patients were moved within the institution, were compared with those for the last 6 months of 1964. His finding that the death rate increased 35 percent for the 1965 period may support his conclusion that relocation causes trauma for older patients and that this in turn decreases their chances for survival. On the other hand, the increased death rate may have been a function of other changes brought about by the reorganization of the institution, such as different admission policies or changed patient services. Similarly, Aleksandrowicz's report of increased mortality rates following relocation can be subject to a number of different interpretations. An examination of the death rate after a fire had necessitated the moving of a ward of 40 geriatric patients, revealed an increase to 20 percent mortality for the 3 months after the fire, as compared with only 7.5 percent for the 3 months preceding the fire. The increased death rate could be attributed not only to the stress of relocation but also to possible deterioration of medical and nursing care, to seasonal changes, or to trauma caused by the fire and evacuation. Although both of these studies revealed large increases in death rates following the relocation of patient groups, they both lacked controls that could rule out the effect of other changing conditions.

In another study, Aldrich and Mendkoff (1963) avoided many of these biasing factors and still found a significantly higher death rate after relocation. All of the 182 patients of a nursing home were transferred, primarily to other nursing homes of the same or better quality in the same communi-

**Data are
beginning to
accumulate that
suggest that the
way the relocation
process is
managed may
affect how well
the patient is able
to handle the
move.**

ty, when the home in which they were living closed as a result of administrative necessity. The fact that all of the patients were moved without regard to their state of health minimizes the chances that the increased death rates after relocation could have been due to selection factors. Further, since patients were moved to nursing homes of equal or better quality, the possibility of declining medical care is not very likely. Finally, because the nursing home closed for administrative reasons rather than because of some disaster, as in Aleksandrowicz's (1961) study, the reason for closing does not in itself present a factor in the decline in physical health of the patients. Aldrich and Mendkoff reported that the effects of relocation on the mortality rate were concentrated in the first 3 months following departure from the nursing home and that after that the rate returned to what it had been for the past 10 years. This study offers strong support for the connection between relocation and increased chances of death for the elderly patient.

Other researchers, in comparing pre- and postrelocation mortality rates, have produced less clear-cut findings (Markus et al. 1970, 1971; Novick 1967; Zweig and Csank 1975). The Markus et al. studies are based on the transfer of the entire populations of two homes for the aged from old downtown buildings to new suburban plants. Erratic changes in mortality rates were observed: At one home, females of ages 75–79 had significantly higher mortality rates after relocation, whereas those 80 and over experienced significantly lower rates; at the other home, males 80 and over and females under 75 died at significantly higher rates, and males under 75, at lower rates. The authors explained that these inconsistencies could be due to chance variability or different admission policies at the two homes.

In the Novick (1967) and Zweig and Csank (1975) studies, patients were also moved from old buildings to new buildings with more modern facilities. The researchers' failure to find increased mortality rates after relocation may have been due to the improved living conditions given the patients. In the Zweig and Csank study, for example, the patients were moved in July from an old building to a new facility with central air conditioning. In the old building the highest monthly death rates had occurred in July and August—a fact that the authors admitted could be due to the hot climate alone. Thus, with the relocation came an improved climate, and the effects of the two variables were inextricably intertwined. In the Novick study, the postrelocation death rate was actually found to be lower than the rate at the old hospital. Although these results are at odds with the more general finding that relocation increases mortality, it is not clear to what extent the results were due to improved surroundings.

Because there are contradictory findings from these studies of the effect of relocation on mortality rates, one would suspect that there are other variables involved that might influence how relocation affects an elderly person. Data are beginning to accumulate that suggest that the way the relocation process is managed may affect how well the patient is able to handle the move. Jasnau (1967) reported that patients who were transferred en masse within the hospital with little or no preparation had higher death rates than did those patients receiving casework service preparation who were transferred individually to nursing homes. Aside from the amount of preparation received, the two groups unfortunately differed in a number of other ways, including their financial status, whether they wanted to move or not, and the type of institution in which they were finally placed. In the Novick (1967) study, in which mortality rates were found to be lower after relocation, the hospital administrators made elaborate efforts to prepare each patient for the move. They scheduled frequent bus trips to the new site so that patients could watch the new buildings being built, and constructed at the old hospital a life-size model of one of the new rooms so that patients could become accustomed to them. Additionally, patients chose the fixtures for the new building, participated in discussions with the social service staff about the move, and were involved in both the packing and unpacking of their personal belongings. Novick (1967) and Zweig and Csank (1975)— who found that the death rate of their group did not increase after relocation—attributed the success with which their groups relocated to the well-managed preparation programs. However, neither study had a control group of patients not receiving this preparation, which could have assured that the way in which the relocation was handled was the crucial factor.

Other investigators have attempted to show that whether the elderly person views the move as voluntary or involuntary will influence the mortality rates. In a report on her dissertation, Ferrari (1963) asserted that among institutionalized women there was a higher mortality rate after admission for those who felt they had no alternative but to move to the institution than for those who felt they had other alternatives. Unfortunately, it is likely that those who perceived a lack of choice may have initially been in poorer health than were the others. Without an attempt to measure health status, it remains unknown how much of the difference in mortality rates was accounted for by the lack of alternatives. In two other studies (Lawton and Yaffe 1970; Wittels and Botwinick 1974) it was reported that when healthy elderly voluntarily moved into a senior citizen apartment building, there was no change in mortality rates. Neither study specifically tested the hypothesis that a greater mortality risk was associated with involuntary rather than voluntary change of residence, however, since all subjects moving did so voluntarily. The fact that mortality rates were not affected could have been because the type of relocation (from one private dwelling to another) did not involve the same loss of social ties or familiar surroundings.

Lieberman (1969)[2] has argued that the type of environment to which the elderly person is relocated is crucial in determining whether the event will be stressful for the person. The larger the difference between the old and new situations, the greater the possibility that the aged individual will need to develop adaptive responses, often beyond his capacity. However, Markson and Cumming (1974) found no differential mortality rate associated with the type of hospital to which patients were transferred. Each hospital was rated on activity, in terms of patient involvement in decision

Other investigators have attempted to show that whether the elderly person views the move as voluntary or involuntary will influence the mortality rates.

. . . for which elderly is relocation most likely to predict death?

making and number of patients discharged. When patients were moved from low-activity hospitals, their mortality rates did not seem to be affected by the level of activity in the new environment. Further research examining the amount of change involved in the relocation as a predictor of death should focus on other more specific aspects of the patient's environment, such as space, schedule of activities, or amount of interpersonal contact.

It has been suggested that the way the relocation process is managed, whether the move is considered voluntary by the elderly person, and the amount of change between the old and new environments are all factors that might influence whether an elderly person will die after relocation. Yet the obvious fact that not all elderly die following relocation has led to the question, for which elderly is relocation most likely to predict death?

In comparing survivors and nonsurvivors following relocation, Wittels and Botwinick (1974) and Markus, Blenkner, Bloom, and Downs (1972) found that those who died after the move were in poorer health initially. These unsurprising results give no information about the effects of relocation; in any group of people, those who are most likely to die are those in poor health. Of more interest are the studies of Goldfarb et al. (1972) and Killian (1970), in which relocated patients in poor health showed a higher mortality rate than patients in similar health who were not moved. The increased death rates in the moderately and severely functionally impaired, as measured by physical examination and physical limitations, were not found among the relocated with little or no impairment (Goldfarb et al.). In fact, Goldfarb and his colleagues suggested that for those who are relatively well physically, relocation may be beneficial. On the other hand, although healthy elderly are not likely to die after relocation, there is some evidence that they too may suffer adverse effects. In their study of healthy elderly being relocated into an apartment complex, Lawton and Yaffe (1970) found that the relocated group showed a greater decline in functional health rating than did the nonrelocated group, even though mortality rates for the two groups were the same. Thus the available research leads to two divergent views on the relationship between physical health status and relocation effects. One view would describe relocation as a process producing declines in all elderly: Those in relatively good health get sick, and those who are severely physically impaired become sicker and are likely to die. The other view, suggested by Goldfarb et al. (1972), proposes that relocation has differential effects depending on the initial condition of the elderly person, that is, relocation may hasten decline in aged persons who are already seriously physically impaired, but for those who are relatively well physically, health is not adversely affected and may even be benefited by the change of scenery. Further research is needed to determine whether an interaction exists between health status and relocation effects. At any rate, relocation seems more likely to predict death for the physically impaired than for those in good health.

Just as physical impairment has been linked with higher chances of death following relocation, so has mental impairment. Aldrich and Mendkoff (1963) found that among their relocated patients, the death rate for the psychotic or nearly psychotic elderly patients was the highest for any group. Markus et al. (1970) reported that persons with severe mental dysfunction, as measured by the Mental Status Questionnaire, had a significantly higher death rate 6 months following relocation than did other relocated residents. An attempt to replicate these results with nursing home residents in another city was unsuccessful, however (Markus et al. 1971). The experimenters speculated that the differences could have been due to different admission policies at the two homes. In a study comparing relocated patients with severe brain syndrome, as evaluated by a psychiatrist, with similarly affected patients who were not moved, Goldfarb et al. (1972) found a higher mortality rate among the relocated. For those with no or mild brain syndrome, relocation seemed to decrease the chances of death. The pattern was also confirmed by the data for number of errors on the Mental Status Questionnaire, although for neither measure of brain syndrome were the differences in mortality rates between relocated and nonrelocated groups statistically significant. Thus, the research on relocation as a better predictor of death for the mentally impaired than for those with no cognitive disturbance remains inconclusive. If such a relationship does exist, the cognitive impairment may simply be a reflection of physical impairment. This possibility is likely among the elderly, for whom arteriosclerosis and other cardiovascular problems often produce altered mental functioning.

There is also evidence that certain personality characteristics of the elderly person may affect the likelihood of his death following relocation. Markus et al. (1970) reported that the degree of perceptual field dependence evidenced by an elderly person predicted his survival after relocation, but a later study (Markus et al. 1971) failed to uphold these findings. Among their relocated patients, Aldrich and Mendkoff (1963) and Aldrich (1964) found that those classified as overtly depressed before relocation had the highest death rate, whereas those whose adjustment was classified as satisfactory or overtly angry died at significantly lower rates. Similarly, Miller and Lieberman (1965) reported that a significantly larger number of elderly who had been depressed before relocation showed more negative reactions (death or development of serious illness) than did those who had not been depressed. Others (Turner, Tobin, and Lieberman 1972; Lieberman[2]) noted that elderly who were aggressive, demanding, active, and narcissistic were found to be most likely to survive relocation.

The relationship between personality traits and incidence of death following relocation is further supported by research assessing the relationship between mortality rates and the patients' response to the news of relocation (Aldrich 1964; Aldrich and Mendkoff 1963). These researchers classified each patient according to his predominant reaction to the news, based on reports obtained from the hospital staff. They reported that the survival rate was highest for patients who took the news in stride or were overtly angry. Patients who become anxious but did not withdraw survived reasonably well, and patients who regressed, became depressed, or denied that the nursing home was closing were least likely to survive.

There is also evidence that certain personality characteristics of the elderly person may affect the likelihood of his death following relocation.

A common factor in these studies has been the description of the elderly person most likely to die following relocation as depressed.

A common factor in these studies has been the description of the elderly person most likely to die following relocation as depressed. This information was derived from studies comparing the survivors and nonsurvivors after relocation; there were no control groups of depressed patients who were not moved. Therefore, data are not available on whether relocation is particularly dangerous for the depressed, or on whether these people would have died at the same rate had they not been moved. Some researchers (McMahon and Rhudick 1964; Nowlin 1974) have found that the elderly living in the community, unaffected by relocation, who are rated as depressed are likely to die sooner than are their nondepressed counterparts. This would suggest that depressed elderly die sooner than nondepressed elderly, regardless of whether they are relocated. Further research comparing the mortality rates of depressed elderly who are relocated with others who are not moved will have to be conducted to determine if relocation selectively affects the depressed.

Another problem with studies linking personality characteristics with mortality rates following relocation is that there have been no controls for physical health status. It could be that the least healthy tend to be depressed and because of their poor health are hastened toward death by relocation, whereas those in good health who happen to be depressed are not affected by relocation. For the diagnosis of depression to be of value in predicting for which individuals relocation will be most dangerous, the physical health status of elderly individuals will have to be controlled.

Before going on to discuss how relocation might act to affect the health of an elderly person, several points will be summarized. The most convincing evidence that relocation does predict death for the elderly comes from studies in which elderly patients have been transferred from one institution to another or from one building to another within the same institution. In these experiments, mortality rates have been compared before and after relocation or between relocated and control groups. The design of these studies is preferable to that of studies in which mortality rates for new admissions have been examined, because the increased death rates after relocation can not be attributed to the harmful effects of institutional life nor to selection factors (e.g., elderly who are seeking admission to an institution may already be approaching death). Of the studies that have looked at transfer effects after entrance into an institution, two stand out as having employed the best experimental design (Aldrich and Mendkoff 1963; Killian 1970). Both found that transfer to another institution is associated with an increase in mortality rates.

It is likely that relocation does predict death for the elderly, but only for those already in poor health. The Aldrich and Mendkoff (1963) study involved the relocation of 180 nursing home patients, all of whom required some type of nursing care. In the Killian (1970) study, mortality rates for nonambulatory patients were especially higher than expected. The findings of Goldfarb et al. (1972) also supported the likelihood that relocation predicts death only among the elderly in poor health; these researchers reported that only relocatees with considerable functional impairment had an increased mortality rate. Other investigators (Lawton and Yaffe 1970; Markson and Cumming 1974; Wittels and Botwinick 1974) have suggested that moves made by healthy elderly are not associated with death.

A number of investigators have speculated on how relocation might affect the health and chances of death of an elderly person. The event has been described as a stressful occurrence, involving radical changes in life space (Lieberman)[2] and deprivation of familiar cues and environmental supports (Markus et al. 1972). Killian (1970) explained that the aged individual's increasing dependency on his immediate environment is even more pronounced in the geriatric patient, for whom the institutional environment can foster, perpetuate, and encourage unwholesome dependency. Thus, when the elderly person is moved from his accustomed environment with social ties and familiar surroundings, into a new one, he experiences "transplantation shock," as Blenkner (1967) termed it. The elderly person must respond to the new environment. Lieberman (1969) explained that the move into the new situation forces the person to make new adaptive responses, whereas Markus et al. (1971, 1972) viewed the relocated person as coping with new sets of stimuli in an unfamiliar environment. It is not immediately clear to what extent the stress of relocation is thought to come from the loss of familiar stimuli or from the shock of new stimuli.

According to the relocation-stress-death theory, the stress resulting from the move affects in some manner the physiological functioning of the individual. Unfortunately, there has been only one study in which the reaction to relocation was assessed at the physiological level (Kral, Grad, and Berenson 1968). In this experiment, the levels of cortisol in the plasma of 54 aged subjects was measured daily for a period of 3–8 days before relocation and for 9–16 days after relocation. Production of cortisol, a hormone originating in adrenal cortex, is though to increase during stress (Selye 1956). The results indicated that the plasma cortisol level increased significantly after relocation for both psychotic and normal males, but not for females. The authors also reported that the greatest plasma cortisol changes were observed in the patients with the severest physical symptoms after relocation, suggesting that this measure may be a prognostic indicator of illness that may develop. Because there was no nonrelocated control group of patients in the experiment, the increased plasma cortisol levels could have been a function of the daily blood sampling or of some other event taking place during the time period.

In addition to the theory that health deteriorates as a result of the stress of relocation, there may be other causes of high mortality in the first few months after transfer. Goldfarb et al. (1972) suggested that factors such as inadequate understanding of the physical needs of a new patient, his subjection to excessive physical demands, and the temporary alteration or discontinuity of supportive medical care need to be considered as possible sources of increased mortality. Although it is difficult to rule out the possibility that inadequate care during relocation is responsible for some of the increased

According to the relocation-stress-death theory, the stress resulting from the move affects in some manner the physiological functioning of the individual.

Common in medical folklore is the belief that an individual who is forced to retire will die much earlier than he would if he were allowed to continue working.

mortality, it does seem unlikely that it accounts for all of it. Further research, in which the care given each patient during and after the move is carefully monitored, is necessary to eliminate the possibility that inadequate care produces mortality.

Summary

Relocation seems to predict death for the elderly who are in poor health. Those whose mental functioning is impaired, either through psychosis or severe brain syndrome, and those who are depressed may also be particularly vulnerable to death following relocation. It is not evident from the available research, however, whether the patients with mental impairment and depression are at risk because of these characteristics or because they are also in poor physical health.

By handling the relocation process in such a way that patients are given psychological support and prior familiarity with their new surroundings, it may be possible to eliminate the higher mortality rate following relocation, since studies in which patients who were elaborately prepared for the move did not have higher than expected postrelocation mortality rates. Unfortunately, it is not clear from these studies to what extent the improved surroundings of the new buildings contributed to the lack of increase in death rate.

It is also possible that whether the elderly person views relocation as voluntary or involuntary and the amount of change between the old and new environments will each affect the mortality rates after relocation. Further research will be necessary to substantiate the effect of these factors.

Relocation for the elderly person has been described as a stressful event, which requires that the person mobilize his resources to cope with the loss of familiar surroundings and to adapt to the new stimuli. This explanation fits with the observation that the elderly with the fewest resources— that is, those in poor physical health, with mental impairment, who are feeling depressed—have lower chances of surviving relocation. Also consistent with this view is the finding that there are, in some cases, physiological changes accompanying relocation, suggesting that the event is experienced as physically stressful. It should be noted, however, that although mortality rates have been observed to increase after relocation, there is no clear-cut support for any particular explanation of the phenomenon.

Retirement as a Predictor of Death

Common in medical folklore is the belief that an individual who is forced to retire will die much earlier than he would if he were allowed to continue working. The "retirement impact theory," as it has been called (McMahan and Ford 1955; Tyhurst, Salk, and Kennedy 1957), is based on the assumption that retirement is a stress that frequently results in physical disorders that may prove fatal before adjustment can be made. Some theorists have explained the stressfulness of retirement in terms of the losses involved: loss of income, loss of companionship, loss of activity and stimulation, loss of prestige, and loss of self-identity (Bock 1972; Tronchin-James 1962). Streib and Schneider (1971) described retirement stress in terms of change. They explained that because the organism becomes adjusted to certain behavior patterns, when an abrupt change in activities and pace occurs, as in retirement, the sustaining patterns are disrupted and a physiological collapse may be precipitated. Ellison (1968) proposed that people frequently respond to the stress of retirement by adopting the sick role. He argued that the losses associated with retirement (loss of income, status, social relationships) contribute to the physical and emotional decline of the retiree.

Proponents of the retirement impact theory have cited as statistical evidence the high mortality rates for individuals who had just retired (Myers 1954). Also offered as evidence have been the findings of studies in which the employment status (retirement vs. full or part-time employment) of older persons predicted whether they would be living or dead several years later (Palmore and Stone 1973; Powers and Bultena 1972). These findings provide little true support for the theory that retirement precipitates death, however, since health status is frequently confounded with retirement status. In other words, workers often retire because of poor health, and those who continue to work are able to do so because of their relatively good health (Streib and Schneider 1971). In neither of the studies investigating employment status as a predictor of death (Palmore and Stone 1973; Powers and Bultena 1972) was the health status of the subjects controlled. In fact, Powers and Bultena showed that both health status and employment status could predict to a significant degree whether their subjects would be dead 11 years later, but they made no attempt to assess the independent power of each factor. Thus it is likely that the retired group contained a disproportionate percentage of people who chose to retire or were retired, because of their poor health.

Myers (1954), in analyzing the mortality rates of workers and retirees under various governmental and private retirement plans, found that the "mortality of retired workers during the first year or two of retirement is considerably above the general level which otherwise might be expected but thereafter merges with such general level" (p. 508). However, it appears that there are a number of characteristics of the pension programs themselves that need to be considered in interpreting the differences in mortality rates. For example, those retiring under a plan that does not have compulsory retirement may tend to be in poor health, that is, employees simply continue working until poor health prevents further employment. On the other hand, if a company requires retirement at a certain age, those retiring at that age may be in better health than that of the general population, which includes those who retired earlier because of poor health. Another factor to be considered is whether the plan provides that retirement, although required at a certain age, may be deferred with the consent of the employer. In this case, the older workers may be those in unusually good health, and consequently those with lower expected mortality rates. Still another factor to be noticed is at what age disability payments and retirements are available in the system. For instance, in the railroad retirement program described by Myers, retirement benefits are available at age 65, but individuals may retire before age 65 with larger benefits if permanent and total disability is proved than if retirement is for age. Under such a plan, mortality rates for those retiring at ages 60–64 were lower than expected, according to mortality tables computed by the company; for those retiring at ages 65–69, actual mortality was appreciably higher than was expected; and for those retiring at ages 70 and over, mortality was quite close to that expected. Because of the many conflicting factors involved and because of the unavailability of specific and reliable data, Myers concluded that no clear and definite conclusions can be drawn about the effect of retirement on mortality.

Another study designed to measure the mortality effects of entry into retirement was confronted with many of these same confounding factors (McMahan and Ford 1955). In examining the mortality rates of Air Force officers for 5-year periods after retirement, it was found that for those retiring between ages 50 and 59, mortality rates during the first 5 years of retirement were higher than the average for white American males. For retiring officers 60–69 years old, mortality rates were lower than expected. The authors acknowledged that in the younger age group, the early retirement could have been the result of physical disability and that this same disability could have been responsible for the higher mortality rates. Likewise, the lower mortality rates among the older retirees may be explained by the fact that the officers were a physically select group. Just as Myers found in 1954, no conclusion could be made, based on current data.

In a similar study, Tyhurst, Salk, and Kennedy (1957) concluded that retirement did not hasten death among male Bell Telephone workers. The retirement program in this company was a flexible one, with most employees retiring at between 60 and 70 years of age. This allowed the company to retire an employee when he was no longer able to meet adequately the requirements of any available job. It also allowed the worker to decide, to some extent, when he would like to retire. Actually some people retired before age 60, usually because they were in poor health or because their job became obsolete. With a retirement system that had so many reasons and ages of retirement, it is difficult to feel confident that the retirees were no different from the working controls.

In reviewing the studies that have examined retirement as a predictor of death, it appears that all suffer from serious methodological problems. In each case, retirement status has been confounded with health status. When workers retire under voluntary retirement plans, retirees are frequently less healthy initially than are those continuing to work. The ideal study would compare the mortality rates of two groups randomly selected from the same population—one group forced to retire at a given age and the other group made to work for several more years. From a practical viewpoint, it would be impossible to manipulate the time of retirement of human subjects. The next best solution would be a study using two groups, one from an industry with compulsory retirement at 65 years of age and the other from a comparable industry that has forced retirement at age 70. The mortality rates would then be compared for the 5-year period between ages 65 and 70. It is possible that for different types of people, retirement may have different effects on health and chances of death. It would seem wise, therefore, to measure the subjects on certain characteristics to determine how these variables might mediate the effect of retirement. For example, Botwinick (1973) suggested that adjustment to retirement may be related to three factors: sufficient income, health, and substituted satisfactions. Other variables that might influence retirement predicting death would be the subject's satisfaction with his job and with the organization of his daily activities. It would be predicted that a person who was very committed to and involved in his work might find retirement more stressful than would a person who was not very interested in his job. Similarly, a person with many enjoyable leisure activities could probably better adjust to retirement than could the person whose primary satisfaction was his work.

Although there has been little research on retirement as a predictor of death and no conclusive evidence that it does predict death, one impression emerges from this body of literature. In each study there seemed to be a recognition that a belief in retirement being detrimental to the worker's health was once widely held. At the same time, the idea was discussed as though it was a superstition once believed in, but no longer given any serious consideration. Supporting this observation is the fact that there have been no studies since 1957 (Tyhurst et al.) whose primary aim was the investigation of retirement as a predictor of death. The apparent diminished interest could be explained in a number of ways. Perhaps there once was a superstitious belief that retirement led to death, which was dispelled once researchers explained that poor health is likely to cause retirement, rather than retirement causing poor health. On the other hand, maybe it is true that retirement does sometimes produce a physical decline and that researchers' present disbelief is based on inconclusive research. Either explanation is possible, for although there has been no clear-cut evidence that retirement predicts death, there has also been no demonstration that retirement does not affect subsequent mortality rates.

Another explanation deserves some consideration: Because of societal changes, retirement possibly is no longer as stressful as it once was, and thus it does not produce the lethal effects it once did. Retirement is thought to be stressful because of losses in income, companionship, activity and stimulation, prestige, and self-identity. However, it is probable that many of these losses have been reduced in recent years. As Riley and Foner (1968) pointed out, retirement is more widespread; in the United States the proportion of men over 65 years old in the work force has dropped sharply from approximately two thirds in 1900 to less than one third in 1960 (p. 42). It seems likely that as retirement becomes a common place occurrence it will not be

> . . . in the United States the proportion of men over 65 years old in the work force has dropped sharply from approximately two thirds in 1900 to less than one third in 1960.

associated with a loss of prestige or self-identity. Similarly, the drop in income occurring at retirement has been decreased somewhat by the extension of social security and various pension plans during the past 20 years. Finally, the loss of social ties and activities associated with retirement is probably more easily replaced today. The recent emergence of a large number of organizations providing recreational, social, and educational programs gives the elderly retiree many activities in which to participate. During this century the declining number of hours in the work week and the declining number of working days per year have allowed more time for leisure activities (Riley and Foner 1968, p. 64). This increased leisure time during working years may serve as practice for later retirement. Another development, the establishment of preretirement counseling in many companies, reputedly stimulates employees to think constructively about retirement and to plan for it well ahead of time (Ash 1966).

Summary
Although there have been no conclusive data to show that retirement does predict death, the existing research has not been well enough designed to allow any conclusions to be made. There have been few studies to date, and all have been plagued by selection factors in which health status is confounded with employment status. More research is needed to determine if retirement does predict death and, if so, for what type of people. Research looking at the effects of compulsory retirement, in which retirees and workers are not likely to differ in initial health status, is required so that health status can be controlled.

Conclusion

In reviewing literature on death of significant others, relocation, and retirement, it appears that the ability of these environmental events to predict death for the elderly depends on a number of variables. Death of a significant other, for instance, seems to predict death under certain conditions. The risk of death is probably greatest during the first year of bereavement and may be higher for males than for females. Most of the studies show that death of a spouse increases the chances of death for the elderly person, and there is some indication that the same may be true for the death of parents or siblings. Although there is a scarcity of research demonstrating which elderly are most susceptible to death during bereavement, the suggestion that those who have few contacts with others will be the most likely to die is one deserving more consideration.

As for relocation, this event probably does predict death for the elderly, but only for those already in poor health. Those whose mental functioning is impaired, either through psychosis or severe brain syndrome, and those who are depressed may also be particularly vulnerable to death after a move. It is not clear from existing research what characteristics of the relocation process itself may influence how well it predicts death for the elderly person. Factors such as how the relocation process is handled and whether the move is voluntary or involuntary may affect mortality rates after relocation, but further research is needed to substantiate the effect of these factors.

The third event considered, retirement, differs from the other two in that there has been very little evidence to suggest that it can predict death at all. One problem in this area of research is that health status has often been confounded with retirement. In other words, it has been impossible to determine whether the high postretirement mortality rates are due to the stress of retirement or are simply a reflection of the workers' tendency to retire because of poor health.

It can be seen, then, in examining the present literature, that there are many questions remaining unanswered. Future studies, in attempting to answer these questions, will need to avoid the methodological problems common in the existing research. Careful controls for age and health status between subject groups is necessary, and the need to look at mortality rates immediately after the event, rather than years later, is indicated.

Although the findings in the existing literature suggest that environmental events may predict death, at least for some people under some circumstances, very little is known about how these events physiologically affect the individual. Several theorists have suggested ways in which death might occur. Cannon (1942) proposed that in the face of a threatening event, the individual experiences extreme fear leading to marked sympathetic nervous system stimulation and adrenal hormone secretion. If the fear state is maintained for more than a few hours, especially without water, cardiovascular collapse and death follow. Richter (1957), on the other hand, suggested a reaction of hopelessness and depression rather than fear. He claimed that bodily functions probably dwindle away via parasympathetic overactivation. Finally, Engel (1971) combined the notions of both of the earlier writers to suggest that both sympathetic and parasympathetic arousal are important. He argued that the lethal influences may involve rapid shifts between sympathetic and parasympathetic cardiovascular effects. In other words, death is likely to occur when uncertainty, both in a psychological and physiological sense, is prominent (p. 780). Unfortunately, only one study (Kral 1968) has employed physiological measures before and after one of these environmental events. This is an area deserving of further research.

An individual's response to death of a significant other, relocation, and retirement can be conceptualized by a number of different theories. Each generates many research ideas. One way of viewing a person's reaction to these events is in terms of crisis theory (Caplan 1964; Eisdorfer 1972; Klein and Lindemann 1961; Lieberman[2]). According to this model, the individual is typically in a state of relative equilibrium with his interpersonal environment. This does not mean that his life is static, but that his behavior produces a consistent pattern when viewed over a long period of time. On certain occasions this balance is upset, and the person finds that he is unable to solve his problems via previously successful behavior. During these crisis

An individual's response to death of a significant other, relocation, and retirement can be conceptualized by a number of different theories. . . . Each generates many research ideas. One . . . is in terms of crisis theory.

situations, the individual is "upset," a feeling usually associated with anxiety, fear, guilt, or shame, depending on the nature of the situation (Caplan 1964, p. 40). There is some disorganization of functioning and a feeling of helplessness in the face of the overwhelming problem. Lieberman[2] explained that the individual's ability to cope with a crisis depends on his available psychological and biological resources. More research is needed, aimed at determining the subject characteristics that might render an individual either more immune or more susceptible to death during a crisis. Lieberman suggested, for example, that poor cognitive functioning may limit the individual's ability to assess the possible constraints and opportunities for adaptation within the environment. Another variable suggested by Lieberman as being influential in the outcome of the individual's attempt to cope with the event is the intensity of stress associated with the crisis. He considered the intensity of the stress to be dependent upon the amount of change resulting from the crisis.

In viewing death of a significant other, relocation, and retirement as crises, then, an elderly person's chances of death (or complete failure in coping) would depend on his available resources and on the amount of change in his life brought about by the event. For instance, after the death of a spouse, the remaining partner's chances of death may be in part determined by his ability to take over the functions that had been provided by the spouse (accounting, housekeeping, earning an income) and by his ability to obtain companionship and encouragement from outside social supports. His risk of death would also depend upon the amount of change resulting from his spouse's death, which would probably be related to the degree to which the remaining partner had been dependent on the deceased.

Another way of conceptualizing these events, through a reinforcement model (Eisdorfer 1972), offers more hypotheses for investigation. In this model, the event is examined in terms of its consequent loss of reinforcement. The assumption is made that depression results from the loss of reinforcement, and that depression, in turn, increases the chances of death. Predictions made from this model would thus involve estimates of the amount of reinforcement received both before and after the event.

In predicting death from retirement, for example, one would need to determine the reinforcement received by the individual at work (income, social interactions with co-workers, status) as well as the amount of reinforcement available after retirement. Reinforcement after retirement might depend on factors such as whether the individual had enjoyable leisure activities or friends off the job. Of course, the rewards obtained would vary among individuals and social classes. For instance, Eisdorfer (1972) predicted that for higher income levels, take-home pay becomes progressively less relevant as the primary reinforcement for work, whereas autonomy, recognition, and social power tend to dominate. In contrast, for the individual in the lower socioeconomic classes, salary would represent a major proportion of job satisfaction.

Still another way of conceptualizing these events is through a learned helplessness model (Seligman 1975). Briefly, Seligman espoused the view that when an individual has experienced trauma he cannot control, he may show the symptoms of learned helplessness, that is, lowered initiation of voluntary responses, decreased aggression, loss of appetite, and some physiological changes. His theory suggests that the crucial factor in the effect of an event is not the loss of reinforcement, but the loss of control over reinforcement.

Forced relocation is a case in point. According to Seligman, if a person is in a marginal physical state, removing his last bit of control over his environment (e.g., where he is located) may well kill him (1965, pp. 184–186). This theory, in predicting death from an environmental event, would emphasize the importance of determining if the event is voluntary or involuntary. It would also suggest that an event would be most likely to predict death for those elderly who lack control of reinforcement in other parts of their lives as well, that is, those in poor health, or forced to retire, or whose friends are no longer living.

Each of these models—crisis, reinforcement, learned helplessness—is useful in describing an individual's reaction to environmental events. The theories, although they emphasize different facets of the event and responses to it, are not necessarily opposing. Their usefulness stems from the research ideas generated, rather than from the validity of any particular model. Each offers a coherent structure focusing on variables that might influence the ability of an event to predict death, leads that future researchers will undoubtedly want to investigate.

Finally, if certain environmental events do predict death for the elderly, the logical next step is to question if and how this might be changed. There are several possibilities for investigation. First, following from crisis theory, in which the resources available to the person determine how well he will be able to adapt to the event, some alteration of social supports may help to prevent death. Caplan (1964), in discussing intervention procedures during crises, suggested that during these times the individual is more susceptible to influence from others than he is during periods of stable functioning. The outcome of a crisis may then be influenced by the intervention of family, friends, or mental health professionals.

The reinforcement model supposes that the severity of the event and the chances of death depend on the amount of reinforcement lost. According to this model, it would seem that death could be prevented by assuring that alternative sources of reinforcement were available to the individual after the event.

Seligman's (1975) learned helplessness model assumes that the loss of control of reinforcement is a precipitating factor in death following one of these environmental events. By giving the individual maximum control over all aspects of his daily life, his chances of death may be decreased. Seligman proposed that by giving institutionalized patients control over aspects such

Each of these models—crisis, reinforcement, learned helplessness—is useful in describing an individual's reaction to environmental events.

as choice of omelets or scrambled eggs for breakfast, blue or red curtains, going to the movies on Wednesday or Thursday, sleeping late or waking up early, they may live longer, show more spontaneous remissions, and will certainly be much happier (p. 183).

Each of these interventions is deserving of further research to determine its effectiveness in lowering death rates after death of a loved one, relocation, or retirement.

Notes

1. Casler, L. *Psychosomatic aspects of death: An experiment with suggestive therapy.* Paper presented at the 75th Annual Convention of the American Psychological Association, Washington, D.C., September 1967.
2. Lieberman, M. A. *Adaptive processes in later life.* Paper presented at the West Virginia Life Span Conference, May 1974.

References

Aldrich, C. K. Personality factors and mortality in the relocation of the aged. *Gerontologist,* 1964, 4(2):92–93.

Aldrich, C. K., and Mendkoff, E. Relocation of the aged and disabled: A mortality study. *Journal of the American Geriatrics Society,* 1963, 11:185–194.

Aleksandrowicz, D. R. Fire and its aftermath on a geriatric ward. *Bulletin of the Menninger Clinic,* 1961, 25:23–32.

Ash, P. Pre-retirement counseling. *Gerontologist,* 1966, 6:97–99; 127–128.

Birren, J. E. Reactions to loss and the process of aging: Interrelations of environmental changes, psychological capacities, and physiological status. In M. A. Berezin and S. H. Cath (eds). *Geriatric Psychiatry: Grief, Loss, and Emotional Disorders in the Aging Process.* New York: International Universities Press, 1965.

Blenkner, M. Environmental change and the aging individual. *Gerontologist,* 1967, 7(2):101–105.

Bock, E. W. Aging and suicide: The significance of marital, kinship, and alternative relations. *Family Coordinator,* 1972, 21:71–79.

Bock, E. W., and Webber, I. L. Suicide among the elderly: Isolating widowhood and mitigating alternatives. *Journal of Marriage and the Family,* 1972, 34(1):24–31.

Botwinick, J. *Aging and Behavior.* New York: Springer, 1973.

Brody, E. M.; Kleban, M. H.; Lawton, M. P.; Levy, R.; and Waldow, A. Predictors of mortality in the mentally-impaired institutionalized aged. *Journal of Chronic Diseases,* 1972, 25:611–620.

Butler, R. N. Aspects of survival and adaptation in human aging. *American Journal of Psychiatry,* 1967, 123:1233–1243.

Camargo, O. and Preston, G. H. What happens to patients who are hospitalized for the first time when over sixty-five? *American Journal of Psychiatry,* 1945, 102:168–173.

Campbell, D. T., and Stanley, J. C. *Experimental and Quasi-experimental Designs for Research.* Chicago: Rand McNally, 1963.

Cannon, W. B. Voodoo death. *American Anthropologist,* 1942, 44:169–181.

Caplan, G. *Principles of Preventive Psychiatry.* New York: Basic Books, 1964.

Casler, L. Death as a pyschosomatic condition: Prolegomena to a longitudinal study. *Psychological Reports,* 1970, 27:953–954.

Clayton, P. J. Mortality and morbidity in the first year of widowhood. *Archives of General Psychiatry,* 1974, 30:747–750.

Clayton, P. J.; Halikas, J. A.; and Maurice, W. L. The bereavement of the widowed. *Diseases of the Nervous Systems,* 1971, 32:597–604.

Costello, J. P., and Tanaka, G. M. Mortality and morbidity in long-term institutional care of the aged. *Journal of the American Geriatric Society,* 1961, 9:959–963.

Eisdorfer, C. Adaptation to loss of work. In F. Carp (ed.), *Retirement.* New York: Behavioral Publications, 1972.

Ekblom, B. Significance of socio-psychological factors with regard to risk of death among elderly persons. *Acta Psychiatrica Scandinavica,* 1963, 39(4):627–633.

Ellison, D. L. Work, retirement, and the sick role. *Gerontologist,* 1968, 8(3):189–192.

Engel, G. L. Sudden and rapid death during psychological stress, folklore or folkwisdom? *Annals of Internal Medicine,* 1971, 74:771–782.

Ferrari, N. A. Freedom of choice. *Social Work,* 1963, 8:104–106.

Garrity, T. F. and Klein, R. F. A behavioral predictor of survival among heart attack patients. In E. Palmore and F. C. Jeffers (eds), *Prediction of life span.* Lexington, Mass.: Heath, 1971.

Goldfarb, A. I.; Fisch, M.; and Gerber, I. Predictors of mortality in the institutionalized aged. *Diseases of the Nervous System,* 1966, 27:21–29.

Goldfarb, A. I.; Shahinian, S. P.; and Burr, H. T. Death rate of relocated nursing home residents. In D. P. Kent, R. Kastenbaum, and S. Sherwood (eds), *Research planning and action for the elderly: The power and potential of social science.* New York: Behavioral Publications, 1972.

Jasnau, K. F. Individualized versus mass transfer of nonpsychotic geriatric patients from mental hospitals to nursing homes, with special reference to the death rate. *Journal of the American Geriatric Society,* 1967, 15:280–284.

Jenkins, C. D.; Zyzanski, S. J.; Rosenman, R. H.; and Cleveland, G. L. Association of coronary-prone behavior scores with recurrence of coronary heart disease. *Journal of Chronic Diseases,* 1971, 24:601–611.

Josephy, H. Analysis of mortality and causes of death in a mental hospital. *American Journal of Psychiatry,* 1949, 106:185–189.

Kasl, S. J. Physical and mental health effects of involuntary relocation and institutionalization on the elderly: A review. *American Journal of Public Health,* 1972, 62:377–384.

Killian, E. C. Effects of geriatric transfer on mortality rates. *Social Work,* 1970, 15:19–26.

Klein, D. C. and Lindemann, E. Preventive intervention in individual and family crisis situations. In G. Caplan (ed.), *Prevention of mental disorders in children: Initial exploration.* New York: Basic Books, 1961.

Kral, V.; Grad, B.; and Berenson, J. Stress reactions resulting from the relocation of an aged population. *Canadian Psychiatric Association Journal,* 1968, 11:201–209.

Lawton, M. P. and Yaffe, S. Mortality, morbidity, and voluntary change of residence by older people. *Journal of the American Geriatric Society,* 1970, 18:823–831.

Libow, L. S. Interaction of medical, biologic, and behavioral factors of aging, adaptation, and survival: An 11 year longitudinal study. *Geriatrics,* 1974, 29(11):75–82; 85–88.

Lieberman, M. A. The relationship of mortality rates to entrance to a home for the aged. *Geriatrics,* 1961, 16:515–519.

Lieberman, M. A. Institutionalization of the aged: Effects on behavior. *Journal of Gerontology,* 1969, 24:330–340.

Lieberman, M. A. Some issues in studying psychological predictors of survival. In E. Palmore and F. C. Jeffers (eds), *Prediction of Life Span.* Lexington, Mass.: Heath, 1971.

Markson, E. W. and Cumming, J. H. A strategy of necessary mass transfer and its impact on patient mortality. *Journal of Gerontology,* 1974, 29:315–321.

Markus, E.; Blenkner, M.; Bloom, M.; and Downs, T. Relocation stress and the aged. *Interdisciplinary Topics in Gerontology,* 1970, 7:60–71.

Markus, E.; Blenkner, M.; Bloom, M.; and Downs, T. The impact of relocation upon mortality rates of institutionalized aged persons. *Journal of Gerontology,* 1971, 26:537–541.

Markus, E.; Blenkner, M.; Bloom, M.; and Downs, T. Some factors and their association with postrelocation mortality among institutionalized aged persons. *Journal of Gerontology,* 1972, 27:376–382.

McMahan, C. A. and Ford, T. R. Surviving the first five years of retirement. *Journal of Gerontology,* 1955, 10:212–215.

McMahon, A. W. and Rhudick, P. J. Reminiscing, adaptational significance in the aged. *Archives of General Psychiatry,* 1964, 10:292–298.

Miller, D. and Lieberman, M. A. The relationship of affect states and adaptive capacity to reactions to stress. *Journal of Gerontology,* 1965, 20:492–497.

Myers, R. J. Factors in interpreting mortality after retirement. *Journal of the American Statistical Association,* 1954, 49:499–509.

Novick, L. J. Easing the stress of moving day. *Hospitals,* 1967, 41:64–74.

Nowlin, J. B. Depression and health. In E. Palmore (ed.), *Normal Aging II.* Durham, N. C.: Duke University Press, 1974.

Palmore, E. Predicting longevity: A follow-up controlling for age. *Gerontologist,* 1969, 9:247–250.

Palmore, E. The promise and problems of longevity studies. In E. Palmore and F. C. Jeffers (eds), *Prediction of Life Span*. Lexington, Mass.: Heath, 1971. (a)

Palmore, E. The relative importance of social factors in predicting longevity. In E. Palmore and F. C. Jeffers (eds), *Prediction of Life Span*. Lexington, Mass.: Heath, 1971. (b)

Palmore, E. and Stone, J. Predictors of longevity: A follow-up of the aged in Chapel Hill. *Gerontologist,* 1973, 13:88–90.

Parkes, C. M.; Benjamin, B.; and Fitzgerald, R. G. Broken heart: A statistical study of increased mortality among widowers. *British Medical Journal,* 1969, 1:740–743.

Pfeiffer, E. Survival in old age: Physical, psychological and social correlates of longevity. *Journal of the American Geriatric Society,* 1970, 18:273–285.

Powers, E. A. and Bultena, G. L. Characteristics of deceased dropouts in longitudinal research. *Journal of Gerontology,* 1972, 27:530–535.

Rees, W. D., and Lutkins, S. G. Mortality of bereavement. *British Medical Journal,* 1967, 4:13–16.

Richter, C. P. On the phenomenon of sudden death in animals and man. *Psychosomatic Medicine,* 1957, 19:191–198.

Riley, M. W., and Foner, A. *Aging and Society* (Vol. 1). New York: Russell Sage Foundation, 1968.

Rose, C. L. Social factors in longevity. *Gerontologist,* 1964, 4:27–37.

Seligman, M. E. P. *Helplessness*. San Francisco: Freeman, 1975.

Selye, H. *The Stress of Life*. New York: McGraw-Hill, 1956.

Shurtleff, D. Mortality and marital status. *Public Health Reports,* 1955, 70:248–252.

Streib, G. F., and Schneider, C. J. *Retirement in American Society*. Ithaca, N.Y.: Cornell University Press, 1971.

Tronchin-James, N. *Arbitrary Retirement*. London: Cassell, 1962.

Turner, B. F.; Tobin, S. S.; and Lieberman, M. A. Personality traits as predictors of institutional adaptation among the aged. *Journal of Gerontology,* 1972, 27:61–68.

Tyhurst, J. S.; Salk, L.; and Kennedy, M. Mortality, morbidity and retirement. *American Journal of Public Health,* 1957, 47:1434–1444.

Weisman, A. D. *On Dying and Denying: A Psychiatric Study of Terminality*. New York: Behavioral Publications, 1972.

Whittier, J. R. and Williams, D. The coincidence and constancy of mortality figures for aged psychotic patients admitted to state hospitals. *Journal of Nervous and Mental Disease,* 1956, 124:618–620.

Wittels, I. and Botwinick, J. Survival in relocation. *Journal of Gerontology,* 1974, 29:440–443.

Youmans, E. G. and Yarrow, M. Aging and social adaptation: A longitudinal study of healthy old men. In S. Granick and R. D. Patterson (eds), *Human aging II* (Department of Health, Education, and Welfare Publ. No. 71-9037). Washington, D.C.: U.S. Government Printing Office, 1971.

Young, M.; Benjamin, B.; and Wallis, C. The mortality of widowers. *Lancet,* 1963, 2:454–456.

Zweig, J. P. and Csank, J. Z. Effects of relocation on chronically ill geriatric patients of a medical unit: Mortality rates. *Journal of the American Geriatric Society,* 1975, 23(3):132–136.

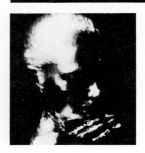

28

Practice

A man has three weeks to live. Do you make him comfortable or do you work like hell? You may think that treatment of dying persons is the same throughout the world. McGrady describes very significant differences across cultures in this chapter. The controversial issues he addresses may leave you with more questions than answers. Any of the following Appendix exercises would be helpful adjuncts to this chapter.

        A.   Announcing One's Own Death

        B.   Appropriate Death Fantasy

        I.   Life and Death Attitudes: Dyadic Encounter

        L.   Privacy Circles

The American Cancer Society Means Well, but the Janker Clinic Means Better

Patrick M. McGrady Jr.

Concerning Bonn, Germany, travel writer Temple Fielding says he'll take downtown Detroit anytime. You visit Bonn, like Detroit, only on business. Unless you happen to be a Beethoven nut. Or unless you happen to have cancer.

In this corrosively frumpy city (population 300,000) is one of the world's least known and most interesting cancer hospitals, the Janker (pronounced Yahnker) Radiation Clinic. It consistently gets better results with its inoperable patients than university hospitals do with many of their operables. And the day my doctor does a double take over the X rays of my lumpy whatever and tenderly inquires if my life insurance and will are in order, I shall arrange for the Red Baron to whisk me off to dreary old Bonn and its dreary old (established 1936) Janker Clinic for treatment.

I had known about the Janker Clinic for five years. I had read its technical publications, interviewed its doctors at medical gatherings and been briefed on its functioning by American cancer specialists who had been there. Finally, I saw for myself. Last year I visited the hospital. For nearly a week, I grafted myself onto my host, Janker medical director Wolfgang Scheef, M.D. I stayed at his home, accompanied him on rounds, shared meals with him, toured the entire hospital, and kept my tape recorder on for hours at a time.

That sojourn gave me an uncomfortable high. Despite walls that needed paint, halls too dimly lit, creaking wood floors and prewar johns, the place thrilled me. The super competence of the Janker staff overwhelmed me. I worried that my report on it would be uncautiously flattering. For a quarter of a century my father wrote press releases on research, especially that sponsored by the American Cancer Society, and he be-

This material was first published in *Esquire,* pp. 111–113, 134, 136, 138, 141, April 1976. Copyright 1976 Esquire, Inc. Reprinted by permission.

queathed to me his dread of being rapidly enthusiastic over *anything* related to cancer. One visit to Bonn clearly was not enough.

I persuaded a steely-eyed, nullifidian American cancer-specialist friend to join me on a second visit to the Janker. If anyone could scare out the bugs from under the chips, he could. I secretly wanted to be proved wrong.

Here was a private hospital (one hundred ten beds) with no government or foundation subsidy that seemed to have developed better cancer treatments than the best of those available anywhere else in the world. A patient at, say, Sloan-Kettering Memorial Hospital in New York (which is funded by practically *everybody*) does not have the benefit of either the professional dedication or several of the techniques available at the Janker. Nor does *any* American patient enjoy the flat sixty-dollar-per-day rate (which covers doctors, nurses, the room, radiation, drugs and good food).

Here was a collection of patients, each of whom had been forwarded by other doctors and institutions with a "hopeless" or "terminal" label on the chart, and all of whom seemed irrepressibly cheerful.

Here were two men, Scheef and his boss, hospital director Dr. Hans Hoefer-Janker (who customarily omits the second half of his surname), who were largely responsible for developing four of the most potent anticancer agents known to the medical world. These include the nitrogen-mustard compound cyclophosphamide (or Cytoxan), the only one of the four that is currently available in the United States; isophosphamide, a nitrogen-mustard compound that is far more powerful than cyclophosphamide and which can be used on a greater range of malignant tumors; A-Mulsin, a highly concentrated vitamin-A emulsion, which is administered in colossal (up to three million units daily) dosages safely; and Wobe-Mugos enzymes, a carefully balanced complex of enzymes that decomposes proteins and fats and is used to prolong remissions obtained with other drugs.

This German hospital seemed just too good to be true. If only my doctor friend would dampen my fervor, he would reaffirm what I wanted to believe and what most American science writers accepted as an article of faith: that the best cancer care is available only in the United States of America. If it isn't available here, then what are the National Cancer Institute and the American Cancer Society spending almost a billion dollars a year on?

Regrettably, my friend was absolutely perfervid in his enthusiasm for the Janker's staff and techniques. In the few days he spent working alongside Drs. Hoefer and Scheef, he experienced a clinical freedom he said he had never known in the United States. I say "regrettably" because his comparisons terrified him. If he were to praise publicly what amounted to a refutation of the bureaucratic system he worked under, it could cost him dearly. He asked that I not mention his name, and I agreed.

He came, in fact, to be in full agreement with the Janker Clinic's flouting of some of the most sacred tenets of the American cancer establishment, to wit:

1. That all radiation or drug treatment must cease if the patient's white blood cell count dips below 1500. The normal count varies between 4800 and 10,800 per cubic millimeter of blood. Scheef will push therapies even with zero counts! He claims that if infections are avoided the count will rebound automatically.

2. That all cancers should be managed either by surgery, radiation, or drugs. Or, if more than one technique is used, they should be used separately. The Janker often uses light radiation to increase the performance of one or more drugs. It also routinely uses immune system stimulants to help the patient's own body to fight the cancer.

3. That postoperative drug therapy interferes with wound-healing and thus should be delayed. The Janker finds this shibboleth unsupported by the evidence and wastes no time in administering drugs after surgery.

For most doctors in the United States, 1984 arrived a long time ago. My oncologist friend[1] has worked under the benevolent gaze of Big Brother for his entire career. He may not touch any drug or technique that has not filtered down through the paper-pushing process at the National Cancer Institute and the Food and Drug Administration. If one of his patients on an experimental therapy takes a turn for the worse, he may not vary the protocol a jot without risking the wrath of his section chief and cessation of government funding. If he tries to import a drug that has proved itself abroad but is not manufactured here, it can be confiscated without notice.

The Janker Clinic is *not* a laetrile mill.

The American Knee-Jerk Objection

The Janker Clinic is *not* a laetrile mill. This needs saying because American doctors doggedly confuse the Janker with the Nieper Silbersee Hospital in Hanover—where laetrile *is* given to cancer patients.

Far and away the most modish of what the American Cancer Society calls unproved methods, laetrile (also called amygdalin or vitamin B-17) is obtained from de-fatted apricot kernels (and, less efficiently, from twelve hundred other plants) by extraction and recrystallization. Amygdalin, some of its proponents maintain, releases cyanide that destroys cancer cells and does not harm normal cells.

Dr. Scheef of the Janker Clinic once tried laetrile orally on twenty patients—with no observable success. Since the presumably more potent injectable laetrile is unavailable in Germany, Scheef is not sure he gave the drug a fair chance. He keeps an open mind on the matter.

You can entertain yourself by asking your family doctor how much he knows about the Janker Clinic.

Chances are no better than one in five that he will confess his ignorance.

Chances are four in five that he will reply in one of three ways: warn you that this is where you're given peach pits for your tumor, or scold you for believing everything you read about old Whatshisname, "that guy who gives goat glands, sheep cells, Novocain, horse piss *and* peach pits for cancer," or tell you brutally that the hospital isn't even in Germany, but somewhere in Mexico or Spain.

1. An oncologist, literally, is a tumor specialist. The term has come to mean a cancer specialist—although most doctors feel that it isn't really a specialty. Too many doctors, here and abroad, feel qualified to treat cancer patients merely by following the directions on the drug company's brochures.

**. . . the Janker
successes are
almost entirely
achieved upon
patients who have
been through one
therapeutic mill
or another and
been jilted by
other doctors.**

What impressed my friend most was the freedom the Janker staff enjoyed. Hoefer and Scheef control their one hundred forty employees with an enlightened paternalism. Decisions are reached by a rapid consensus. Protocols are revised the moment they are perceived to be ineffectual—without any need to kowtow to government kibitzers, medical societies, do-good propaganda and fund-raising agencies, boards of directors or groups of "peer" onlookers.

The Janker Clinic's preemptive focus is the patient. Nothing is permitted to interfere with the primary goal of prolonging the patient's productive life-span. The patients' cheerfulness probably can be explained by their knowledge that this is the one place in the whole world where they will be given the best available combinations of drugs, hormones, biologicals and radiation in the quest to dethrone King Cancer.

The Janker may well be the only cancer hospital where the owner arrives on the scene at five a.m. sharp so that he can get the paper work out of the way early and spend the remainder of his working day (till nine or ten p.m.) with his patients, each of whom he sees twice a week. Scheef sees each patient four times a week.

Scheef's data show that he induces a full or partial remission[2] in seventy percent of the Janker's patients, of whom some 76,000 have been treated since 1936. The clinic gets exquisite results with many tumors that resist any type of treatment elsewhere. These results are more stunning even than the statistics would seem to show because, whereas most compilations of remissions refer to newly diagnosed, primary treatments, the Janker successes are almost entirely achieved upon patients who have been through one therapeutic mill or another and been jilted by other doctors. This fact makes their win-loss ratio almost flabbergasting.

Take pancreatic carcinomas. The mean survival time of patients after diagnosis elsewhere is three months and eighteen days. The Janker treats the most irredeemable of these, most of whom have bloated liver metastases. Of twelve such patients treated so far, the mean survival time has been eight months. One woman patient has had a two-year remission.

At best, some testicular cancers are tantamount to a three-month death notice. All of the Janker's patients with testicular cancers were practically D.O.A., with their tumors spread throughout their lungs. Using two drugs prohibited by the Food and Drug Administration (A-Muslin and the Wobe enzymes) and isophosphamide (available only to five investigators here), Scheef was able to save thirteen of his first forty-three patients—all thirteen, at this writing, alive, working and apparently healthy.

Of twenty patients suffering from a variety of head, neck, and tongue cancers treated exclusively with A-Mulsin, there have been no failures and many complete remissions.

Results consistently better than average are achieved in other cancers, including all cornifying squamous cell carcinomas (mostly cancers of the skin and mucosal tissues), cancer of the penis, pancreatic cancers, all lung cancers, stomach cancers, most sarcomas (which afflict bones, muscles and

2. A full remission is usually defined as the complete disappearance of measurable symptoms for at least a month. A partial remission is the reduction of a tumor by at least half of its diameter for the same period.

connective tissue, mainly in children), and cylindromas (rare honeycomb-like carcinomas).

However, the Janker gets results no better than average with childhood leukemia and Hodgkin's disease (cancerous enlargement of the lymph nodes, spleen and, sometimes, the liver and kidneys)—two forms in which some American centers have made notable progress.

The Janker started its prewar existence as a radiation clinic, pioneering in the development of sophisticated X-ray modalities, including the first use of television X-ray diagnostic work-ups, in 1949. It claims to have the world's largest collection of radiological films, which are distributed to hospitals worldwide. Its X-ray cameras can take up to eight large (35 cm × 40 cm) pictures per second. It has the case histories of 60,000 patients, as well as a mammoth collection of slides classified by patient category, neoplasm, stage, response, and so forth. If some charitable soul ever bequeaths them $250,000, they'll computerize their data.

Nearly a decade ago, the Janker broadened its attack on cancer by hiring Wolfgang Scheef, a chemotherapist then barely thirty years old. Scheef had successfully pushed the highly toxic cyclophosphamide dose levels three times higher than the regulation thirty milligrams per kilogram of patient body weight at his previous hospital.

Almost all cytostatic agents depress the body's immune system, including the white blood cell count. Few or no American physicians knowingly allow the patient's w.b.c. to go lower than 1500. If the count goes lower than 2000, the theory goes, the body will be: (1) unable to fight even slight infections and (2) unable to regenerate white blood cells to a normal level.

Scheef theorized that if care were taken to keep the patient infection-free, the w.b.c. could go down to zero and still come back up. The drug kills only the young cells, leaving mother cells alive to proliferate.

While working at a general hospital in a Bonn suburb thirteen years ago, Scheef asked his chief's permission to increase the cyclophosphamide dose on a cancer patient from 30 to 40 mg/kg of body weight.

"Don't worry," said Scheef, "I'm sure the white blood cells will regenerate."

They did. The stronger dose improved remissions. But when Scheef asked to bump the dose to 50, he was vetoed. This would put the w.b.c. to under 1000. Every manual said that death was a virtual certainty at that level.

One of his patients, a close friend, urged Scheef to give him the higher dose. Scheef agreed, provided the patient tell no one. He then confided his plan to an intern assistant. When the room was finally emptied of hospital personnel, Scheef injected a whopping four grams of the cyclophosphamide and asked the intern to keep a close eye on the situation.

Later the intern asked the patient if he'd been injected. Loyally, the patient said no. The intern, hearing this, injected another four grams.

The w.b.c. plummeted to zero. By the book, he was as good as dead.

> **Scheef theorized that if care were taken to keep the patient infection-free, the w.b.c. could go down to zero and still come back up.**

Proud of his ruse, the intern whispered to Scheef that he'd given the injection without being noticed.

"*What* injection?" asked Scheef.

"The cyclophosphamide."

Frantic, both men devoured the literature on the drug—at that time some four hundred papers—to save the patient's life. The animal work made clear that corticosteroids, usually administered to patients on cyclophosphamide, should *not* be given. They kept their eyes peeled for signs of monilia, a fungus infection, which could have wiped out the patient in days. For three weeks Scheef got practically no sleep, but within the three weeks, as predicted, the patient's white blood cell count rose to normal. Moreover, there wasn't a cancer cell to be found in his body.

Still nervous—but eager—Scheef tried the accidentally found 100 mg/kg regimen on four female patients, two with breast cancers and two with ovarian carcinomas. All got full remissions.

The hospital director was confounded by Scheef's mysterious behavior.

"Why," he asked the young physician, "are you letting the w.b.c. go so low? And why are you doing the counts yourself, and spending your nights in the lab? And why is it that our cancer patients are doing so well?"

Scheef explained the conspiracy—and got his boss's permission to use the higher dosages routinely. Since they did not use corticosteroids, as most other institutions did, they were not plagued with the usual bleeding complications.

In fact, Scheef freely admits that there was an element of luck in his calculated risk. Very quickly, on later patients, he encountered unexpected side effects from the higher dosages. But as they appeared, he found ways of treating them.

His most important find was that bone-marrow poisoning by the drug was reversible as long as corticosteroids were not given. (These hormones— still widely used in general practice—insidiously deactivate the white blood cells. By seducing them away from cancer sites and into the bloodstream— where they show up in blood counts—by reducing inflammation and making the patient feel better, corticosteroids counterfeit evidence of a remission. In fact, however, the white blood cells are careening about like cops on a drunken holiday—disarmed and useless.) Infections were avoided by having the patient keep his mouth clean with antiseptic gargles and warning nurses to give antibiotics the moment any sign of infection appeared.

Bleeding in the bladder, caused by acid urine, was avoided by giving baking soda. Cysteine, an amino acid, gave added protection to the entire genito-urinary system.

Much of any patient's anguish over chemotherapy stems from the temporary baldness that often accompanies use of drugs like cyclophosphamide and isophosphamide. Scheef believed that he might be able to reduce hair loss by getting cysteine into the scalp by electrophoresis.

One day he made an aqueous solution of cysteine with the solvent dimethyl sulfoxide (DMSO) and a dye, indigo carmine. The dye, when it showed up in his urine, would tell him how fast the cysteine had penetrated the system. Urine would show him if the drug was working.

After soaking his scalp in the solution, he attached silver plates to the nape of his neck and forehead and hooked them up to his car battery, which, his slide rule told him, provided the precise voltage required. The second he turned on the current he passed out. Two hours later, when he awoke, he realized that he had misplaced the decimal point on his slide rule and given himself ten times the power necessary for the experiment!

To determine whether the cysteine had been absorbed by his system, he went around the garage to a corner of his garden and sprinkled the posies.

Marveling at the sight of his father pissing deep purple, his four-year-old son exclaimed: "Please, Papa, teach me how to do that. With that trick I can get elected president of the kindergarten!"

When I first visited the Janker Clinic in March of last year, Scheef gave me the guest bedroom in his home in Brühl, a suburb lying halfway between Bonn and Cologne. We spent the whole day of my arrival, Sunday, talking cancer and drinking Schinkenhäger and Beck. His capacity was awesome and his coherence, even by three a.m., never diminished.

But the next morning, his left foot had swollen monstrously. Next to the bitchy blights of Venus, no ailment so mortifies the victim as flaming gout—particularly when he is a hospital medical doctor. As he hobbled past terry-clothed patients and starch-smocked nurses and doctors, he uttered brief explanations, sometimes with the old doggerel: *"Des kleinen Mannes Sonnenschein ist Fressen und Besoffensein!"* (Roughly: "The little man finds his sunshine in eating and drinking like swine.")

Scheef is a chunky, balding man with a black-bramble beard and soft hazel eyes; he is given to ebullient laughter and ebullient scowls. He picks occasionally from a tin of menthol snuff that serves as surrogate for the cigarettes he gave up in 1974. After the Sunday bout he never drank during his work-week. Instead, he took Antabuse, whose threat of violent nausea powered his will from Monday through Friday.

"I must constantly ask myself," Scheef told me, " 'Am I really giving this patient what I would take myself—or give to my father or to my daughter?' It's not always easy to answer.

"Treating a cancer patient is like preparing food. Each patient requires seasoning to taste. You must rationalize each ingredient from your data. But no two patients are alike. Each is special.

"The *only* way I can learn about cancer is by spending a lot of time with my patients. I talk to them about themselves, their families, anything and everything. Often, in the middle of conversation, an idea will come to me. Out of the blue I hit the proper therapy. But I can't learn unless I see patients every day. What I call 'mathematical doctors' don't do this."

"I must constantly ask myself," Scheef told me, " 'Am I really giving this patient what I would take myself—or give to my father or to my daughter?' It's not always easy to answer. . . ."

"That son of a bitch, Dr. So-and-so. He dropped a patient he had no business dropping. He was concerned about his success statistic. That's all he thinks about."

Our chat is interrupted by a phone call from a physician who asks if his sister can be treated at the Janker. Her doctor, a high official of the German cancer society, had sent her home with palliatives—to die.

"Yes," says Scheef, "we can treat her here. We've had considerable success with ovarian cancer—even with metastases to the liver. Get her here quickly, though."

After hanging up, he fumes: "That son of a bitch, Dr. So-and-so. He dropped a patient he had no business dropping. He was concerned about his success statistic. That's all he thinks about."

When I returned for my second visit to the Janker, in the company of my specialist friend, the news from Scheef was the he had become teetotal. He missed the beer and schnapps, he said. Hugely. They always brought him his best ideas.

"I only need moments to know that something is true. Maybe five seconds. I might need weeks to understand why it's true. But when I'm sure, I'm completely sure. And I *have* to be drinking to come up with the idea."

A case in point was his first approach to the cyclophosphamide problem. The doses were too small. How to raise them, safely?

One night he brought home a pile of books and periodicals. He poured himself a drink, several drinks. Then he noticed a technical paper from the Ministry of Defense archives on skin conditions afflicting workers engaged in deactivating mustard gases stockpiled during World War II. His eyes widened when cysteine was mentioned as a prophylactic. Further on into his nocturnal swill, he read another technical paper on the skin irritations caused by cyclophosphamide, a nitrogen-mustard compound. Eureka!

"I said to myself: 'Okay, Mensch, now I know that we can deactivate *all of these mustards* with cysteine.' We began a big investigation. And today cysteine is the major protection we have against all the alkylating cytostatic agents. Without it, we couldn't use them as we do so routinely everywhere. And I got this idea while drinking."

The Janker's most formidable weapon is isophosphamide, a sister nitrogen mustard with more indications than any other cytostatic drug—thanks to Scheef's own ingenuity.

First introduced in 1967 at an International Congress for Chemotherapy, isophosphamide began most impressively on the basis of eye-popping results on animals. But clinicians quickly found that the drug was death on patients' kidneys. It annihilated the small distal tubules, causing hemorrhagic cystitis. Patients on more than 50 mg/kg of body weight became gravely ill. Many died.

In 1969, at a Congress for Internal Medicine at Wiesbaden, the Asta Company convened representatives from the twelve European clinics researching isophosphamide to eliminate the drug. (Anticancer drugs are a notoriously unprofitable item.) One by one, they all voted to stop their research—except Scheef and Hoefer.

"It's too good *not* to use," Scheef told Asta official Professor Norbert Brock. "Moreover, we have solved the kidney and bladder problems. Let me prove it to you."

Asta replied that it was too late. The company had stopped production. Moreover, in the whole world there were only seven pounds left.

"Okay," urged Scheef. "Give us those seven pounds and let us do a clinical study. If this were merely an insecticide, you'd have solved them already. But because it's a cancer drug, *nobody's* bothered to. This drug knocks out tumors that fail to respond to any other drug."

Brock gave in—but there was one problem. All the drug companies, including Asta, refused to give Scheef animals to work with. The drug was dangerous. The animals were, ah, too expensive. And since all the university clinics had given up on isophosphamide, how could the Janker hope to succeed anyway?

Scheef was forced to work with his patients as his guinea pigs. He chose only volunteers whose cancers could not be remitted by any other therapy and who had a maximum three-week life expectancy.

In the fall of 1975, Hoefer and Scheef published a landmark four-year study on isophosphamide, showing it to be the most useful anticancer drug known to man. Not only did it have a wider application than its sister cyclophosphamide, but it could be used on previously treated patients who were resistant to any further therapy. If scrupulously monitored, it was also less toxic than cyclophosphamide.

What made the results even more significant was the fact that most of their patients were terminals for whom the potential of surgery, radiation, and cytostatics had been exhausted. The majority had cancers that had spread so gruesomely that the grave seemed at most a few days or weeks away. Indeed, sixteen of the first patients kept their rendezvous with death within the predicted three-week period.

The isophosphamide power-boosting process involved several steps:

• By merely keeping the urine alkaline with baking soda, they boosted the maximum tolerated dose from 50 to 70 mg/kg body weight.

• Giving the patient up to six quarts of liquid a day brought it up to 120.

• By protecting the bladder with cysteine and spreading the injections over five or ten days, it went up to 300. At around 400, however, the isophosphamide began to kill the bone marrow and there the dose-raising had to stop.

They devised still more tricks to increase its cancer-killing ability. They avoided the infections that could have been lethal during the low white blood cell stage by instructing the patient on the importance of oral hygiene and the high liquid intake. They used vincristine to synchronize the cancer cells' mitotic division so that the drug would strike them all at the most vulnerable point (the so-called G2 phase) in cell replication. They gave a little radiation, wherever possible, to increase cell absorption of the water-soluble drug.

Of their 360 patients, 101 had a full remission, 150 a partial remission, and only 79 were complete failures. Thirty cases were not evaluated.

Extraordinarily good results were seen in ovarian carcinomas, breast cancers and small-cell bronchial (lung) carcinomas. Equally striking were remissions in the nigh untreatable pancreatic carcinomas, various testicular tumors, osteosarcomas (bone), chondrosarcomas (cartilage), myosarcomas (muscle), and gastrointestinal adenocarcinomas.

The investigators warned, however, that owing to the danger of complications the drug should only be given at special cancer hospitals equipped to administer the complicated treatment of its side effects.

Five years ago, the Janker system of using isophosphamide was disclosed at a chemotherapy congress in Prague. Just before Scheef delivered his paper, the N.C.I.'s Stephen Carter, deputy director of cancer treatment, walked out of the room, muttering to a colleague that he had no interest in the drug since it was "just another cyclophosphamide" and that he was perilously swamped with new drugs anyway. Although Milan Slavik, chief of the N.C.I.'s investigational drug branch, has reported those results to American investigators, they have been met with disbelief. Admittedly, use of the drug is so delicate an undertaking that the Asta firm will supply it to German clinicians only if they have worked with it at the Janker Clinic. Yet it seems nothing short of scandalous that neither the American Cancer Society nor the National Cancer Institute has been able to spare a couple thousand dollars to send one American investigator to Bonn to learn how isophosphamide (and the other Janker therapies) could save the lives of thousands of American cancer patients.

Ever since 1966, when I began researching a book on medical work relating to the prolongation of youth, I have known the two men responsible for creating the Janker's special vitamin-A and enzyme preparations. Max Wolf, M.D. concocted the original formula of proteolytic (protein-decomposing) and lipolytic (fat-dissolving) enzymes he registered under the label Wobe (an acronym for Wolf and his assistant, Mrs. Helene Benitez). Karl Ransberger, president of the Munich pharmaceutical firm Mucos, strengthened the formula until it became a powerful agent in the treatment of various inflammations, including cancer. Later, he turned his attention to developing for veterinary use an old German World War II vitamin-A emulsion formula. The enzymes and vitamin formulas have since made him one of Germany's leading cancer-drug manufacturers.

To date more than two thousand patients have used the high-concentrate A-Mulsin for their cancers at the Janker. The little green and white aerosol cans (for oral administration) adorn approximately one-third of the patients' night tables.

At the suggestion of a veterinarian, Scheef experimented with the Mucos A-Muslin to increase cancer cells' vulnerability to cyclophosphamide. Prior to these tests, he had already tried every other available form of the vitamin with varying degrees of unsuccess. But with the new emulsion, cancers formerly resistant to chemotherapy began to respond. Lung metastases vanished. Scheef wondered it the vitamin A alone might be responsible.

When an order from the hospital for two hundred twenty pounds of the vitamin crossed Ransberger's desk, he called Scheef to ask why an oncologist wanted a veterinary product. Scheef said he wanted to use it clinically on cancers—but wished that it were more potent. Extrapolating from animal data, he said, a cancer patient should be receiving up to thirty million units.

Ransberger prodded his chemists to come up with a more concentrated product. After several weeks, he delivered to Scheef several bottles labeled A-MULSIN, HOCHKONZENTRAT.

Once again, as he had done with the cysteine to prevent balding, Scheef tried the preparation on himself first. It almost killed him. In five days he swallowed thirty million units of the emulsion. His hair fell out; his skin peeled; his lips and mouth fissured into a miniature Grand Canyon. But he survived—and learned that dosages should start low and increase gradually.[3]

One day, Scheef found himself confronted with an octogenarian patient with cancer of the penis. The conventional treatment—excision—was a loathsome notion for the old man.

"Anything but surgery," he told Scheef. "It's been my best friend for as long as I can remember. I'm not going to let it go now. I shall die with it as I've lived with it."

Scheef began a topical treatment with vitamin-A acid and systemic treatment with the A-Mulsin orally, bracing them with small amounts of radiation. The tumor disappeared totally.

Three years later, the patient died—his treasure still secure and intact—of cancers elsewhere in the body.

When he was still unsure about A-Mulsin for lung cancer, Scheef put fifty bronchogenic-carcinoma patients from one floor on a vitamin-and-radiation combination. He also put eight-two comparable patients from another floor on radiation alone. In September, 1972, after a year of the trial, the results conclusively favored the new therapy: in the experimental section, eighteen out of the fifty patients were still alive, while only seven of the eighty-two on conventional radiation had survived. Thirty-six percent versus 8.5 percent. Moreover, the mean survival time of patients in the experimental section who did not live out the year was sixty-seven percent better than the controls.

The Wobe enzymes are as beguiling as the vitamin-A preparations. Scheef is convinced of their value as adjuvant therapy in pancreatic cancers, adenocarcinomas, and malignant melanomas, even though they have not been submitted for solid, controlled testing. He also puts many post-intensive-care patients on enzymes in the belief that they may prolong remissions. They have earned themselves a niche as treatment of choice at the Janker in many inflammations, hematomas, thrombophlebitis, even

3. Caution: Vitamin-A preparations available in the U.S. cannot be taken in these high dosages without grave risks. Even A-Mulsin therapy requires monitoring by a physician.

cold sores and herpes zoster, of which Scheef says: "We don't know of anything that works as well as enzymes for herpes zoster. We've treated at least twenty-five or thirty patients with them. If you catch it in the first three or four days, the patient will be cured without further pain, lesions, and so forth. The best modality is an intramuscular injection of two hundred milligrams."

In Scheef's home, the enzymes are standard medicine-chest fare. "If I get a runny nose, bronchitis, pneumonia, or a sore finger, I first take a handful of enzymes. Often I need nothing else."

The enzymes, when injected, occasionally devastate certain solid tumors that have not spread. Six years ago, Scheef injected several ampuls of liquid enzymes into a fifty-five-year-old woman's adenocarcinoma of the uterine corpus. The cantaloupe-size tumor promptly liquified, oozing forth three pints of a dark muck, populated by dead cancer cells. As of two years later, when she last checked in, the woman was totally cancer free.

Most beguiling of all is the question of whether the enzymes alone can destroy benign and/or cancerous lumps in a woman's breast.

Several uncontrolled tests on women who rejected biopsies and surgery seem encouraging, if inconclusive. With twenty such women, whose mammographies were extremely ominous, Scheef administered thirty Wobe pills daily to each over a period of three or four months. In well over half of the group, the lumps vanished permanently. Those women whose lumps remained were treated conventionally.

The successes achieved at the Janker are, as I have said, the more noteworthy for the fact that it is, almost always, a hospital of last resort. It is far more difficult to heal cancerous lesions that have metastasized after the second or third go-round with conventional therapies. A case in point is that of a Spanish actress who, midway through her third pregnancy, observed hard, menacing lumps nudging through the soft contours of her right breast. In a short time, she was unable to lift the breast from her rib cage. She panicked.

A Madrid surgeon took a biopsy of the breast. It was positive. If he operated, an abortion would have been necessary. On those grounds alone, she refused surgery. But the cancer had spread so far that the surgeon would have achieved little but a grand and useless mutilation.

She then booked in at a London hospital and was given a drug combination that did not work. Within days, she was told that her case was hopeless.

Then she flew to New York and was checked out at Sloan-Kettering Memorial Hospital. After examining the scans, the X rays and the by now grotesque right breast, the doctors there refused to proceed with treatment.

Before leaving New York, friends urged her to consult Max Wolf. Wolf, they said, had a knack for bizarre treatments which, often amazingly, got the job done. This seems to be the case. One of Wolf's patients was W. Somerset Maugham, who had suffered from an intractable malaria for fourteen years. The condition had been treated unsuccessfully by twenty-two doctors. Maugham told Wolf that if the torment was not exorcised, he would commit suicide. Wolf brazenly replied that he would give him the largest dose of quinine ever injected into a patient. "It's the only thing I can think of," Wolf told the writer. "It will either kill you or cure you." It cured him.

Wolf sent the Spanish actress straightaway to the Janker Clinic.

Treating a celebrity is one thing. Treating a celebrity with a rampaging, widespread cancer, who had been abandoned by the best specialists of three countries, was another. Scheef did not welcome the challenge.

They waited till she had given birth to her baby, a girl. Then Scheef began an aggressive therapy of low-dose radiation to synergize the various drugs they would use: cyclophosphamide, trophosphamide, isophosphamide, A-Mulsin and the enzymes. It would be impossible, of course, to know which parts of the therapy were the most effective. But that, of course, was of secondary importance to getting her better.

Within six weeks, the actress was well enough to leave the hospital. She continued on the enzymes, which Scheef advised her to stay on the rest of her life. In months, the breast returned to normal. Every palpable abnormality had disappeared.

Three years later, she revisited her Madrid surgeon. He could not believe that anything had "cured" her cancer—and told her so. (Most surgeons seem to believe that cancer can only be cured by cutting it out with cold steel.) He informed her that biopsies would be unnecessary, since the presence of the cancer had been established unquestionably three years ago.

"At least your breast is now operable," he said. "I can remove it without difficulty."

Which he did. Interestingly, the pathologists were unable to find a single cancer cell in the mastectomied breast, although its tissues had seriously degenerated because of the radiation and chemotherapy assaults.

The efficiency and absence of political backbiting at the Janker is due to the unique climate created by its owner, Hans Hoefer-Janker M.D. Twice married, with five children, Hoefer, fifty-four, works eighty hours a week and is the very antithesis of the classical German hospital director who often vanishes for weeks without explanation, spends inordinate time with his private patients, never inconveniences his career, and generally plays the role of tyrant.

"In most hospitals," explains Hoefer, "the cleaning women are the soldiers; the nurses the corporals and sergeants; the doctors the commanding officers. In our clinic we have no ranks. Too much democracy is better than too little—but you can only have it with good and intelligent people. In certain situations, you have to rule like a despot. Such as with young doctors, fresh from the university, who tell you that you're all wrong because Professor So-and-so from some university has written the contrary in his book on the subject. But they learn."

"In most hospitals," explains Hoefer, "the cleaning women are the soldiers; the nurses the corporals and sergeants; the doctors the commanding officers. In our clinic we have no ranks. . . ."

Dr. Hans Hoefer-Janker will probably die of leukemia. His death will be a long-term, self-contrived suicide. He will die of leukemia because of his regular, prolonged exposure to radiation incurred in a therapeutic technique he has evolved for treating cancers of the anal-rectal area.

He places radium in a bronze capsule, which is then inserted by hand between the tumor and the intestinal wall. Precision of placement of the capsule is all-important, and it can only be done manually, its location determined by a TV screen's projection of the fluoroscope. Placement may require up to twenty minutes, and there is no possible shielding. With the capsule finally in place, the patient's tumor is then bombarded with X rays in the radiation room.

For the patient, the double-barreled attack is a dream. Survival rates on inoperable patients are at least as good as any other institution's results on operable patients (i.e., a five-year survival rate, without recurrence, of forty-five percent, which is half-again better than plain cobalt treatment).

When Scheef tried the technique on a patient once, Hoefer was furious.

"Please do not do this again, Wolfgang. You know how dangerous it is. I am the only person in this clinic permitted to perform it."

With each five minutes of exposure, Hoefer absorbs from five hundred to one thousand millirads. The procedure is done about twenty times per year.

An American surgeon watching Hoefer in the radiation room cringed: "Dr. Hoefer, this is insane. If you continue this, you will certainly die from leukemia. Surely with all your ingenuity you should be able to find a way to protect yourself."

"Maybe," replied Hoefer. "If you can think of something, let me know. But aren't the results beautiful?"

One wonders why the Janker's work should have eluded the powers that be in the United States. The answer is that it hasn't—not completely. However, the few physicians who have taken the trouble to investigate the clinic usually have spent no more than a day or two there. To my knowledge, there is but one institution here seriously investigating the gamut of the Janker's methods: the Whitestone General Hospital in Whitestone, New York.

I asked a National Cancer Institute official who had visited the Janker why American patients could not get isophosphamide, A-Mulsin, Wobe enzymes, and the various Janker techniques that had proved so superior. His replies were disturbing: five investigators were trying isophosphamide clinically but hadn't found it too promising. Were they using the Janker's aggressive, fractionated high dosages? No, small, intermittent dosages. Why? Every doctor could use a drug as he saw fit.

Almost certainly the investigators will find isophosphamide "unpromising." The chances are high that Mead Johnson—the pharmaceutical company that is experimenting with the drug here—will propose euthanasia for it, discreet burial and no flowers.

The N.C.I. official was waiting for Scheef to send him the result on A-Mulsin therapy, but he suspected that the most useful part was the radiation. He had been unaware that A-Mulsin could be used without radiation. In any event, there was no rush.

The enzymes he had no interest in, based on "insufficient documentation" provided by the Janker.

That the National Cancer Institute, with a several-hundred-million-dollar budget, should insist that two overworked German oncologists should be versed in the American medical establishment's talent for paper work seems unreasonable.

The American Cancer Society is even more rigid. It prides itself on keeping the Janker techniques out of the United States. At its inception, the society should have played the role of ombudsman for cancer victims, keeping researchers and doctors on their toes, calling foul when new drug development is roadblocked by the F.D.A., testing unusual methods that showed some promise.

Instead, it has become a major part of the problem. It eschews sponsorship of clinical and research innovation and instead goes in for propaganda (cigarettes are harmful, the seven danger signals, celebrity radio, and TV spots) and it ritually condemns and suppresses unorthodox methods which, incidentally, it does not even trouble itself to investigate thoroughly.

Under vice-president Arthur Holleb M.D., who appears to delight in criticizing out-of-town techniques, the A.C.S. wages a covert and effective campaign to keep methods it disapproves of from seeing daylight in the research it funds.

Owing perhaps to an oversight in Holleb's department, I was offered access to the "Unproven Methods" files for a half hour. When the powers that be learned I was reading their correspondence, I was ordered to leave the premises. I did have time, however, to copy some interesting documentation.

Of some personal interest was a letter Holleb had sent to New York's late-night radio-talk-show host Long John Nebel just after the appearance of Karl Ransberger, the purveyor of the enzymes and the vitamin-A emulsion, and myself.

The note included a "resume" which pointed out that Ransberger once had received a doctorate from an English diploma mill. Since I was on the show with Ransberger, I was surprised Holleb didn't mention the fact that I once had been sent an unsolicited degree in naturopathy (an honor I returned promptly to the bestower). In any event, Holleb did not bother to discuss the merits of Ransberger's work or his preparations. He closed his briefing with a plea for Nebel's discretion: ". . . We would prefer that the A.C.S. not be referred to by name, since this might lead to legal action. We would rather spend our time, energy, and funds on continuing cancer research, education and service."

Later, in a letter to Robert A. Good, Ph.D., M.D., who heads research at the Sloan-Kettering Institute, Holleb warned Good about monkeying with these "unproven methods":

The American Cancer Society . . . eschews sponsorship of clinical and research innovation and instead goes in for propaganda (cigarettes are harmful, the seven danger signals, celebrity radio, and TV spots). . . .

"The other night the Long John Nebel radio show (WMCA) carried a several-hour interview with Karl Ransberger. He and Dr. Max Wolf are promoters of the 'Wobe Enzymes-Vitamin-A Emulsion' treatment for cancer. Both men have been well-known to us for many years. Our extensive files may contain information which can be helpful to you if Karl Ransberger's comment that 'Dr. Lloyd Old of the Sloan-Kettering Institute is testing my treatment' is true. The prior training of Karl Ransberger makes for interesting reading. . . .

"I wish I knew how one could better control the unfortunate and premature publicity which links my distinguished alma mater to the promotional side of these unproven methods. We have both agreed that the public will be best served if tests are properly conducted in a prestigious institution, but the exploitation of the good name of the Sloan-Kettering Institute is becoming embarrassing. Perhaps your staff would be willing to consult with us and review our files before commitments are made."

Interestingly, despite the considerable millions in annual funding received by Sloan-Kettering, Max Wolf was asked two years ago to donate $15,000 to defray the costs of doing animal research on his Wobe enzymes—which he promptly paid.

Drs. Good and Old, once fair-haired hopes of the cancer-research vanguard, particularly for their interest in new forms of immunotherapy for cancer, have declined categorically to answer any questions regarding Wolf or their interest in the Janker therapies.

Poor America. Its money-fat, guts-thin biomedical research establishment has more and more to do with paper and abstract mathematics and fear and less and less to do with new therapies or even with people suffering from cancer.

If it would only send some good doctors to the Janker Clinic, it might not only learn something about cancer care, but it might get a good lesson or two on freedom.

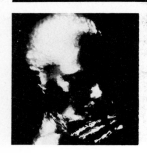

29

Practice

Your wife or boyfriend is dying from cancer. You find yourself emotionally tied in a knot. Or perhaps you are a nurse, social worker, or physician who treats terminally ill persons. You too find yourself feeling helpless, frustrated, and alone in agony. Where can you go in your community to discuss your concerns? Garfield and Clark provide one effective example of how innovative thinking can provide a much needed service to a variety of persons. When you have completed your reading, the following Appendix exercises are recommended:

        C.   Awareness of Grief Process

        D.   Awareness of Losses

        H.   Fantasizing Grief Reaction of Significant Others

        M. Saying Good-bye to a Loved One

The SHANTI Project: A Community Model of Psychosocial Support for Patients and Families Facing Life-Threatening Illness

Charles A. Garfield

Rachel Ogren Clark

Introduction

Recent advances in medical knowledge and technology have produced profound qualitative changes in the nature of dying and chronic illness. The increasing sophistication of therapeutic measures capable of prolonging life has lengthened the average time between the onset of fatal illness and the termination of life. That added time could be a great blessing, allowing the dying person and those he or she loves the possibility to renew their intimacy, be together, share their sorrow, anger, fears, and the joy that comes from the experience of their loving. This time is a potentially powerful opportunity for growth and resolution. However, because our culture has taught us to deny and camouflage dying and death, few of us—patients, families, friends, and medical personnel—know how to use this gift of time in a positive way. The majority of patients still face the dim prospect described by Aldous Huxley: "increasing pain, increasing anxiety, increasing morphine, increasing demandingness, with the ultimate disintegration of personality and a loss of the opportunity to die with dignity."

We organized the SHANTI Project as a response to the realities of social distancing and emotional alienation. Our hope was to develop an effective model of health-care intervention for dealing with some of the psychological and social needs of people facing life-threatening illness—patients, their families, and the professionals who serve them. In developing this model we had three specific aims: (1) to offer *direct community services* consisting of counseling and companionship for patients and families facing life-threatening illness, and grief counseling for survivors of a death; (2) to provide opportunities for *professional training and public education* on relevant issues that arise in ministering to the psychological and social needs

This material was first published in the authors' book *Psychosocial Care of the Dying Patient*, pp. 355–364, McGraw-Hill Book Company, New York, 1978. Copyright 1978 McGraw-Hill Book Company. Reprinted by permission.

of the dying and their families; and (3) to conduct substantive *research* to evaluate the impact of the SHANTI Project as a community service, using research methodology from clinical and social psychology and sociology.

What Human Problems Come to Our Attention?

Who calls the SHANTI Project? Our basic operating principle concerning calls is that we will respond to requests for assistance from anyone dealing with a life-threatening illness.

In general, calls to the project fall into two major categories: (a) requests for information and (b) requests for services. Calls for information come primarily from people who want to know how they can become volunteers in the project, where they can attend professional training programs, or how they can get a SHANTI volunteer to address their group or provide in-service education.

Following a call from the head nurse of a hospital coronary care unit, several volunteers visited the unit to discuss the SHANTI Project. The initial meeting was set up to explore the possibility of making referrals to the project. Soon after the joint discussions began, it became clear that the nurses on the unit had personal issues to discuss. Many acknowledged the tremendous emotional stress of their work and spoke more about their own reactions than about the needs of their patients. The volunteers assumed the role of consultants and tried to point out the covert norms operating in the social system of this unit. For instance, one of the powerfully enforced contextual rules was that anyone expressing strong feelings related to patient care or requesting help with a given patient was less than fully competent. That is, although individual nurses paid lip service to the team approach and to cooperative endeavor, there were very stringently enforced rules about individual responsibility that practically excluded collaborative effort. Many nurses experienced considerable distress because they felt unable to request legitimate support even in near-emergency situations. One SHANTI volunteer pointed out that the senior nurses on the unit, who had less direct contact with patients, were enforcing these norms covertly while never admitting to them verbally. Each of the staff nurses admitted to strong negative feelings about particular senior nurses stemming from situations in which the staff nurse had been chastised for requesting assistance in what should have been a routinely collaborative task. One nurse, who had recently completed what she later described as a totally inadequate orientation, broke into tears when she realized that some of her "failures" were due not to incompetence but rather to inadequate introduction to specific procedures. She received much support from her fellow staff nurses, who acknowledged that she had been victimized by an inappropriate orientation.

The nurses soon changed their request to the SHANTI Project and inquired about the possibility of having one or two volunteers serve as facilitators of a support group for staff nurses. A volunteer recommended that the meeting also be opened to senior nurses so that clear and direct communication could be established within the unit to the benefit of nursing staff and patients alike.

The nurses also spoke of their frustration in dealing with contradictory inputs from medical staff. For example, one specialist might recommend a set of procedures indicating an aggressive approach to therapy, while a second might conclude that there is nothing more to do for the patient. The nurses expressed tremendous dismay at having to deal with these contradictory opinions. Therefore, they said that another item on their agenda for these group support meetings would be the development of more effective communication with medical staff.

The calls for services are usually from one of four kinds of clients. First there are calls from *patients who desire in-person counseling, companionship, and emotional support from a volunteer.*

A SHANTI volunteer who had been regularly visiting an elderly patient in a nursing home learned that Becky, her client, was expected to die very soon. When the volunteer visited Becky it was clear that she was not fully aware of the severity of her condition, although physically she had deteriorated appreciably. Becky was confused about her medical status and was receiving little accurate information from her physician or the nursing staff. Her belongings had already been packed in cardboard boxes in expectation of her death. Her family and friends had not been notified about the gravity of the situation. With Becky's permission and encouragement, her volunteer called the physician, who had known his patient for many years, and requested that he visit with Becky. He promptly came and expressed to Becky and the volunteer his own sad feelings about the impending loss of his friend and patient. The volunteer called Becky's best friend, her younger brother, and her niece to tell them Becky was dying. During the next few hours, all three came to see Becky for the last time. None of them, however, felt comfortable staying more than a few minutes. The nursing staff was willing to allow the volunteer as much time as she needed, and she decided to stay with Becky throughout the night. They spoke at length and Becky revealed that she was aware of her situation because of the discussions with her doctor and the volunteer. She indicated that she felt far better now that the ambiguity of her condition had been reduced. She was able to say goodbye to several of the people most important to her and later that evening, with the SHANTI volunteer holding her hand, Becky died.

Many callers are quite specific about their needs. Some ask for a volunteer who can teach them relaxation techniques to help reduce their pain or anxiety; someone who can help them deal with breaking the news of their illness to other members of the family; someone who will listen without being frightened away like family and friends who change the subject at each mention of death or when fear or anger arise. Although occasionally the requests are for a limited number of visits, the vast majority of contacts have developed into close relationships between volunteer and patient, lasting from several weeks to many months.

The members of the SHANTI Project are aware of the value and effectiveness of peer counseling. Some of our volunteers are dealing with cancer, heart disease, or other chronic life-threatening illnesses. They have been trained to counsel other patients and to apply what they learn from these interactions to their own situations. Peer counselors are often unusually effective because they have access to perspectives unavailable to the rest of us.

Barbara, a woman with seriously advanced uterine cancer, requested a counselor who was knowledgeable about her specific illness. When the opportunity to meet with a peer counselor was presented, Barbara agreed and an on-going relationship was established. Because she was anticipating continuing chemotherapy treatments of the sort that her volunteer had also experienced, much useful ex-

> **Peer counselors are often unusually effective because they have access to perspectives unavailable to the rest of us.**

The help that Paula received in recognizing her own strength allowed her to make it possible for Jim to die at home as he wished.

change of information took place between volunteer and client. The volunteer agreed to accompany Barbara to her chemotherapy treatments, and encouraged her to discuss openly with her physician any aspect of the treatment or the disease that concerned her. The two developed an extremely strong bond based primarily on their joint efforts in fighting a common illness. Later, when Barbara's husband requested support, a second SHANTI volunteer was sent to assist him. This conjoint model—i.e., more than one volunteer working with a single family—has been employed quite successfully. This case is still in progress. The first volunteer, her own health permitting, intends to remain with Barbara throughout the course of her illness. The second volunteer is prepared to provide support to Barbara's husband and, in the event of her death, to be available through the period of grief.

The second group of requests for service comes from people close to a patient. They may ask for a *volunteer to spend time with an entire family* in which one member is suffering from a life-threatening illness; or for a *volunteer to work with just one member of a patient's family—often a spouse.* The patients for whom these people are caring either (a) have not requested the help of a volunteer, (b) live outside the geographical range of the SHANTI Project (whereas the relative lives in the San Francisco Bay Area), or (c) are already seeing another volunteer (in which case, one volunteer would serve primarily as the patient's advocate and companion and the other as advocate and support for the patient's spouse or family).

Following an introductory call from a well-known oncologist in the Bay Area, Paula, the wife of a thirty-five-year-old man with acute leukemia, called the SHANTI Project to ask for help. As a nurse, Paula recognized the importance of emotional support for cancer patients, but her husband, Jim, was not interested in talking with anyone, even his wife. Paula found the impact of living with the threat of Jim's impending death increasingly difficult to bear and had become extremely anxious and unsure of her ability to care for and relate to her husband. The side-effects of Jim's chemotherapy treatments, remissions followed by recurrence of symptoms, the change from out-patient to in-patient status were all causing confusion for Paula and jeopardizing her relationship with Jim. Paula communicated all of this information during her initial phone call to the SHANTI Project and requested a volunteer who could help her separate the realities of the situation from the morass of confusion. She especially wanted to plan a strategy for coping with her own feelings while reestablishing communication with Jim. Paula asked for a woman volunteer who was about her age and who understood Catholicism, as she felt her religion to be her primary source of support. A volunteer fitting that description was available and met with Paula that evening. After this initial meeting, the volunteer saw Paula often, sometimes accompanying her to the hospital to visit Jim. They spent many additional hours consulting by phone.

Upon realizing how important the volunteer was to his wife, Jim requested another volunteer as his own advocate. He had many unexpressed feelings that he felt he could not communicate to Paula. Most were related to his fear of death, his feelings about the possibility of survival, and his relationship with his parents and brother in Indonesia. Another volunteer was sent to serve as a primary support for Jim. As time progressed, the volunteer-client relationships evolved into a conjoint format in which the four individuals would meet together as well as in pairs. The help that Paula received in recognizing her own strength allowed her to make it possible for Jim to die at home as he wished. It also made it possible for her to be with him in a loving, calm, and supportive manner during his final hours, even though her pain was great. Both SHANTI volunteers were with Paula and Jim when he died.

More than six months later, and in the midst of grieving, Paula and her SHANTI volunteer still meet frequently. They are attempting to help Paula work through her grief, discussing various aspects of their shared and separate experiences with Jim. They have become close friends and seem likely to continue their relationship throughout the grieving period and beyond.

It is important to recognize that the strain of an extended life-threatening illness can be enormous for patient and family and that few adequate emotional supports are available. Most dying people desperately want and need the presence and affection of those whom they love. Yet without caring support for themselves and validation of their rights and feelings, those loved ones, because of their own fear, sorrow, frustration, and sense of helplessness, often withdraw and become emotionally and physically inaccessible to the patient. The presence of emotional support can help generate that degree of hope and strength necessary for patient and family to deal with the seemingly overwhelming burdens of a terminal illness.

The third group of callers who request volunteers are *people who have survived the death of a family member or close friend.* They are often experiencing the trauma of separation, including loneliness, profound sadness, and a sense of loss and disorientation.

Jane, a single parent, called the project to request a volunteer to help her through her grief. Her only child, a ten-year-old boy, had died two weeks earlier after open-heart surgery that had a 90 percent chance of success. Jane had no family support, and while her friends were good listeners, they were unable to provide her with useful feedback. She needed to talk with someone who understood the psychological aspects of grief and who could point out that her reactions were normal. She was very relieved to learn that her feelings were not predictors of imminent and irreversible mental breakdown.

A volunteer whose primary expertise is grief counseling was selected and has spent many hours with Jane. At Jane's request, they have discussed the horror of watching her child attached to tubes and monitors and not being allowed to hold him. Even worse, the anguish of not being with her son when he died. This occurred because caring but misguided medical staff felt it would be too painful, and therefore sedated her heavily and put her to bed in a room down the hall. Jane has talked with her volunteer about the need to redefine her own identity (she has seen herself as a mother for ten years, and suddenly is without a child to mother); about the changes in her lifestyle and perspective that have occurred now that no one depends upon her, waits for her, loves her completely; about letting go of any possibility of seeing her son grow to adulthood; about her sleeplessness, her loss of appetite, her inability to concentrate, and her sudden bouts with depression, all of which are typical symptoms of grief. Jane's volunteer provided loving and practical support throughout potentially suicidal situations brought on by the depths of existential despair. They were able to view the severe depression as a sign that Jane had accepted her son's death and was beginning the slow, undeniably painful process of adjusting to that sad reality.

Jane and her volunteer have agreed to work together for as long as they both feel that the relationship is a supportive one. In putting together the pieces of her life, Jane is attempting to map out her plans for the immediate future and, with the help of her volunteer, has developed a more satisfactory social life.

Most dying people desperately want and need the presence and affection of those whom they love.

Unfortunately, survivors of a death must suffer their anguish in a death-denying society whose principal messages are: "Don't let it get you down. Cheer up. Be brave. Forget the past—it's over. Just throw yourself into living." These messages clearly say: "Don't show me your pain; it frightens me." Our culture encourages us to short-circuit emotional suffering at every opportunity. For the grieving person, this means there is little chance for working through the pain of loss, because what is in reality a psychological necessity is seen by others as morbid self-indulgence. SHANTI volunteers look upon grief counseling and continued emotional support for survivors as an integral function of their work. The project offers help during the period of grieving to survivors of our own clients (those with whom we have worked prior to their deaths) and to survivors of persons with whom we had no contact before they died.

The fourth type of call for services consists of *requests for backup consultation and/or emotional support from people who work with the dying outside the usual institutional settings.* Private duty nurses who care for terminally ill patients at home, clergy who are called upon to counsel dying members of their congregations, teachers who work as home tutors to children with potentially terminal illnesses, visiting homemakers, and others who work along with the dying frequently encounter the psychological conflict and emotional anguish that accompany terminal illness. However, they often have no readily accessible colleagues with whom to discuss their reactions and feelings and the cumulative emotional impact of their work. SHANTI volunteers can share the personal understanding they have gained through similar contact with the dying as well as general information on specific issues related to dealing with life-threatening illness.

History and Operation of Project

In June 1974, Dr. Garfield and several colleagues were discussing possible alternative support systems for the dying. They talked of hospices and the expense and organizational expertise that would be needed to form such an institution in the Bay Area. They also explored the feasibility of using volunteer counselors to provide support for those dealing with life-threatening illness. Dr. Garfield was hoping to find an alternative requiring less long-term planning and fewer financial demands—a way to bring help to people *now.* Stewart Brand, who developed the *Whole Earth Catalog,* came up with the uniquely simple concept that formed the functional basis of the SHANTI Project. Brand's suggestion was to make it possible to reach a group of volunteers at one central telephone number who had the interest, ability, and time to work with the dying. These volunteers, when contacted, would go out into the community to visit with patients in their homes, in hospitals and nursing homes, or in any other mutually agreeable location.

On February 1, 1975 an answering machine was attached to a telephone in the home of Rachel Ogren Clark, Co-Director of the SHANTI Project.

Anyone who wants to use the service can call and leave a message. Mrs. Clark returns the calls, discusses the client's situation and needs in detail, and then relays that information to the SHANTI volunteer best equipped to meet the needs of the caller. That volunteer then sets up a time to meet the client as the beginning, it is hoped, of an on-going one-to-one supportive relationship. Only first-hand referrals are accepted—which means that work is only with those people who themselves request a volunteer. The only exception to this principle of operation is, if a person is too ill to talk on the phone, referral is accepted from nursing, medical, and social work staff, or from a family member, with the assurance that the patient has knowledge of the project and has asked to see a volunteer. This policy usually prevents situations in which patients agree to see a volunteer when they would really rather not.

Each volunteer becomes an advocate through a commitment to "doing what needs to be done" as determined by both patient and volunteer.

A psychologist from an oncology unit at a major hospital called the project to request a volunteer for Steven, a terminally ill man with lung cancer. It was learned that in two weeks' time Steven would be leaving for an extended-care facility. The psychologist realized that a volunteer who could provide continuity of care might be a valuable asset to his patient. Steven was having tremendous difficulty acknowledging the emotional impact of his illness. He was extremely frightened by the prospect of dying and the flood of powerful feelings it threatened to release. After clearly determining Steven's interest and obtaining his permission, the psychologist introduced the SHANTI volunteer to Steven, and the three of them engaged in conversation. When Steven left the acute-care hospital for the extended-care facility, the volunteer accompanied him and continued to visit throughout his stay at the new institution. Later, when Steven returned home, he asked his volunteer to continue visiting him. The volunteer was able to provide on-going support for Steven as well as periodic feedback to the staff members of the acute-care and extended-care facilities. The volunteer will remain with Steven until he dies, and then will be available to Steven's wife for grief counseling, should she request it.

A record is kept of initial calls to the project and volunteers keep notes on all contacts with their clients. These records are kept confidential and are used only for purposes of evaluating our work. To date, the telephone service has worked efficiently, and this mode of operation will be continued.

The SHANTI Volunteers

SHANTI volunteers are client advocates. The word "advocate" literally means "supporter, favorer, and friend." It also means "Holy Spirit" and "Spirit of Truth." In serving as a client advocate, the SHANTI volunteer is not bound by a rigid definition of his or her role, as are most professionals and family members. Each volunteer becomes an advocate through a commitment to "doing what needs to be done" as determined by both patient and volunteer. At times volunteers clean ashtrays or make phone calls; at other times they consult with medical and nursing staff or family members, and still other times they serve their client as companion and friend. The SHANTI volunteer is not a professional psychotherapist or member of the

The SHANTI Project   407

clergy, although some function elsewhere in these capacities. However, each volunteer must sometimes deal with psychological and spiritual issues in the interests of the client. Volunteers are aware of the importance of knowing when to involve specific health professionals—for example, psychotherapist, physician, nurse, social worker, or clergy. While patient advocacy often calls for a high tolerance for ambiguity, it allows for a considerable flexibility in the service of client and family. As volunteers learn to avoid the trap of "addiction to action" and thereby discover the art as well as the science of helping another human being, they frequently find that "the experience of being cared for may benefit the patient more than the direct effect of the care" (Quint 1967). Volunteers therefore find it easier than they expected to maintain the compassionately caring and empathic attitude that impelled most of them to enter the project in the first place.

Volunteers realize that the likelihood of their providing meaningful emotional support to patients is based on the facts that they are willing advocates and that they possess considerable expertise in the psychosocial aspects of life-threatening illness. Because they consider themselves to be guests in the hospital rooms or homes of their clients, volunteers recognize that their continued presence may be directly connected with their physical, emotional, and spiritual usefulness. For many volunteers, an additional revelation has been that caring for another human being can be as emotionally rewarding for the helper as for the recipient.

The SHANTI Project is committed to providing continuity of care for all clients. Once a client-volunteer relationship is established, the SHANTI volunteer's primary allegiance is to the client rather than to any single institutional setting. The volunteer continues to work with his or her client whether the client is at home, agrees to a series of hospitalizations, or is moved to an extended-care facility. This continuity of care is one of the major factors differentiating the SHANTI Project from other existing social services.

Volunteers come to the client's bedside as patient advocates, but also with the wish to cooperate as fully as possible with professional staff. As facilitators of communication between their client and various health professionals, volunteers are often in a position to offset the all-too-frequent lay perception that hospital professionals are insensitive automatons performing esoteric physiological rites on the bodies of their patients. They can recount experiences in which professional staff emerged as kind, sensitive human beings forced to work under extreme stress, and who possessed vital information about the client's emotional needs. The volunteers remain open to full cooperation with staff in the service of the client's needs.

Most people approach helping services in one of three ways—through self-initiated action, through the advice of others (physician, nurse, family, friends, the clergy), or by coercion. Because the SHANTI Project only accepts first-hand referrals, health professionals and others can obtain the services of a patient advocate only by first getting acquainted with the project themselves. They can then tell the patient about the SHANTI Project as well as about other community resources so the patient can evaluate his or her own needs and decide on the advisability of contacting the project.

As the project has progressed, we have learned to predict what kinds of people will make the most effective volunteers. All prospective volunteers send us a statement describing why they want to work with patients and families facing life-threatening illness. They are subsequently invited to an interview with one or two experienced volunteers and the co-directors of the project. In addition to an evident sense of compassion, the qualities looked for include a high tolerance for ambiguity; an ease in talking about dying (as evidenced by discussion that is personalized rather than predominantly philosophical); capacity for introspection as reflected in extensive self-knowledge; a healthy sense of self-confidence; high tolerance for frustration; a degree of psychological mindedness; a sense of humility that allows one to view sharing in someone else's dying as a joint process with learning occurring on both sides; the ability to speak in and understand various metaphors (religious, cultural, or symbolic); and relevant professional training in counseling, psychology, social welfare, nursing, or medicine. SHANTI volunteers do not pretend to be totally altruistic; all admit that the work brings them valuable rewards and enhances their personal growth. However, a prospective volunteer who sees working with the dying primarily as one more event in a series of personal-growth experiences would not be accepted into the project. Neither would someone whose religious convictions included the need to proselytize. Other characteristics that would exclude a prospective volunteer from the project are a powerful need to control and a strong belief that there is a "right way to die."

Each SHANTI volunteer makes a commitment to work at least one year with the project, and expects to spend eight to ten hours per week with clients. The individualized training, supervision, and support considered necessary for all volunteers begins with each volunteer attending one or more training seminars before being accepted into the program. Among the various training seminars offered by the SHANTI Project is a five-day national conference conducted yearly at the University of California, Berkeley. The training programs are designed to acquaint volunteers both with the skills required of volunteers and the basic orientation of the project.

To make volunteer training an on-going process, frequent contact between experienced project members and new volunteers is encouraged. At regular weekly meetings volunteers freely share professional and personal expertise in an unusually supportive emotional milieu seldom found elsewhere. We generally follow case-conference format, occasionally inviting guest consultants to speak on training issues of particular interest. All volunteers also have easy access to the project's co-directors and staff throughout the week. The directors meet frequently with volunteers to maintain an awareness of the particular needs, skills, and development of each volunteer.

. . . a prospective volunteer who sees working with the dying primarily as one more event in a series of personal-growth experiences would not be accepted into the project.

> **". . . stand rather in the face of death together with those who grieve."**

The idea behind the SHANTI Project was a new concept, and the perseverance of the SHANTI volunteers has made it a workable one. The volunteers are a heterogeneous group, both in philosophical orientation and in personal background and experience. Almost every religious belief (including nonbelief) is represented among the volunteers. Many come from the helping professions: social workers, psychologists, teachers, gerontologists, and the clergy. Others are housewives, architects, students, artists, secretaries, and musicians. Their ages range from 22 to 73. What our volunteers have in common is the willingness, emotional strength, and trained sensitivity to confront humanely the realities of death and dying without resorting to the evasion and denial so often apparent. Almost all the volunteers have experienced profound personal loss and have gained considerable psychological maturity as a result. They are hardworking, deeply committed people—sometimes prone to compassionate overwork— who have exhibited the courage to provide consistent support to clients faced with the enormous emotional burdens resulting from serious illness. At present the volunteers are providing more than 3,000 hours of counseling per month—services that did not exist prior to the establishment of the SHANTI Project.

To say we are pleased with what we've learned and done would be an understatement; to say we have completed our development would be incorrect. We will continue our efforts to *"not* run away from the pain, to *not* get busy when there is nothing to do and instead stand rather in the face of death together with those who grieve" (Nouwen 1974).

References
Nouwen, Henri. 1974. *Out of Solitude.* Notre Dame, Indiana: Ave Maria Press.
Quint, Jeanne. 1967. *The Nurse and the Dying Patient.* New York: Macmillan.

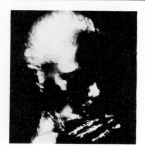

30

Practice

T he relationship between law and medicine is an important one as exemplified in the Natural Death Act passed in the State of Texas in 1977. Bugen, Tullos, and Bolton challenge us to understand our legal and moral rights regarding our eventual deaths and review one means of safeguarding these rights. Knowing that one of the authors is terminally ill while the other two are caregivers helps to underscore the importance of looking at an issue from "both sides." The following Appendix exercises will help foster understanding of the issue:

A. Announcing One's Own Death

B. Appropriate Death Fantasy

G. Funeral Fantasy

K. Planning for Living

L. Privacy Circles

N. The Final Rite of Passage: A Technological Update

Control, Quality of Life, and "The Right to Die"

Larry A. Bugen

Sally Tullos

Zorena S. Bolton

How can death as the "ultimate indignity" be humanly dignified? A momentous debate rages on in this regard! Our dilemma lies in part in our confusion between event and process. The sting of death as a final event or state of being is perhaps an indignant possibility. To think of unyielding forces from within or without determining our finitude is a blow to our need to have a say in the matter. This is particularly true in situations involving sudden and unexpected death.

Death, however, may also be viewed as a process or transition between the state of being alive and being dead. For many persons death does not come swiftly. The transition between life and death may be prolonged. This transitional period has been receiving a great deal of attention, especially with respect to two issues: (1) To what extent should a dying person have *control* over this transitional period of time? And (2) how should quantity of life be balanced against *quality of life*?

Control

Many human functions—like the birth process, for example—are undergoing a kind of "deprofessionalization" and concomitant personal involvement. Expectant parents attend Lamaze classes, support one another through labor and delivery, and request Leboyer delivery methods. As a result, less medication is being requested for pain control, the entire family is becoming involved in both delivery and rearing practices, and doctors are being screened in regard to their willingness to share control.

Similarly, the issue of control is being reexamined with respect to the dying process. Symbols of this new kind of "declaration of independence"

. . . issues will be
elaborated . . .
with respect to
the "Natural
Death Act" of
the State of
Texas.

include the living will, Laetrile, funeral prearrangement, and right-to-die legislation. Public discussion of each of these matters demonstrates the increasing desire of people to have more input—more control—and is affecting medical treatment and human behavior throughout the land.

The Laetrile controversy appears to set the scientific community, i.e., the Food and Drug Administration, against the lay community. Does the extract from apricot pits really have any value as a cancer combatant? As the *Wall Street Journal* points out, "The Laetrile boom is based on far more than a desperate grasp by dying cancer victims for a medical miracle. It springs from a deep disenchantment with the medical profession and a powerful resentment against big government" (July 21, 1977, p. 12). Control is clearly the issue!

Along with an increase in control comes a responsibility to make just and valid decisions. In the case of "right-to-die" legislation, the directive to withhold or withdraw life-sustaining procedures requires a decision running counter to the norms of most health-care providers and health-care delivery systems. Providers will certainly question the wisdom of such choices. Are terminal patients and their families in their "right minds" when they pursue such a commitment? Aren't persons who are threatened with life-threatening illnesses already burdened to the hilt with decisions? Perhaps it is the right to make such decisions and not the ultimate correctness of them which matters.

Quality of Life

The variety of drugs, mechanical devices, and other measures available today often have the effect of postponing death more than prolonging life. Biomedical ethics, which implore us to value the mere summation of chronological years, are being seriously questioned. Assumptions regarding the sanctity of life "at any cost" are crumbling under increasing concern about *quality of life.*

Our definitions of life and death must conceptually change in order to keep abreast of new realities. Health, for instance, must be seen more holistically as a "personal function" and not just a "biological function." If a team of medical experts defines a comotose patient as being alive and "healthy" because his or her heart still beats and the brain continues to manifest monitored waves, biomedical progress will falter. We all are more than an integrated sum of autonomic functions. We have personalities, emotions, behaviors, attitudes, and beliefs that sustain and nourish us. The highest form of biomedical ethics recognizes that quality of life is dependent upon all of the above.

In the following pages these issues will be elaborated more fully and interpreted with respect to the "Natural Death Act" of the State of Texas. This recent legislation, printed below, has implications for both health-care consumers and providers involved in the delivery of health-related services. Both consumer and a provider will respond to the bill.

The Natural Death Act is a written document voluntarily executed by a patient to give a directive to an attending physician to withdraw life-sustaining procedures in the event of a terminal condition. The act thus represents an "elective death" and most closely approximates *negative euthanasia*—planned omission of therapies or treatment which would "probably" prolong life. In contrast, *positive euthanasia* would mean planned implementation of therapies or treatment intended to speed up the process of death.

Joseph Fletcher (1964) distinguishes four forms of elective death which reflect varying degrees of choice, purpose, and responsible freedom. (a) Euthanasia is *voluntary* and *direct* if chosen and carried out by the patient. Suicide would certainly be an example. (b) Euthanasia is *voluntary* but *indirect* if an individual makes a decision well in advance of a terminal illness that someone should carry out his or her predetermined wishes if the patient is not able to do so. The Natural Death Act would most appropriately be placed here. (c) Euthanasia is *direct* but *involuntary* if "mercy killing" occurs without the person's request at the time or previously. (d) Finally, euthanasia is *indirect* and *involuntary* if nothing positive is done to benefit the patient or if anything negative is done without the patient's consent and appears to be a passive act.

The true power and beauty of the Natural Death Act of Texas lies in its reliance upon the values of the dying person. Leon Kass (1974) has eloquently stated that "we might say that the possibility of a humanly dignified facing of death can be destroyed from without (and, of course, from within), but the actualization of that possibility depends largely on the soul, the character, the bearing of the dying (person) him or herself—i.e., on things within." The Natural Death Act permits such actualization. It reads as follows:

> **The true power and beauty of the Natural Death Act of Texas lies in its reliance upon the values of the dying person.**

ENROLLED
AN ACT

relating to the Natural Death Act and a procedure for a person to provide in advance for the withdrawal or withholding of medical care when the person has a terminal condition; providing certain immunities; making certain provisions as to the effect on insurance of the making of or carrying out a directive as defined in this Act; defining offenses and providing penalties; and declaring an emergency.

BE IT ENACTED BY THE LEGISLATURE OF THE STATE OF TEXAS:

Section 1. This Act shall be known and may be cited as the Natural Death Act.

Sec. 2. In this Act:

(1) "Attending physician" means the physician selected by, or assigned by the physician selected by, the patient who has primary responsibility for the treatment and care of the patient.

(2) "Directive" means a written document voluntarily executed by the declarant in accordance with the requirements of Section 3 of this Act. The directive, or a copy of the directive, shall be made part of the patient's medical records.

(3) "Life-sustaining procedure" means a medical procedure or intervention which utilizes mechanical or other artificial means to sustain, restore, or supplant a vital function, which, when applied to a qualified patient, would serve only to artificially prolong the moment of death and where, in the judgment of the attending physician, noted in the qualified patient's medical records, death is imminent whether or not such procedures are utilized. "Life-sustaining procedure" shall not include the administration of medication or the performance of any medical procedure deemed necessary to alleviate pain.

(4) "Physician" means a physician and surgeon licensed by the Texas State Board of Medical Examiners.

(5) "Qualified patient" means a patient diagnosed and certified in writing to be afflicted with a terminal condition by two physicians, one of whom shall be the attending physician, and the other shall be chosen by the patient or the attending physician, who have each personally examined the patient.

(6) "Terminal condition" means an incurable condition caused by injury, disease, or illness, which, regardless of the application of life-sustaining procedures, would, within reasonable medical judgment, produce death, and where the application of life-sustaining procedures serves only to postpone the moment of death by the patient.

Sec. 3. Any adult person may execute a directive for the withholding or withdrawal of life-sustaining procedures in the event of a terminal condition. The directive shall be signed by the declarant in the presence of two witnesses not related to the declarant by blood or marriage and who would not be entitled to any portion of the estate of the declarant on his decease under any will of the declarant or codicil thereto or by operation of law. In addition, a witness to a directive shall not be the attending physician, an employee of the attending physician or a health facility in which the declarant is a patient, a patient in a health care facility in which the declarant is a patient, or any person who has a claim against any portion of the estate of the declarant upon his decease at the time of the execution of the directive. The signature of the declarant shall be acknowledged, and the witnesses shall subscribe and swear to the directive before a notary public. The directive shall be in the following form:

DIRECTIVE TO PHYSICIANS

Directive made this _____ day of _____ (month, year).

I _____ , being of sound mind, willfully and voluntarily make known my desire that my life shall not be artificially prolonged under the circumstances set forth below, and do hereby declare:

1. If at any time I should have an incurable condition caused by injury, disease, or illness certified to be a terminal condition by two physicians, and where the application of life-sustaining procedures would serve only to artificially prolong the moment of my death and where my attending physician determines that my death is imminent whether or not life-sustaining procedures would serve only to artificially prolong the moment of my death and where my attending physician determines that my death is imminent whether or not life-sustaining procedures are utilized, I direct that such procedures be withheld or withdrawn, and that I be permitted to die naturally.

2. In the absence of my ability to give directions regarding the use of such life-sustaining procedures, it is my intention that this directive shall be honored by my family and physicians as the final expression of my legal right to refuse medical or surgical treatment and accept the consequences from such refusal.

3. If I have been diagnosed as pregnant and that diagnosis is known to my physician, this directive shall have no force or effect during the course of my pregnancy.

4. I have been diagnosed and notified at least 14 days ago as having a terminal condition by _____ , M.D., whose address is _____ , and whose telephone number is _____ . I understand that if I have not filled in the physicians name and address, it shall be presumed that I did not have a terminal condition when I made out this directive.

5. This directive shall have no force or effect five years from the date filled in above.

6. I understand the full import of this directive and I am emotionally and mentally competent to make this directive.

7. I understand that I may revoke this directive at any time.

Signed _____

City, County, State of Residence _____

The declarant has been personally known to me and I believe him or her to be of sound mind. I am not related to the declarant by blood or marriage, nor would I be entitled to any portion of the declarant's estate on his decease, nor am I the attending physician or declarant or employee of the attending physician of declarant or an employee of the attending physician or a health facility in which declarant is a patient, or a patient in the health care facility in which the declarant is a patient, or any person who has a claim against any portion of the estate of the declarant upon his decease.

Witness _____

Witness _____

STATE OF TEXAS

COUNTY OF _____

Before me, the undersigned authority, on this day personally appeared _____ , _____ , and _____ , known to me to be the declarant and witnesses whose names are subscribed to the foregoing instrument in their respective capacities, and, all of said persons being by me duly sworn, the declarant, _____ , declared to me and to the said witnesses in my presence that said instrument is his Directive to Physicians, and that he had willingly and voluntarily made and executed it as his free act and deed for the purposes therein expressed.

Declarant _____

Witness _____

Witness _____

Subscribed and acknowledged before me by the said Declarant, _____ , and by the said witnesses, _____ and _____ , on this _____ day of _____ , 19 _____ .

                                    _____
                                    Notary public in and for _____
                                    County, Texas

Sec. 4. (a) A directive may be revoked at any time by the declarant, without regard to his mental state or competency, by any of the following methods:

(1) by being canceled, defaced, obliterated, or burnt, torn, or otherwise destroyed by the declarant or by some person in his presence and by his direction;

(2) by a written revocation of the declarant expressing his intent to revoke, signed and dated by the declarant, such revocation shall become effective only on communication to an attending physician by the declarant or by a person acting on behalf of the declarant or by mailing said revocation to an attending physician. An attending physician or his designee shall record in the patient's medical record the time and date when he received notification of the written revocation and shall enter the word "VOID" on each page of the copy of the directive in the patient's medical records; or

(3) by a verbal expression by the declarant of his intent to revoke the directive. Such revocation shall become effective only on communication to an attending physician by the declarant or by a person acting on behalf of the declarant. An attending physician or his designee shall record in the patient's medical record the time, date, and place of the revocation and the time, date, and place, if different, of when he received notification of the revocation and shall enter the word "VOID" on each page of the copy of the directive in the patient's medical records.

(b) Except as otherwise provided in this Act, there shall be no criminal or civil liability on the part of any person for failure to act on a revocation made pursuant to this section unless that person has actual knowledge of the revocation.

Sec. 5. A directive shall be effective for five years from the date of its execution unless sooner revoked in a manner prescribed in Section 4 of this Act. Nothing in this Act shall be construed to prevent a declarant from reexecuting a directive at any time in accordance with the formalities of Section 3 of this Act, including reexecution subsequent to a diagnosis of a terminal condition. If the declarant has executed more than one directive, such time shall be determined from the date of execution of the last directive known to the attending physician. If the declarant becomes comatose or is rendered incapable of communicating with the attending physician, the directive shall remain in effect for the duration of the comatose condition or until such time as the declarant's condition renders him or her able to communicate with the attending physician, but in any event shall terminate at the end of five years from the date of execution.

Sec. 6. No physician or health facility which, acting in accordance with the requirements of this Act, causes the withholding or withdrawal of life-sustaining procedures from a qualified patient, shall be subject to civil liability therefrom unless negligent. No health professional, acting under the direction of a physician, who participates in the withholding or withdrawal of life-sustaining procedures in accordance with the provisions of this Act shall be subject to any civil liability unless negligent. No physician, or health professional acting under the direction of a physician, who participates in the withholding or withdrawal of life-sustaining procedures in accordance with the provisions of this Act shall be guilty of any criminal act or of unprofessional conduct unless negligent. No physician, health care facility, or health care professional shall be liable either civilly or criminally for failure to act pursuant to the declarant's directive where such physician, health care facility, or health care professional had no knowledge of such directive.

Sec. 7. (a) Prior to effecting a withholding or withdrawal of life-sustaining procedures from a qualified patient pursuant to the directive, the attending physician shall determine that the directive complies with the form of the directive set out in Section 3 of this Act, and, if the patient is mentally competent, that the directive and all steps proposed by the attending physician to be undertaken are in accord with the existing desires of the qualified patient and are communicated to the patient.

(b) If the declarant was a qualified patient at least 14 days prior to executing or reexecuting the directive, the directive shall be conclusively presumed, unless revoked, to be the directions of the patient regarding the withholding or withdrawal of life-sustaining procedures. No physician, and no health professional acting under the direction of a physician, shall be criminally or civilly liable for failing to effectuate the directive of the qualified patient pursuant to this subsection. A failure by a physician to effectuate the directive of a qualified patient pursuant to this subsection may constitute unprofessional conduct if the physician refuses to make the necessary arrangements or fails to take the necessary steps to effect the transfer of the qualified patient to another physician who will effectuate the directive of the qualified patient.

(c) If the declarant becomes a qualified patient subsequent to executing the directive, the attending physician may give weight to the directive as evidence of the patient's directions regarding the withholding or withdrawal of life-sustaining procedures and may consider other factors, such as information from the affected family or the nature of the patient's illness, injury, or disease, in determining whether the totality of circumstances known to the attending physician justifies effectuating the directive. No physician, and no health professional acting under the directive of a physician, shall be criminally or civilly liable for failing to effectuate the directive of the qualified patient pursuant to this subsection.

Sec. 8. (a) The withholding or withdrawal of life-sustaining procedures from a qualified patient in accordance with the provisions of the Act shall not, for any purpose, constitute an offense under Section 22.08, Penal Code.

(b) The making of a directive pursuant to Section 3 of this Act shall not restrict, inhibit, or impair in any manner the sale, procurement, or issuance of any policy of life insurance, nor shall it be deemed to modify the terms of an existing policy of life insurance. No policy of life insurance shall be legally impaired or invalidated in any manner by the withholding or withdrawal of life-sustaining procedures from an insured qualified patient, notwithstanding any term of the policy to the contrary.

(c) No physician, health facility, or other health provider, and no health care service plan, or insurer issuing insurance, may require any person to execute a directive as a condition for being insured for, or receiving, health care services nor may the execution or failure to execute a directive be considered in any way in establishing the premiums for insurance.

Sec. 9. A person who willfully conceals, cancels, defaces, obliterates, or damages the directive of another without such declarant's consent shall be guilty of a Class A misdemeanor. A person who falsifies or forges the directive of another, or willfully conceals or withholds personal knowledge of a revocation as provided in Section 4 of this Act, with the intent to cause a withholding or withdrawal of life-sustaining procedures contrary to the wishes of the declarant, and thereby, because of any such act, directly causes life-sustaining procedures to be withheld or withdrawn and death to thereby be hastened, shall be subject to prosecution for criminal homicide under the provisions of the Penal Code.

Sec. 10. Nothing in this Act shall be construed to condone, authorize, or approve mercy killing, or to permit any affirmative or deliberate act or omission to end life other than to permit the natural process of dying as provided in this Act.

Sec. 11. Nothing in this Act shall impair or supersede any legal right or legal responsibility which any person may have to effect the withholding or withdrawal of life-sustaining procedures in any lawful manner. In such respect the provisions of this Act are cumulative.

Sec. 12. The importance of this legislation and the crowded condition of the calendars in both houses create an emergency and an imperative public necessity that the constitutional rule requiring bills to be read on three several days in each house be suspended, and this rule is hereby suspended, and that this Act take effect and be in force from and after its passage, and it is so enacted.

The Natural Death Act in Texas: A Patient's Perspective

My name is Sally Tullos, and I have leukemia. During the 1977 session of the Texas legislature, the Natural Death Act was introduced in both the House and the Senate. As a terminally ill patient, I testified before the Senate Jurisprudence Committee in favor of this bill. The Natural Death Act passed out of the Senate and the House committees, passed through both houses of the legislature, and became law on August 29, 1977. My purpose here is to consider the effects this bill will have on society, especially hospitals and members of the helping professions, and its implications for the terminally ill patient, his or her family, and his or her doctor-patient relationship.

I remember March 15, 1977 well. That Tuesday afternoon I testified before the Senate Jurisprudence Committee. Earlier that morning I was in Houston, Texas. Monday I had been to M.D. Anderson hospital for my regular checkup and was returning home Tuesday to begin chemotherapy that afternoon. It was during all of this that I realized that I could testify if I drove home like hell. Somehow I felt that I belonged at the hearing.

When I arrived home, I managed to postpone my chemotherapy until as late as possible (which was a blessing to me), and drove to the state capital.

I felt excited and somewhat hesitant about speaking at the hearing. I wondered who would be there, that is, who else would testify, and whether these people were for or against the bill. My most pressing concern was how the legislators would react to me, a terminally ill patient, expressing my views about the bill. While I was waiting to begin my speech, I had the feeling that many of the legislators were thinking of death in purely intellectual and philosophical terms. They seemed to consider the proposed bill in an impersonal manner, thinking only in terms of vague ethical questions. They seemed to look at the matter in a "what if" framework. When I spoke, however, there was a stunned, shocked silence. I do not believe anyone actually thought that I, as a dying patient, would be willing to testify about my impending death.

The Natural Death Act is now law. One of my concerns is how many terminally ill patients are aware of this existing law. A second concern is the manner in which the Natural Death Act will be distributed or be available to patients throughout the state. The Natural Death Act will not benefit patients if it is hidden or put away on some back shelf in the courthouse.

Since the manner of distribution is not outlined in the bill, I offer the following suggestions. It seems to me that a hospital is the most obvious place to distribute copies of the bill. Copies of the Natural Death Act could be placed in waiting rooms of hospitals, in outpatient clinics, and doctors' offices, in chaplains' offices, and in social service departments. It might even be possible for patients to be given a copy of this bill in an orientation package when they are admitted to the hospital. Another option is that offices be maintained 24 hours a day in hospitals with staff available to talk with patients and their families about the Natural Death Act. This is feasible and necessary since death-related crises occur around the clock.

These "death counselors" would be people who are very comfortable in their role. The salaried staff would include professional social workers, psychologists, chaplains, and, possibly, medical doctors. In addition to professional staff, trained volunteers might be recruited from the community. These people could be students, persons who just want to help, and others who have been through a death-related experience. If the patient is well enough, the counselor will talk with him or her and the family about the choice of maintaining or withholding life support equipment. The Natural Death Act would be explained to the family and the patient. Ultimately, the decision is the patient's, but ideally families should be involved in the decision-making process. I strongly believe that death counseling must be available to patients and their families in order that a rational decision be made. Hopefully, with the passage of the Natural Death Act and the services of death counselors, families will not be forced to make the difficult decision regarding life supports during times of panic and trauma.

There is, though, one serious problem in having death counseling in the hospital setting. The Natural Death Act specifically states that a notary public sign the declaration, and that the two witnesses to the declaration "not be the attending physician, an employee of the attending physician, or a health facility in which the declarant is a patient. . . ." Therefore, it is imperative that the death counselors serve only in a *counseling* capacity and hence cannot witness the patient's document. Hospitals cannot use their own notary publics, and the two required witnesses would have to be brought in from outside the hospital setting. It is important to note that, though a patient may want to sign the Natural Death Act, he may be physically unable to leave the hospital, and thus the notary public and the two witnesses would have to come to him.

> **I strongly believe that death counseling must be available to patients and their families in order that a rational decision be made.**

Today . . . it is in vogue to talk about death and dying. Yet . . . it is still taboo to mention one's own impending death and admit how out of control it makes us feel.

Obviously, the procedure would be facilitated if the patient would sign the Natural Death Act when less seriously ill, aware of the diagnosis, and more mobile.

Today in our society it is in vogue to talk about death and dying. Yet beneath all the professional jargon, it is still taboo to mention one's own impending death and admit how out of control it makes us feel. Sometimes it is felt that terminally ill patients are not able to deal with the knowledge of their true condition. The family often carries the burden of knowing how sick the patient actually is. I feel that a patient is aware of how sick he or she is even if this is not expressed verbally.

A patient's awareness is due to several factors: painful procedures, length of hospitalization(s), nonverbal cues from family, friends, and medical personnel (the sicker one is the more people stay away), physical deterioration such as weakness and fatigue, and knowledge of one's diagnosis. It is difficult to imagine submitting to chemotherapy month after month and failing to grasp the implications of my diagnosis as a leukemic.

With the knowledge of my diagnosis, I now know intellectually that my disease is terminal. No one had to tell me I was dying. I knew it. Now I have to accept it at the gut level. Since death is a subjective experience, I have to decide what my death means to me. I feel that the problem for both patient and physician is acknowledging this reality of death and the feelings which accompany it. It is difficult to place total responsibility on the doctor or on the patient. In order for patients to be prepared to sign the Natural Death Act, both patient and doctor must be encouraged to see the patient's condition as it actually is. By the time a patient is willing to sign the Natural Death Act and confronts the physician, he or she has worked through many feelings of grief and is at least beginning to accept their death. With the signing of this document, the patient is publicly accepting responsibility for a decision regarding the withholding of life supports.

My final concern is whether the Natural Death Act will indeed be a viable option for the terminally ill patient. The Natural Death Act applies only to those patients who do not want to be maintained on life supports when death is imminent. On the other hand, there are dying patients who *do* want to be maintained on life supports. It is imperative that each patient have the right to make a personal decision. The Natural Death Act gives terminally ill patients an opportunity to make a decision. Without the passage of this law, patients would have no legal option in the present health care system.

As this article asserts, the Natural Death Act must be widely distributed. It is necessary for members of the helping professions and community planners to develop ways of distributing this bill so that patients will be aware of their choices. Doctors will perhaps begin to talk more openly with patients about terminal illness, and will stop seeing a patient's death as a personal defeat but rather as a biological process that the patient may choose to hasten by relinquishing life supports. In either case, the choice is still the patient's.

Reflections on "Natural Death" and Natural Death Directives: A Care-Giver's Perspective

We experience our ideas, beliefs, and expectations about death as simply reflecting the way things are and always have been. Actually, our expectations about death and the process of dying have changed greatly over time and have been influenced, like most of our life, by growing technology. Our expectations are likely to continue to change.

Historians and philosophers tell us that the meaning of "natural death" has changed over the years. Only four hundred years ago when few people lived to an old age, a "natural" death came early and it was "unnatural" to grow old. Later, to die "naturally" meant that one got one's proportionate share of medical care, avoided early "untimely" death, and died in old age. Today, it means not receiving an "undue" amount of medical care which will "unduly" prolong a life that would otherwise end more quickly (Illich 1974).

What are our expectations? That death is to be feared. And, for most of us, even more fearful than death is the period in which we are neither dead nor alive, but lingering. What we fear most is the emotional, physical, and financial drain on our survivors, a drain that serves no meaningful purpose. If we have accumulated any money to leave to those we love, we fear it will be spent on our care at one hundred times the speed it took to save it. What we fear most is the helplessness and dependency, the confusion, the pain, and the discomfort, the not being ourselves, the total dependence on others for physical care—in short, a period of life which can be stretched out, as the years go by, for longer and longer periods by the use of modern technology.

Why do we need "Natural Death" legislation? Without it none of us can say we do not want our lives stretched out (should it be clear that we will soon die anyway) and know that our wishes will be respected. Physicians, because of legal liability and an unclear mandate from the patient, may feel constrained to keep a person technically "alive" longer than it makes any sense to do so. Relatives—feeling guilty because they will go on living, fearing they have not done everything they can, fearing to wish for such a thing as death for someone they love, and wanting to keep from feeling the loss which awaits them—cannot let go. We ourselves may be unable any longer to ask that machines not be employed. A "Natural Death Act," one of what might be termed "right-to-die" bills, was first passed in California in 1976 and was considered and passed in a variety of forms in rapid succession by other state legislatures. As passed in Texas (closely modeled after the California law), it provides that a person may, fourteen days or more after certification of terminal illness has been made, sign a directive to physicians which stipulates that under certain conditions his or her life will not be prolonged with the use of artificial life-sustaining procedures when death is imminent.

> **Why do we need "Natural Death" legislation? Without it none of us can . . . know that our wishes will be respected.**

A "natural death" directive means one must really come to terms with dying.

The act has its limitations. Like all legislation, the act is the result of a political process. It contains many "safeguards" necessary to insure passage by those who would otherwise fear its implications. Its "safeguards" pose significant drawbacks to its usefulness. For example, the fourteen-day waiting period between a patient's receiving a terminal diagnosis and signing the directive is designed to ensure a reasoned decision. Many people, however, are struck down suddenly by strokes, heart attacks, and traumatic accidents that render them unconscious and unable to execute such a directive. The act has, in fact, very limited applicability.

Perhaps the Act is most useful because it legally and publicly establishes that withdrawal of life-sustaining procedures is justified under certain circumstances—that is, people need not be kept alive to the last possible moment. Further, passage of the Act raises such issues to the level of conscious thought and public discussion.

Use of the directive is not without difficulties as well as rewards. To sign such a directive following the diagnosis of a terminal illness is different from signing a "living will" when one is healthy. A "natural death" directive means one must really come to terms with dying. It also necessitates clear, unambiguous communication between the physician and the patient. Who is to raise the issue initially? To spell things out so directly is perhaps to invade an individual's private space and hasten the emotional process of dealing with dying. We fear both subjecting people to unnecessary or premature pain and having to experience that pain with them. The directive presents both a problem and an opportunity.

Because an individual knows (after hospitalization, if not before) that no one cares about his or her life as much as he or she does and because one may hold out hope of an intervening, albeit "scientific," miracle, it may be frightening to sign such a directive. People feel ambivalent about such essential things. They want to know that they will not be asked to suffer unnecessarily, but they also want to know that, if there is still hope, they will receive the support and encouragement they need to keep fighting for life. Such ambivalence is the stuff of which inaction is made. Helping a patient make such a choice as a directive poses may prove to be an opportunity to confront and relieve the fear it brings to the surface.

"Natural death" legislation is not a panacea, but neither does it represent a static concept any more than biomedical technology does. We must expect that all will undergo change as the years go by.

References

Fletcher, J. Anti-dysthanasia: the problem of prolonging death. *Journal of Pastoral Care,* 18, 1964, 77–84.

Illich, I. The political uses of natural death. In P. Steinfels and R. Veatch, eds. *Death Inside Out: The Hastings Center Report.* New York: Harper & Row, 1974.

Kass, L. Death as an event. In P. Steinfels and R. Veatch, eds. *Death Inside Out: The Hastings Center Report.* New York: Harper & Row, 1974.

Structured
Exercises for
Death Education

Appendixes

The following appendixes are sixteen structured exercises that may be used in conjunction with the assigned reading. In more and more classes in death and dying, both instructors and students are recognizing the important role of experiential learning and therefore use group experiences to complement reading and/or didactic presentations. These exercises are designed to relate to specific chapters. In the introductory paragraph that precedes each chapter in this book, two or more of these exercises are recommended as helpful adjuncts to the reading. The exercises may be incorporated in a number of ways.

Guidelines for the use of structured exercises

1. Class members could form permanent support groups that meet during each class session. Exercises congruent with the reading for any class session would then be experienced during the allotted class time (perhaps half the period).
2. Classes meeting more than once a week could devote an entire class session to the exercises relevant to that week's assigned reading.
3. Some instructors may choose to build in three one-day workshops during the course of the semester. A workshop devoted to attitudes might begin the semester, while a grouping of exercises devoted to funeral preplanning or intervention may close out a semester.
4. The exercises may also be ordered so that an entire weekend marathon is possible.

The implementation of any structured experience requires careful thought and planning because of the sensitive nature of attitudes and feelings. Instructors must take some precautions so that the following conditions are established.

1. Class members should be encouraged to participate with the same group members so that a feeling of trust and cohesion develops.
2. Members should understand that their participation in experiential learning is purely voluntary and that a choice not to participate will in no way be reflected in their grade.
3. Members should understand that they may withdraw from any experience for any reason.
4. Members should be aware of helpful resources, both on and off campus, which they may use if needed.
5. Members should understand how each experience is related to the goals of the course, the reading assigned, and other exercises already presented.

Instructors may feel ill-prepared to facilitate group experiences themselves and yet see the value of incorporating them. If this is the case, instructors might consult with the university counseling center, psychology department, or community agencies. Qualified facilitators are available in most communities. At all times it should be remembered that the goal of the group facilitator is to assist each participant in a group to achieve fuller development as an effective human being. The following attributes for a facilitator seem particularly important.[1]

1. Personal qualifications. A group facilitator should:
   a. Be aware of his or her needs, motivations, strengths, weaknesses, values, and the impact he or she may have on others.
   b. Be able to monitor himself/herself and work through personal problems.
   c. Be able to learn from personal feedback.
   d. Believe in his or her self-worth and accept responsibility for what is done.
   e. Be able to empathize with the feelings of others.
   f. Be genuinely concerned for the needs and welfare of others.
2. Knowledge and skill. A group facilitator should possess:
   a. Knowledge and understanding of human behavior.
   b. Knowledge and understanding of group dynamics and group behavior.
   c. Knowledge and skill about how to design group experiences.
   d. Training in specific skills—e.g., listening and other communication skills and nonverbal behavior.
   e. Knowledge of ethical practice involved with group facilitation.

[1] In large part they represent guidelines for the preparation of group facilitators proposed by a task force of the American College Personnel Association in 1976.

Announcing One's Own Death

Appendix A

Goals

1. To recognize participant's own mortality.
2. To become aware of expectations and assumptions about death.
3. To desensitize participants to thinking about their own death.

Rationale   American customs and rituals ignore and deny that death is an inevitable part of life. This exercise invites participants to confront their death and to become aware of their expectations about how they will die, (e.g., young, violently, painfully), to lessen the awesome, mysterious quality of death.

Group size   Five to fifteen people.

Time required   One hour and a quarter.

Materials   Pencil and paper and a 4x8'' index card for each participant.

Physical setting   Quiet classroom or group room.

Process

1. Short group discussion on ways American society denies and ignores the fact of death (e.g., people die in hospitals instead of at home; children are not allowed to see dying people or to attend funerals). (Approximately 10 minutes.)
2. It is normal for people to imagine dying in different ways (e.g., violently in car accident; alone in their sleep; after a long illness). After assuring participants that imagining different ways of dying is normal, ask them to share the different ways they have imagined their own death. (Approximately 10 minutes.)
3. Ask participants to imagine that they have the power to plan their own death. Have them elaborate on their plan by writing the answers to the following questions: How old will you be? Where will your death occur? What will you be doing? Who will be there with you? What will the cause of death be? (Approximately 15 minutes.)

Contributors:
Rick Bradstreet and Anna Marie González, University of Texas at Austin, Texas.

4. Pass out index cards. Invite participants to design an announcement of a landmark personal event: their death. The announcement may include the information from the above questions. It should include how widely they wish to publicize the event and who (if anyone) they will invite to be present at the announcement. (Approximately 15 minutes.)

5. Invite participants to share their announcements with the group. (Approximately 10 minutes.)

Evaluation   Ask participants to evaluate experience and the exercise.

Appropriate Death Fantasy[1]

Goals

1. Conceptualization of personal appropriate death.
2. Isolation of factors necessary for an appropriate death.
3. Recognition and acceptance of variation between individuals regarding what is appropriate for them.

Rationale   Students are asked to apply materials previously addressed in deciding on an appropriate personal death, in Weisman's terms. The exercise also facilitates recognition and acceptance of personal mortality.

Group size   The first part (fantasy) of the exercise should be conducted in a large group. Follow-up discussion of the experience should occur in small groups of six to ten members.

Time required   One and one-half to two hours, depending on number of members in the discussion groups.

Preparation   Prior readings and class discussions (e.g., chapter 2, Kübler-Ross's stages; Weisman's[2] appropriate death, description of dying in hospitals, etc.)

Physical setting   The fantasy may be conducted outside or inside in a larger group. Participants should be comfortable and have sufficient space so as not to disturb each other. Following the fantasy exercise, space should be available to allow participant to meet in separate discussion groups.

Process

1. The goals of the exercise are explained and the procedure to be followed described.
2. Participants are instructed to make themselves physically comfortable, to close their eyes, not to talk, and to eliminate external distraction. Two minutes of silence precede initiation of the fantasy to facilitate focusing on relevant issues.

Contributor:
Judith Olson, University of Wyoming, Laramie, Wyoming.
[1]It is suggested that this exercise be used as the first of three units. The recommended second and third units are, respectively, Appendix G.,Funeral Fantasy and Appendix H., Fantasizing Grief Reaction of Significant Others.
[2]A. D.Weisman, *The Realization of Death: A Guide for the Psychological Autopsy* (New York: Jason Aronson, 1974).

3. Participants are allowed approximately twenty minutes to develop a fantasy of their own appropriate death—the death they would choose for themselves. In structuring the fantasy, participants are asked to make it as realistic as possible. The facilitator may suggest including such details as the following to enhance the realism:

> Age at dying/death
> Nature of death (accident, suicide, illness, etc.)
> Location of death (auto, hospital, home)
> Association of location and sights, smells, people, etc.
> Emotions experienced (fear, anger, acceptance, etc.)
> Physical decline and loss of control to point where life leaves the body
> Handling of pain (drugs, etc.)
> Unfinished business
> Intrapsychic deathwork (denial, etc.)
> Relationships—interpersonal death work—with whom, issues addressed, issues avoided, comfort levels
> Concerns about finality of death, immortality, survival of significant others, etc.
> Duration of the dying interval, effects of illness, etc.

The emphasis throughout should be on the experiences of the self, not the perspective of others.

4. The facilitator announces the conclusion of the fantasy. Participants are asked to open their eyes and, when ready, move to their discussion groups for the remainder of the period.

5. Discussion foci include the difficulty of imagining one's own death (primary paradox); reasons for selection of individual appropriate deaths; difficulties encountered in the fantasy (e.g., desire for a clear mind but inability to tolerate pain); factors necessary for an appropriate death (e.g., at home, with friends, accidental death, etc.) and their implications. In addition to illuminating in a very personal sense one's approach to death, the exercise is highly productive in delineating areas or relationships important to living.

Awareness of Grief Process

Goals
1. To help participants become aware of and experience the feelings associated with the loss of someone close to them.
2. To allow participants to become aware of the sense of grief and the various stages and emotions associated with grief.

Rationale Through sharing and reexperiencing the loss of a loved one, participants will have a better understanding of the grieving process.

Group size Twenty to twenty-five people; for group activities, no more than four per group. (It is important that these participants have some trust for one another.)

Time required Thirty minutes.

Physical setting Room with movable chairs.

Process
1. This exercise can occur at the beginning or end of a didactic presentation or discussion of the grief process.
2. The following instructions should occur slowly with enough time between questions to allow participants to fully explore and experience the exercise:

"Sit back, relax, and close your eyes. Take a couple of minutes to think of a person who has been close to you—a spouse, parent, child, sibling, friend—whom you have lost recently. How did this loss occur? Was it through death, divorce, change in relationship of some kind? What are your feelings now in the moment about that person? Do you feel sad—lonely—angry—numb—peaceful—guilty?

"How did you feel at the time of the loss? What feelings and thoughts do you remember at different times since then? What helped you account for feelings and attitudes at the time, and what now?"

Contributors:
Patsy Mendoza and Melba Vasquez, University of Texas at Austin, Texas.
Reference:
Elisabeth Kübler-Ross, *On Death and Dying* (New York: Macmillan Publishing Co., Inc., 1969).

3. Discuss with partner or small group as much as you wish to share.

Variations   Before discussion in small groups, a handout on the stages of death can be distributed to help participants define their feelings, relate them to the stages presented, and identify what stage they are in at the moment.

Awareness of Losses

Appendix D

Goal
To help people become aware of the various types of loss.

Rationale   It is important that participants be aware of the various types of losses that can contribute to the grief process.

Group size   20 to 25 people.

Time required   45–60 minutes.

Materials   Paper and pencil for each participant; handout copies of *"Losses Checklist,"* printed below.

Physical setting   Any room with movable chairs.

Process
1. Have participants make a quick list of all the things they have experienced as "losses"; e.g., someone or something no longer available or attainable.
2. Hand out the "Losses Checklist" and ask participants to check off the losses they have experienced; and also to add any not on the list that they have experienced. Have them make a special notation of some kind (two checks instead of one) of those that had not occurred to them.

Variation   Share and process with a partner and/or a small group.

Contributors:
Melba Vasquez and Patsy
Mendoza, University of
Texas at Austin, Texas.

Losses Checklist[1]

Obvious Losses
____ death of a loved one
____ the breakup of an affair
____ separation
____ divorce

Related Losses
____ loss of job
____ loss of money
____ moving
____ illness (loss of health)
____ change of teachers; change of schools

____ robbery
____ success (the loss of striving)
____ loss of a cherished ideal
____ loss of a long-term goal
____ change in relationships with children

Losses Related to Age
____ childhood dreams
____ puppy love
____ crushes
____ adolescent romances
____ leaving school (dropping out or graduation)
____ leaving home

____ change of jobs
____ loss of "youth"
____ loss of "beauty"
____ loss of sexual drive (or worse, the drive
remains but the ability falters)
____ menopause
____ retirement

[1] Melba Colgrove, Harold Bloomfield, and Peter McWilliams, *How to Survive the Loss of a Love* (New York: Bantam, 1977), pp. 2–3.

Confronting the Realization of Death

Appendix E

Goals

1. To get the participant in touch with the reality of his or her own death.
2. To pinpoint a person's particular difficulties about facing the reality of his or her own death.

Rationale   The fear of dying can be amorphous and elude a person who has not actually taken the time to think about what it is he or she really fears. If the exact fear or area of difficulty can be identified, it can be worked on to the person's satisfaction—which is far better than leaving the person in the state of fear or nonacceptance of his or her fate.

Group size   The exercise should be done with groups of four to six members. A group this size is large enough for the participants to experience the variety of their individual fears as well as the support of learning that others have similar ideas. It is also small enough to allow the intimacy of a small group and the security of a safe place to share, to exist.

These smaller groups can be part of a larger group which, after the exercise, can reconvene to discuss common fears. The larger group should not be larger than thirty or forty, to enable all groups to participate in discussion.

Time required   Approximately forty-five minutes. However, the time will, of course, depend on the length of discussion within the smaller and larger groups.

Materials   Paper and pencil for each participant.

Physical setting   Room with chairs or pillows to seat participants comfortably. There should be enough space for the participants to have some privacy when they break into small groups. They should be able to talk within their groups without disturbing or being disturbed by other groups. They may either sit in chairs pulled into a circle or on the floor with pillows, but they should be comfortable.

Contributor:
Caren Gertner, University
of Texas at Austin, Texas

Process

1. The larger group should divide into smaller groups of four to six persons. If other exercises have been done in small groups, the same groups should be retained.

2. The person in charge of the larger group should present the exercise after the groups have been formed.

3. An introduction and explanation of the exercise should be along these lines (with variations as the leader sees appropriate for the particular group):

   "We all know on one level that we are going to die someday. It may be later or sooner, but it will happen.

   "When we think of death, and in particular our own death, various thoughts come to mind on many different levels—some negative, some positive.

   "What I would like you to do in your groups now is to take some time, around five or ten minutes, for thinking about your own death. Each of you write down some of the points surrounding death that are negative to you, from your own particular view. These could be fears or disappointments, feelings or more cognitive thoughts. They may seem realistic to you or silly, but consider them 'worthy,' for you may be surprised to find that others have the same 'weird' fears you do.

   "After taking this time to yourself to write down the various things that come to you, I'd like you to share your list with your group for fifteen minutes [flexible] or so."

4. After the time for group sharing in the smaller groups, the larger group is called back together to discuss what points seemed to be common to people in all groups and what it was like to share these fears and thoughts with others.

Variations Step 4 of Process may be changed as follows: (1) Remain in the small groups and continue with other exercises. Or (2) return to the larger group without sharing particular experiences from the smaller groups, hence retaining the privacy of the smaller groups.

Euthanasia Exercise

Appendix F

Goals

1. To familiarize students with the concept of euthanasia.
2. To confront students with the difficulty of decision making in this area.
3. To offer students a variety of situations relating to euthanasia decisions that may help them to differentiate active from passive approaches.

Rationale   The American culture is a death-denying one in that most people desire a sudden rather than a prolonged death. However, many persons find themselves in situations that allow varying degrees of choice or decision. These choices may relate to the dying process or to death itself, as in the case of suicide. These decisions merit a simulation requiring participants to explore problem situations that call for active decision making on the part of the caregivers.

Group size   Five to eight people.

Time required   Thirty to forty minutes.

Materials   Pencil and a copy of the Euthanasia Worksheet (printed below) for each individual.

Physical setting   Quiet classroom with movable chairs.

Process

1. The instructor should make a brief presentation on the nature and forms of euthanasia to introduce the concept.
2. The presentation should be followed by a discussion of associated problems.
3. Participants may then form groups of approximately seven members.
4. Each participant completes a copy of the Euthanasia Worksheet.
5. A facilitator or natural leader should lead a discussion relating to the exercise. The following questions are suggested as guidelines.
    a.   How did you feel about the exercise?
    b.   What difficulties underlie our decisions regarding euthanasia?

Contributor:
Larry A. Bugen, Ph.D.,
St. Edwards University,
Austin, Texas.

c. What forms of euthanasia were you most willing to advocate?
d. Which problem situations were the most difficult for you to deal with personally?
e. Under what circumstances would you be most willing to advocate euthanasia for yourself or a close family member?

6. The instructor should then lead a discussion with the entire class so that individual groups might have an opportunity to hear a broader range of reactions.

Euthanasia Worksheet

For the next few minutes you are the physician-in-chief of a large hospital. Each day at this time you are handed a list of case histories which all present questions of euthanasia, now that euthanasia—or mercy-killing of any type—has been legalized and the legality upheld by the U.S. Supreme Court. You are in no danger of lawsuits from any source because the American Medical Association inserted as part of the bill an amendment stating that the physician-in-chief is always correct in his or her decision in such cases and no one else has any legal say in the matter. Some of the cases you read each day are of patients known to you; others are of strangers you have no time to meet.

Sign your name at the bottom of this page in both places. Indicate your decision for each patient by putting a check or X in the appropriate place to signify active euthanasia, passive euthanasia, or continuation of life. Then rank-order the patients you put into either euthanasia category to show who is to be killed first, second, third, etc. by your subordinate physicians. You will have no part in the actual euthanasia unless you specifically request to perform the medical action.

I, _____ , M.D., as Physician-in-Chief of this hospital, do hereby make the following judgments in the following cases, to be fulfilled to my satisfaction by Drs. Acevedo, Barringer, and Cordoba.

Signed,

_____ M.D.
Physician-in-Chief

Date _____

Case Number 66078

Infant male, born of 23-year-old mother; questionably desired pregnancy. Severe anomalies noted at birth; cleft face extending up through frontal bone, with no nasal bone and no medial orbits; eyes on stalks; microcranium; webbing of hands and feet. Child cannot survive without nasogastric tube-feeding, gastrostomy (incision into the stomach), or intravenous fluids. The parents have not yet seen the child.

Active _____ Passive _____ Life _____ _____

Case Number 66079

Infant female, born of 29-year-old mother; not desired pregnancy. Patient born with inoperable spina bifida [a congenital spinal deformation]. Child will never walk, may be able to live 7 or 8 years in a wheelchair. Parents cannot afford expensive drugs and treatment for the child; have 3 other children at home. Child's reflexes normal; intelligence appears normal.

Active _____ Passive _____ Life _____ _____

Case Number 66080

Infant female, born of 35-year-old mother; first child, desired pregnancy. Child exhibited at birth characteristic signs of Down's syndrome [mongolism]. Can expect no higher than 4th grade scholastic achievement during child's life. May need sheltered workshop in adulthood. Child also has a duodenal atresia, correctable by surgery. Parents request that surgery not be done so the child will die, although they could easily afford the surgery as they have a high income from husband's work: executive manager of a profitable international business firm.

Active _____ Passive _____ Life _____ _____

Case Number 66081

Infant female, born of 22-year-old mother; desired pregnancy. Initial neonatal life normal. Child discovered in crib at home not breathing and blue at 7 days of life. Rushed to hospital, which was near the home. Immediate action taken to resuscitate child in emergency room—successful. Parents are now in the emergency room waiting room, awaiting news. Child will be profoundly retarded, never exceed intelligence level of an infant; will probably die at age 10–20 from infection. What is your decision before parents are informed? They can be told the resuscitation was successful or not.

Active _____ Passive _____ Life _____ _____

Case Number 66082

Female, age 30, suffering from acute leukemia. She is presently in the sterile bubble, medically doing well but subjectively experiencing acute nausea, vomiting, and mental distress. There is no cure for the disease at present, but the patient's chances for a remission are high. She may live up to 3 more years. The last few days she has been asking for the treatments to stop, and occasionally for death, since her agony is so great. Her family agrees with any decision she makes. Hospital personnel enjoy her as a patient because she is so friendly and so good with the other patients when she feels good.

Active _____ Passive _____ Life _____ _____

Case Number 66083

Male, age 37, suffering from cancer of the stomach. Symptoms occurred suddenly at work one day and since then he has been in surgery 6 times over a period of 8 months. The family, a wife of 34 and their four children, cannot afford cobalt treatment as prescribed, or the family will need welfare. Without the cobalt treatment the disease will progress rapidly. Any more surgery is also out of the question because of its expense. The patient asks to be released from the treatments in order to be allowed to die at home with dignity, surrounded by his family. The wife wants the patient to live, but with some counseling she would probably change her opinion. With treatment, the man could live with relatively constant pain another 8–10 months.

Active _____ Passive _____ Life _____ _____

Case Number 66084

Female, age 24, in a coma since March, 1975. She can periodically breathe without a respirator but is usually dependent on one. She can take in nourishment only through nasogastric tubes or intravenously. She apparently has no consciousness left and is essentially a human vegetable. Her family begs for the respirator to be turned off and given to another patient somewhere; and even if she lives without the respirator, for her to be killed mercifully, for her sake and for their peace of mind.

Active _____ Passive _____ Life _____ _____

Case Number 66085

Female child, 6 years old, an only child, with acute leukemia. She can still walk around the unit, but her stomach is swollen to twice its usual size from the medication, and she is apparently in some pain all the time. Her 28-year-old parents are unable to visit her except on weekends, since they live 75 miles away and both have to work to pay for the treatments. She is resigned to hospital life, having almost grown up here, with treatments since age 3. She pathetically asks the nurses: "How long will I live? Will I ever see Johnny and Edward again?" (Two children who died recently.) She has seen death almost since her birth. Some hospital staff members and the parents of other children are asking why she can't be released from her suffering.

Active _____ Passive _____ Life _____ _____

Case Number 66086

Male, age 64, in intensive care unit with liver shutdown as a result of chronic cirrhosis of the liver. Patient has a history of being in jail for petty crimes, vagrancy, and alcoholism. This is his 8th admission for an alcohol-related bodily dysfunction. The patient wants to live. If he does, however, he will have nowhere to go. He will probably hang around the hospital waiting room, as he often has in the last few years, begging money for alcohol or food and harassing women. The hospital staff resents him, he has been disowned by his parents, deserted by his wife and children, and neither welfare nor the social service agencies wish to work with him any longer. Certain community workers and citizens are asking for his euthanasia, as he has an expected life span of only 3 years anyway.

Active _____ Passive _____ Life _____ _____

Case Number 66087

Female, age 59, recently having gangrene of both legs causing their amputation, as a result of lifelong diabetes. She has lost all hope for life. She feels she has nothing to live for, as her children rarely visit her and she doesn't feel close to anyone. Her husband died 8 years ago, leaving her to live alone in their small cottage in the country. After she leaves the hospital she will be placed in a local nursing home on the edge of the city, called a "concrete jungle" by many. She says the country is the only place for her to live a happy life, but her children feel it is better for her to be in the nursing home closest to their homes. She displays symptoms of severe depression, bewailing her fate, and she begs the doctors constantly for death.

Active _____ Passive _____ Life _____ _____

Case Number 66088

Female, age 89, in the hospital for kidney disease. She must spend several hours each day attached to the local kidney dialysis machine, which is very frightening and therefore a painful experience for her. She knows her condition will be fatal and asks her doctor why she can't be taken off these new-fangled machines and be allowed to die in peace at home. She fights the treatments, refuses her medications, and calls her children frequently (both of whom want her to be given the *best* of treatments until the very end).

Active _____ Passive _____ Life _____ _____

Case Number 66089

Male, age 55, conscious and communicative, dependent upon a heart-lung machine for life, after below-the-arm paralysis from an auto accident. He was a famous folksinger of a past generation. He requests repeatedly that the machine be turned off. His family, he says, is well provided for, his relatives have all had time with him, he has discussed his euthanasia with all of them and they all see it as the best action for his life. They have all grieved and are finished with grief, including him. He is confident of a happy after-life with his perceived God. He feels ready.

Active _____ Passive _____ Life _____ _____

Appendix G   Funeral Fantasy

Goals

1. To define and distinguish between personal and societal preferences for and functions of the funeral or memorial service.
2. To consider alternatives of burial, cremation, body donation, etc.
3. To understand and appreciate differences between individuals in choices made.

Rationale   By relating prior exposures (e.g., readings, lectures, visits to funeral homes) to oneself, people can clarify intellectual vs. emotional preferences and the role of self, others, and society in decisions regarding disposition of the body.

Group size   The fantasy may be conducted in a larger group, and subsequent discussion with small groups of six to ten members.

Time required   One to two hours.

Physical setting   Larger room for fantasy experiences and adequate space for smaller discussion groups to meet without distracting each other.

Process

1. Instructor describes procedure to be followed and explains goals of the exercise.
2. Participants are requested not to talk and to make themselves comfortable, close their eyes, and eliminate distractions.
3. Participants are given approximately 15 to 20 minutes to fantasize arrangements and ceremony related to disposition of the body following their appropriate death (Appendix B). The fantasy should include: length of time following death until service and burial/cremation; location of service; who is present; what is said and by whom; nature of the eulogy; flower or memorial arrangements; casket open or closed; embalming; clothes worn; preparation of the body; selection of grave marker; and burial, or cremation and handling of ashes, or donation of the body; etc.

Contributor:
Judith Olson, Ph.D.,
University of Wyoming,
Laramie, Wyoming

4. Conclusion of the fantasy is announced and participants are asked to form into discussion groups.

5. Discussion includes the range of options available and reasons for the choices made. The significance of disposition arrangements to the "deceased" vs. significant others vs. society should be differentiated. Whose preferences are most relevant to the decision process? Do the results capture the life and person of the "deceased"? What is the desired function of arrangements in the eyes of the "deceased" and others? What details of arrangements were surprising (e.g., preference for religious services with respect of the survivors, decision not to give body to science, choice of a large, impressive tombstone, etc.)? What attitudes and values are reflected, and how do they vary among group members?

Variations The exercise may be expanded to include the writing of a personal obituary. In conjunction with the eulogy, this encourages discussion of life plans and goals.

Contributor:
Judith Olson, Ph.D.,
University of Wyoming,
Laramie, Wyoming

Appendix H   Fantasizing Grief Reaction of Significant Others

Goals

1. Exploration of dynamics of grief.
2. Consideration of problems faced and resources available to significant others.
3. Contemplation of life continuing for significant others without the physical presence of the individual conducting the fantasy.

Rationale   By applying reading and lecture material related to grief to somone close, the less acceptable (and socially sanctioned) aspects of the grieving process are more readily understood.

Group size   The fantasy portion of the exercise may occur in a larger group. Discussion of the experience should occur in groups of six to ten members.

Time required   One and a half to two hours, depending on size of discussion groups.

Preparation   Previous readings and lecture material related to stages of bereavement, relation of nature of death to the grieving process, typical and atypical grief reactions, illness and grief, etc.

Physical setting   Comfortable setting for a large group and adequate meeting space for small discussion groups to meet without distracting each other.

Process

1. Instructor explains goals of the exercise and describes procedures to be followed.
2. Participants are requested not to talk and to make themselves physically comfortable, close their eyes, and eliminate external distractions.
3. Participants are given approximately 20 minutes to fantasize the reaction of their most significant others to their own appropriate death (Exercise B). They are instructed to initiate the fantasy at the point where the significant other

receives news of the death and then to follow the ensuing life of the significant other for a period of six months after the death.

4. The conclusion of the fantasy is announced; participants are asked to open their eyes and move to their discussion groups.

5. Discussion of the fantasy continues for approximately one hour following the fantasy period. Impact of the fantasy on participants typically necessitates discussion of their personal reactions to the experience before they address aspects of the fantasy itself. Additional areas of discussion usually include the survivor's manner of expressing emotions; the supportive individuals who are available to the survivor; unresolved issues in the relationship with the "deceased" which remain troublesome for the survivor; the range of emotional reactions evidenced in the survivor, including anger and guilt; internal and external resources that facilitate the grieving process and re-establishment of living; and concerns regarding the survivor's need to establish new significant relationships. Participants are frequently aware of issues which need to be addressed in their relationships with potential surviviors (ranging from financial provisions to resolution of conflicts).

Appendix I

Life and Death Attitudes: Dyadic Encounter

Goals

1. To compare and contrast life and death attitudes and discuss those attitudes with another person.
2. To experience individual feelings about death and verbalize these feelings.
3. To reduce the ambivalence most people have toward death-oriented discussion.

Rationale   Death in America is a cultural taboo and the subject is often avoided. Through an awareness of death we can become more perceptive toward life and its meaning to us. This exercise attempts to probe our feelings about life and death in order to help us verbalize and express both positive and negative attitudes.

Group size   A maximum of twenty people is recommended, because of the extraordinary nature of the material presented.

Time required   A minimum of one hour should be allotted to complete the exercise booklet. It is recommended that no time limit be set for the ensuing discussion, to allow full expression of individual reactions and subsequent closure of the group experiences.

Materials   For each participant, one Exercise Booklet (printed below), sheet of plain white paper, and pencil or pen. The exercise should be reproduced in a form that presents one question at a time to ensure that the participants concentrate on one question at a time. All necessary instructions are contained in the booklet.

Physical setting   The paired participants should be comfortably seated, facing each other.

Process

1. The group should be divided into pairs.
2. Participants are requested to read the instructions in the booklet and proceed at a comfortable pace.

Contributors:
William J. Soboter, Robert Rosand, and Connie Schick, Ph.D., Bloomsburg State College, Bloomsburg, Pennsylvania
Reference:
S. Pfeiffer and J. Jones, *Handbook of Structured Experiences for Human Relations* (Palo Alto: Human Relations Press, 1975).

3. The dyads should be advised that they can discontinue the exercise if either partner becomes anxious or uncomfortable.
4. The facilitator should be available to answer any questions that may arise during the exercise.
5. Each person is requested to write down, after completing the booklet, any thoughts, emotions, or reactions experienced.
6. The dyads are reconvened into the larger group, and individual reactions to the process are discussed.

Life and Death Attitudes

Read silently. Do not look ahead in the booklet.
A theme that is currently gaining interest is death. Death attitudes are frequently a reflection of life attitudes. The two often go hand in hand.

Despite the increased amount of printed material available, people still tend to shy away from death-oriented conversations. In the course of a dyadic discussion many similar ideas and attitudes can surface.

This encounter is designed to facilitate communication between two people concerning their attitudes toward life and death. It is hoped that openness and honesty will permit an interesting discussion which will show the similarity of ideas.

Please observe the following rules.
Don't look ahead in the booklet. Both partners should proceed through the questions at the same pace.

Both partners should complete each statement in the order presented and discuss their responses with each other before continuing.

You may discontinue the exercise if you become uncomfortable or anxious.

Turn the page and begin.

1. Life is . . . . . .

2. The thing I want to *do* most during my life . . . . . .

3. The most important thing in life . . . . . .

4. My life up to now . . . . . .

5. In the future I . . . . . .

6. At the moment I feel . . . . . .

7. I'm happiest when . . . . . .

8. When I'm alone I . . . . . .

9. I believe strongly that . . . . . .

10. What really turns me on . . . . . .

11. Right now I'm feeling like . . . . . .

Stop and take a moment to consider your responses up to this point. Try to relate your feelings to your partner, being sure to provide feedback to each other.

12. Consider for a moment:

Have I answered honestly??
Are we communicating??
Do I want to continue the dyad??

Answer the following questions.

13. Death is . . . . . .

14. What frightens me about death is . . . . . .

15. A corpse makes me feel . . . . . .

16. Our methods of burial are . . . . . .

Stop and consider your answers. Are you being as honest as before? If not, why not? Again, be sure to give your partner feedback.

17. Cemeteries are . . . . . .

18. Mourning about the dead is . . . . . .

19. What really depresses me . . . . . .

20. I could accept death when . . . . . .

21. Right now, I feel . . . . . .

Consider again: Honesty and communication. Share what you have learned about yourself and your partner. Do you wish to continue?

Answer the following questions.

22. Life after death . . . . . .

23. Reincarnation is . . . . . .

24. The soul is . . . . . .

25. Heaven is . . . . . .

Stop and consider the interaction up to this time. Do you consider it to be a positive or negative experience? Have you learned something about your partner? Have you learned something about yourself? Has discussing death increased your awareness of life? Does it help to discuss death?

Appendix J   Mortuary Form

Goals

1. To familiarize students with the variety of options available at the time of death.
2. To encourage students to plan their own funerals NOW in conjunction with others who might help implement preferences.
3. To encourage a review of the life-planning process based on clarification of values and attainment of goals.

Rationale   It is not uncommon to find that students enrolled in death and dying seminars have not been to funerals or have not attained an understanding of mortuary considerations. This is of some concern since these individuals may be called upon to make important decisions during the death crisis of a relative or friend. By completing the following questionnaire, students will have an opportunity to prepare and discuss personal preferences relating to the disposition of the body, the mortuary service, and life values and goals.

Group size   Group size may vary between five and eight members.

Time required   The exercise will typically be completed within 40 to 60 minutes.

Materials   One copy of the Mortuary Form for each participant and a pen or pencil.

Physical setting   A room with movable chairs is needed so that participants can face one another during the sharing process.

Process

1. The facilitator should present a brief rationale for the exercise.
2. Participants should then be encouraged to reflect and respond to each of the items without discussion.

Contributor:
Author unknown.

3. When all members of a group have completed the questionnaire, members should be encouraged to share with one another any insights or emotional reactions experienced while completing the questionnaire.
4. When all groups have processed the exercise independently, the facilitator may lead a general discussion on mortuary procedures.

Mortuary Form

Personal Preference and Vital Statistics

Name _____ Age at death _____

1. Cause of death _____
2. Place of death (if nonaccident); i.e., home, hospital, other institution

_____

3. I will be survived by _____

_____

4. At my death I was _____

_____

5. I will be mourned by _____

_____

6. I always wanted but was never able to _____

_____

7. I was a member of (community, and/or social groups, religious affiliation, if any) _____

_____

8. My educational background included _____

_____

As each of you completes the following sections, try to think and decide what you really want for your death. The following are some of the general questions that are asked and some of the conventional alternatives. Some of these alternatives may or may not really meet your needs.

Disposition of the Body

My body will be shipped to _____

Remains to _____

I want my body to be: Cremated ____   Buried ____   Donated to science ____

I want my remains placed in an: Urn ____   Cemetery plot ____   Mausoleum crypt ____   Elsewhere

(please describe) _____

_____

I would like my casket hermetically sealed [airtight]:   Yes ____   No ____

I would like my casket to be made of: Zinc ____   Steel ____   Hardwood ____   Redwood ____ Pine

____   Other ____   Undecided ____

Caskets range in price from $100 to $2,750. I would like my casket to cost in the range of $ _____ to

$ _____ .

I would like my body to be embalmed: Yes ____   No ____

I would like to have special cosmetics used in preparing my body: Yes ____   No ____   (Please specify) ____

_____

I would like my hair to be arranged in a certain way: Yes ____   No ____   (Please specify) _____

_____

I would like my body to be viewed with the following accessories: (Jewelry? Watches? Glasses? etc.; be

specific) _____

_____

I'd like my body to be buried with the following accessories: (Jewelry? Watches? Glasses? etc.; be specific)

_____

My mortuary preference is _____ . Undecided ____

I would like an autopsy to be performed: Yes ____ No ____ Undecided ____ . If undecided, under what conditions would you want the autopsy to be performed? _____

Memorial Service

I would like a memorial service: Yes ____ No ____

I would like a memorial service after disposition of the body: Yes ____ No ____

I would like the following individual or individuals to conduct my memorial service: Family ____ Minister ____ Friend ____ Fraternal ____ Mortician ____ Other _____

_____

Describe the type of memorial service you would like. _____

_____

_____

_____

Flowers may be sent to: _____

_____

In lieu of flowers, I would like a contribution made to: _____

_____

I would like my service to be conducted without my casket present: Yes ____ No ____

I would like my casket open ____ closed ____ at the memorial service.

I would like the visitation in my home: Yes ____ No ____

I would like visitation for the family prior to the service: Yes ____ No ____

I would like my casket to be open ____ closed ____ during the visitation.

I would like my body to be viewed by: Family only ____ Friends and Acquaintances ____

I would like to have the following casketbearers: _____

_____

_____

I would like a limousine for my immediate family: Yes ____   No ____

I would like a casket coach: Yes ____   No ____

I would like music: Yes ____   No ____

I would like the following musical selections for my memorial service:

_____

_____

I would like a vocalist for my memorial service: Yes ____   No ____   If yes, what selections? _____

_____

I would like to have a eulogy in my memorial service: Yes ____   No ____   If yes, given by whom? _____

_____

What things do I not want at my service? _____

_____

_____

_____

_____

_____

_____

_____

_____

_____

Life/Values/Goals

As you think about your death and as you see your life now, try to answer the following:

1. What three things would be said about you and your life if you died today?

    a.

    b.

    c.

2. Given the likelihood that you will not die today, and have time left to change some things in your life, what three things would you most like to have said about you and your life?

    a.

    b.

    c.

3. If someone were to witness a week of your life, what assumptions would that person make about your values—what matters to you?

    a.

    b.

    c.

4. What values do you hold that are not evident from the way you live your life?

    a.

    b.

    c.

5. What three goals are important to you as you plan your life?

    a.

    b.

    c.

6. What keeps you from achieving what you want for your life?

    a.

    b.

    c.

Appendix K Planning for Living

Goals

1. To provide participants an opportunity to review their lives as experienced to date.
2. To provide participants an opportunity to plan for the future.
3. To provide participants an opportunity to determine what resources are needed to accomplish future plans.

Rationale To develop in participants an awareness that each person can actively plan and choose new patterns of living NOW.

Group size Groups should be kept to a maximum of seven.

Time required The entire exercise can take from two and a half to five hours, depending upon the facilitation available and/or the willingness of the participants to share with one another.

Materials One copy of "Planning for Living" instruction booklet (printed below) for each participant and pen or pencil.

Physical setting Any setting that allows a group of six or seven participants to face one another will be acceptable. Deeper levels of sharing will occur in informal settings that incorporate pillows, rugs, etc.

Recommended variation Participants might be encouraged to postpone waiting and sharing their eulogies until the following class session. A subsequent class session may then take place at a cemetery, at which time each participant asks another group member to read his or her eulogy.

Process

Contributor:
Author unknown

1. Participants complete the "lifeline" and share their drawings with one another.
2. Facilitator leads a general discussion on the lifeline.

3. Participants complete "Who am I," "Identity Review," and "Sharing."
4. Facilitator then leads a general discussion on role identities.
5. Participants write their "eulogies" silently and then share emotional and cognitive reactions with one another.
6. Facilitator leads general discussion on eulogies.
7. Both "Fantasy Day" and "Life Inventory" are each completed as above. Each are then followed by discussion within groups and as a total group.

PLANNING FOR LIVING

Introduction
America is not a traditionalist or fatalist society, yet most of us often act as though we think the future is something that happens to us rather than something we create every day. Partly because the field of psychology emphasizes how childhood experience determines later adult behavior and partly because most of us accumulate obligations as we go through life, we often explain our current activities in terms of where we have been rather than where we are going. Because it is over, the past is unmanageable. Because it has not happened, the future is manageable. The following exercises are designed to help you think about where you are, where you want to go, and what resources you have for getting there.

Lifeline.   Use the lower half of this sheet of paper to draw a line representing your lifeline, and put a check mark on it to show where on the line you are right now. The line can be straight, slanted, curved, convoluted, jagged, etc.; it can be "psychological" or "chronological." It is a subjective thing—it represents how *you* think about *your* life. After you've drawn it, share what it means to you with others in your group.

Who am I?   This exercise is designed to explore the check mark on your lifeline. Write ten different answers to the question "Who am I" in the space provided below. You may choose to answer in terms of the roles and responsibilities you have in life, in terms of groups you belong to and beliefs you hold, in terms of certain qualities or traits you have as a person, in terms of behavior patterns, needs, or feelings that are characteristic of you, etc. Try to list those things which are really important to your sense of yourself—things that, if you lost them, would make a radical difference to your identity and the meaning of life for you.

Silent, individual reflection is necessary while doing this exercise. When you are finished, go right on to the next item, Identity Review.

(1)	
(2)	
(3)	
(4)	
(5)	
(6)	
(7)	
(8)	
(9)	
(10)	

Identity Review.   Consider each item in your "Who am I" list separately. Try to imagine how it would feel if that item were no longer true of you. (For example, if you put "husband" or "wife" as one of the items, what would the loss of your spouse mean to you? How would you feel? What would you do? What would your life be like?) After reviewing each item in this way, rank-order the items in the list by putting a number in the box to the right of each item. Put "1" beside the item which is most essential to your sense of yourself, the loss of which would require the greatest struggle to adjust to. Put "10" beside the item which is least essential to your sense of yourself. Try to rank-order all items in this way, without any items tying for first place, second place, third place, etc. If some items in your list are aspects of you that you dislike and would like to be rid of, they don't necessarily fall in the lower end of the rank order. The question for rank-ordering is, how big would the adjustment struggle be if you lost that item? Some aspects of yourself that you dislike might be very hard to give up!

Sharing. Share your "Who am I" and "Identity Review" exercises with the rest of your group. No one should be forced to share his or her list, and no one *can* be forced to share all the thoughts and feelings that occurred, but be as open as you can. If you are willing to share your list, take the initiative and share it with the others; invite their comments and questions; invite comparison with theirs.

Eulogy. Through the two above exercises, you've explored the check mark on your lifeline. This exercise is designed to explore the future end of your lifeline. The task is to write the eulogy that you wish would be a possible and realistic one to be delivered about you at your funeral. Don't write the eulogy that could realistically be delivered if you died tomorrow, unless that represents all you want to be in the future. So allow yourself future time, and even indulge yourself in some fantasy and wishful thinking when composing a eulogy to your life. As in the "Who-am-I" exercise, this exercise requires reflection, silence, being alone with yourself.

Use the rest of this sheet and the back of it to write your eulogy.

Fantasy Day. Having explored the check mark and the future end of the lifeline, now sample the space in between. To do this, construct a "fantasy day" sometime in the future. The day can be a "special day" that you would really love to experience. Or it can be the kind of "typical day" that you really wish would characterize your life. Or you can create a week instead of a day, etc. The important thing is to create an experience you really want some time in the future.

You may find it helpful to make notes about your fantasy day. If so, use the space below for that purpose. Or you may find it works better to just close your eyes and let your imagination roam.

When you're finished, share your fantasy with the rest of the group!

Life Inventory. In this exercise you generate as many answers as you can to a list of seven questions about your values and the resources you have for realizing those values. The seven questions are listed below.

A good procedure for constructing your life inventory is as follows. First, take a few minutes alone to write down as many answers to the seven questions as come to mind quickly, without thinking too deeply. In fact, the more spontaneous you can let yourself be, the better. Second, compare your answers with those of the other members of the group. Additional answers may thus be suggested to you, which you can add to your own list. Third, use the other group members as consultants to take a more searching look at your life inventory, to help you discover still more answers.

1. When do I feel fully alive? What things, events, activities, etc., make me feel that life is really worth living, that it's great to be me and to be alive?

2. What do I do well? What have I to contribute to the life of others? Over what skills do I have mastery? What do I do well for my own growth and well-being?

3. Given my current situation and given my aspirations, what do I need to learn to do?

4. What wishes should I be turning into plans? Are there any dreams I've discarded as "unrealistic" that I should start dreaming again?

5. What underdeveloped or misused resources do I have? (Resources might be material things or talents or friends, etc.)

6. What should I start doing *now*?

7. What should I stop doing *now*?

Privacy Circles   **Appendix L**

Goals

1. To help participants become aware of how sensitive people are to issues related to death and dying.

2. To make participants confront the issue of whom they would reach out to for help in situations involving death and dying.

3. To prepare participants to give or seek needed help in death-related rites of passage.

Rationale When faced with his or her own death, the individual often finds himself/herself unprepared and ill-equipped with the social and interpersonal communication skills to accept or help friends and relatives to accept the circumstance. Most people enter stages of bargaining and rejection of the inevitable before they can accept death. Generally, people avoid preparation for aiding another or seeking aid for this critical rite of passage.

Privacy circles can be used effectively to stimulate consideration of the persons who can be most helpful or can use the most help in death-related circumstances.

Group Size Groups of any size can participate in this activity. It can even be broadcast by radio or television to reach vast audiences.

Time Required Twenty to thirty minutes.

Materials The teacher or facilitator needs a chalkboard and chalk, and the participants each need a sheet of paper and a pencil or pen. Copies of a set of five concentric circles can be preprinted for distribution, or members of the group/class can draw them (see figure 1).

Physical Setting Virtually any setting can be used. Ideally, a classroom large enough for the group or class to be seated comfortably would serve as the setting.

Contributor:
William B. Cissell, Ph.D.
University of Texas at
Austin, Texas

Process

1. The facilitator distributes sheets of paper already printed with a set of five concentric circles—or, if blank paper is used, instructions are given to draw them. When the participants are prepared, the facilitator instructs them to write something about themselves (a belief, a feeling, or an action) in each band of the set of circles. For example, a person who has a secret desire to become an actor may be unwilling to share that secret with any other person. That secret desire would belong in the "Self" band. The same person may have a desire to possess a poster of Robert Redford. If he or she is willing to share that desire with anyone, including a clerk at a record shop, then it would belong in the "Strangers" band.

2. Once the participants understand the relationship among the bands, the facilitator should introduce hypothetical death-related desires or feelings or planned actions. A key word or phrase for each of these should be placed in the appropriate band. Some examples of the situations facilitators may use are as follows:

    a. You choose to request that no life-sustaining equipment be attached to your body should you suffer a terminal illness.

    b. You believe life-sustaining equipment attached to your terminally ill mother should be removed.

    c. You have occasionally felt a strong urge to commit suicide.

    d. You have just killed, through a negligent act, a strange hunter. No one has witnessed this act.

    e. You have just killed, through negligent driving, a small child. This occurred in a remote location and there were no witnesses.

    f. You need money to finance an expensive but questionable medical procedure that may save your life.

    g. You need money to finance pain-relieving and life-sustaining medicines and equipment while you suffer the discomforts of a terminal disease. You have been informed you can survive for several months, but there is absolutely no chance you can survive the illness. The cost of treatment will be extremely expensive.

3. When the participants have completed writing key words or phrases in the appropriate bands, the facilitator places them in small groups of three to five. Members of the groups are instructed to report, in rotation, what they placed in each band and explain why to the other group members.

4. After reporting has been completed in the small-group setting, the facilitator asks for a spokesperson from each group to report to the entire group. Common and uncommon experiences are discussed.

Variations

1. A series of five concentric rectangles (see figure 2) can be used instead of circles.

2. A letter keyed to each statement rather than a key word or phrase can be placed in a band.

3. Process step 3 can be eliminated when time does not permit all steps to be used.

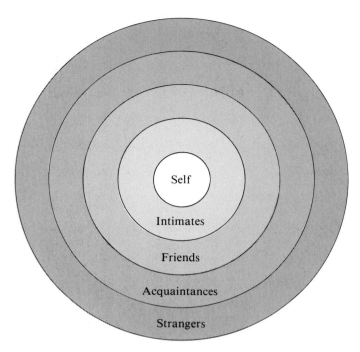

Figure 1

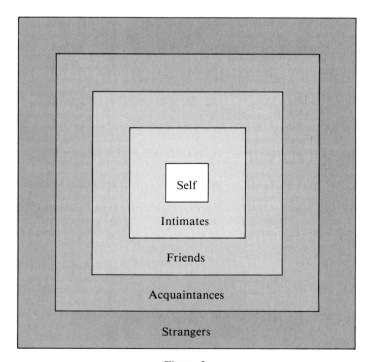

Figure 2

Appendix M Saying Good-bye to a Loved One

Goals
1. To become aware of important thoughts and feelings which had not been expressed to the dead loved one.
2. To facilitate expressing important thoughts and feelings.
3. To offer opportunities to complete relations with dead person.

Rationale Often when a loved one dies, the survivors feel stuck—unfinished and helpless to complete some important aspects of their relationship. Many survivors continue to feel frustrated, sad, and angry unnecessarily. By expressing whatever they want to say to the dead person, the survivor is able to complete the relationship and move on through the grief process.

Group size Eight to twelve persons.

Time required One and a quarter hours.

Physical setting Comfortable, quiet group room with pillows to allow people to sit or lie on floor if they wish.

Process
1. Ask participants to get into a comfortable posture and relax and close their eyes. Taking several deep breaths often helps people to relax. (three minutes)
2. Invite participants to keep eyes closed and recall a dead loved one with whom they still feel unfinished. A sign of being unfinished is if the person would like to have one more visit with the dead person. (five minutes)
3. Invite participants to fantasize a final visit with the loved one in a familiar setting (e.g., home, hospital, garden). Have participants fantasize the actual scene. (five minutes)
4. Have participants begin talking silently to the loved one in the fantasy and instruct them to watch and listen to what the loved one says and how he or

Contributors:
Anna Marie González and
Rick Bradstreet, University
of Texas at Austin, Texas

she looks while talking. Instruct the participants to continue the conversation until all that needs saying has been said and all the loved one says in return has been heard. (ten minutes)

5. Instruct participants to say good-bye in any way they want to when the conversation is finished. Also, suggest that, as part of the fantasy, participants find a place, person, or group of persons with whom they can feel comforted. (five minutes)

6. Invite participants to gradually come back from their fantasy when they are ready. (five minutes)

7. Invite participants to share their experience with other members of the group. (thirty minutes)

Evaluation   Ask group members to evaluate the experience. What parts were helpful? What parts were not useful? Was the timing good? Did participants gain a new perspective on the relationship with the loved one?

Variation   Have participants imagine a loved one who is not dead but likely to die soon.

Appendix N The Final Rite of Passage—A Technological Update

Goals

1. To take a new look at an old tradition. This new look is from the vantage point of the new audiovisual technology that is widely available. As an alternative to the traditional practice of viewing the body, this exercise suggests that mourners view an audiovisual tape.

2. To individualize the funeral procedures in such a way as to put the "atmospheric control" in the hands of the deceased. Atmospheric control is the same thing you notice when you go to a funeral home. For example: (1) notice the quiet; (2) notice the mannerism of the personnel; (3) notice the smell; (4) notice the decorum; (5) notice the difference in your own behavior. That's "atmospheric control." Through the use of audiovisual technology you can create your own atmosphere at your funeral; you can have your own control. The point here is that the atmosphere is within your control. If you want to swing through several moods, or just one mood, you can do so by theatrics. The use of content, music, voice inflections, etc., effects the audience's emotional state. This manipulation of emotional effect is done professionally by funeral directors. Some funeral directors have developed their theatrics into an art form.

3. To give the deceased a tool by which relatives, friends, and acquaintances can be brought into a single shared communion.

Rationale The terminal stage of life can be a period during which the individual "self actualizes," achieves integration, and explores the limits of personal potential. This exercise explicity suggests that the individual, the community, and the culture might facilitate the manifestation of spiritual and psychological growth of the terminal stage of life by (1) recognizing the potential for growth that exists during the terminal states of life, regardless of age; (2) understanding that the prevailing values of this society do not allow for the accurate description of potential growth that exists; and (3) recognizing that although death is the final crisis to be faced, it is still just one of the major crises that a full life brings.

Contributor:
James Brooks, University
of Texas at Austin and
Austin-Travis County
Mental Health/Mental
Retardation Center

Group size This exercise is for the individual and therefore should center around just one person. However, this does not preclude other persons having active or passive roles in the audiovisual tape (either on tape or in its production).

Time required Reflection time, anywhere from a half-hour to a few days. Recording time, approximately one to one-and-a-half hours. Playback time (optional), approximately a half-hour.

Materials Audiovisual recording equipment; audiovisual playback equipment (optional); record player and/or cartridge (optional); memorabilia (optional), i.e., photographs, awards/trophies, heirlooms, ad lib material.

Physical setting The physical setting should be subjectively chosen. Ideally, it should reflect the personality of the individual doing the exercise and be consistent with the content of the material being presented. The range of physical settings possible include recording in an apartment or studio to recording at the top of Mt. Everest. The intensity or depth of the content could range from sitting in front of the equipment and talking to having a cast and renting a major movie studio complete with props and writers.

Process
1. The individual contemplates his or her termination (no *ifs* or *buts*).
2. Now that you are terminated, put the salient pieces of your life together from beginning to end.
3. Assign priorities to current roles.
4. Collect memorabilia (optional).
5. Decide on visual setting to shoot tape.
6. Decide on audio background for tape; i.e., music, waterfalls, urban noises, etc.
7. Roll the tape while you give the camera a *recapitulation* of the salient points of your life history (include current goals and future expectations).
8. Give the tape to a person who will take responsibility for presenting it at your funeral.

Sample Monologue I was involved in various varsity sports in high school. Sports accounted for much of my popularity. I dated a number of girls who probably would not have given me the time of day if I had not excelled in sports. One of the girls I eventually married. I went to college for two reasons: (1) everyone said I should, and (2) I could continue to participate in competitive sports. It was during college that I married the girl I dated in high school. Although I went to college primarily to continue in sports, I soon began to realize the value of a college education. I began to set my sights on graduate school. Now in graduate school, studying to be a sociologist, I am anxiously awaiting my first child.

Variations
1. The tapes could be saved to create a library for the family.
2. Tapes of particular individuals might be stored at community libraries or recreation centers.
3. The tapes could be stored much more efficiently and economically than bodies.

Appendix O Values Grid

Goals
1. Develop within the participant an understanding of seven processes.
2. Make participants aware that few people have clarified their values regarding death-related issues.
3. Provide participants with a tool for clarifying values.

Rationale   In general people tend to avoid confronting issues related to death. Few have developed beliefs and actions related to death that fit all seven of the valuing processes basic to values clarification standards. The values grid developed by Simon, Howe and Kirschenbaum is an effective tool for helping people develop stronger and clearer values regarding death-related issues.

Group size   This works best with groups of six to sixty. It can be used effectively with groups of large sizes but attention would need to be given to such factors as appropriate facilities and control of the teaching-learning environment. Large groups are more apt to become distracted from the learning activity than are small groups. A group of less than six is apt to be so small that the benefits of group interaction would be lost.

Time required   The goals of this teaching-learning strategy can be realized in one 45–50 minute session. However, greater benefit can be gained from two 45–50 minute periods.

Contributor:
William B. Cissell, Ph.D.,
University of Texas at
Austin, Texas
Reference:
Sidney B. Simon, Leland
W. Howe, and Howard
Kirschenbaum, *Values
Clarification* (New York:
Hart Publishing Company,
1972).

Materials
1. Hand-out copies of a grid like that printed below, reproduced on full-size sheets of paper: i.e., a list of issues to be considered followed by seven lettered columns.
2. Chalk and chalkboard or overhead projector and marker.

Physical setting   A classroom is the optimal setting; however, out-of-doors sites can be utilized effectively as well. Furniture should be mobile to allow participants to move chairs into small groups.

Issues	a	b	c	d	e	f	g
1. Suicide							
2. Euthanasia							
3. Death Penalty							
4. Abortion							
5. etc.							

Process

1. The facilitator distributes copies of the grid and asks participants to glance down the list of issues and to note the seven columns. Next, the facilitator writes the following questions on a chalkboard or overhead projection transparency:

    a. Are you *proud* of your position?

    b. Have you publicly *affirmed* your position?

    c. Have you chosen your position from *alternatives*?

    d. Have you chosen your position after *thoughtful consideration* of the pros and cons and consequences?

    e. Have you chosen your position *freely*?

    f. Have you *acted* on or done anything about your beliefs?

    g. Have you acted with *repetition* or *pattern* or *consistency* on this issue?

2. After the participants have read the questions, the facilitator asks them to place a check mark opposite each issue in each column whose corresponding question can be answered affirmatively. For example, if the participant can answer, "Yes, I am proud of my position on suicide," a check mark is placed in column *a*. If the participant can answer, "Yes, I have publicly affirmed my position on suicide," a check mark is placed in column *b*. And so forth for all seven questions.

3. Members of the group can be asked to suggest some issues to be added to the list. Issues such as murder, war, death through self-defense, negligent homicide, funeral customs, and high-risk sports and recreational activities are worthy issues for consideration. The facilitator can expand or limit the list of issues to suit his or her purposes.

4. Place the participants in small groups of threes, fours, or fives. Instruct members of each group to discuss, in turn, each of the issues listed. Each participant should: (a) state an issue; (b) describe his/her position on that particular issue; and (c) discuss how his/her position did or did not meet the seven valuing processes.

5. When all of the issues have been reported within the groups, the facilitator should ask spokespersons from several groups to report upon the observations they noted regarding the process used. The facilitator should guide discussion at this point to emphasize how the approach used differs from the discussions group members had probably experienced previously. Participants should become aware that this activity did not require a defense of their beliefs. Rather, it requires them to consider the manner in which they arrive at their convictions and note how firmly they hold their beliefs.

6. If used early in a course on death education, this exercise can be followed by the nominal group process.[1] The nominal group process provides a mechanism for selecting the issues that participants consider most important for attention.

[1] J. Pfeiffer and J. Jones, *The 1975 Annual of Structured Experience for Human Relations Training* (La Jolla, Calif.: University Associates, 1975), p. 35.

Variations

1. All of the death-related issues can be generated from the group.

2. Step 4, placement in small groups, can be eliminated if there is insufficient time. A few individuals in the group can be called upon to report their reactions to the exercise. However, it must be recognized that eliminating step 4 reduces some significant group interaction benefits that can be gained from this exercise.

Warm-up Exercise

Goal   To enable participants to become acquainted with the concept of death and become aware of the importance of living in the present.

Rationale   To have meaningful participation with the intense subject of death, participants must be gradually desensitized to the subject.

Group size   Twenty-five to thirty people.

Time required   Twenty to thirty minutes.

Materials   Paper or index cards for participants to write on and pens or pencils.

Physical setting   Any room with movable chairs

Process
1. Have participants imagine and respond briefly in writing to the following stimulus questions (allow a few minutes for each set of questions):
   a. What do you see yourself doing, being involved in, five years from now? What kinds of things are you spending your time and energy on? What are you like?
   b. What are you like ten years from now? What kind of people are in your life? What kind of quality of interaction do you have with those people?
   c. Picture yourself twenty years from now. What do you see yourself doing? What are your roles? What is your physical appearance like? How is your health? Who is in your family? Who is not in your family? Are you doing what you want to be doing?
   d. Knowing all this about yourself, what is the span of life that remains to you? In view of how you want to be and who you want to be, what are you doing now to move toward that image? What are you doing now that is detrimental to attaining that ideal?
2. Have participants stop writing and think quietly for a couple of minutes about this exercise. How was it for you? Did you have any blocks or prob-

Contributors:
Melba Vasquez and Patsy Mendoza, University of Texas at Austin, Texas

lems with any part of the exercise? What parts did you enjoy? What did you not enjoy?

3. Have participants share as much of this experience as they wish with a partner or a small group (no more than three or four) for about five minutes apiece.

Variations   Have the group members share their ages with one another. Have them then discuss how their age may be related to their responses to the stimulus questions. Have them identify (*a*) which questions were most important to them, and (*b*) which questions were most difficult for them to respond to.

Name Index

Friedman, S., 104, 112, 153
Friesen, S. R., 186, 188
Fulton, R., 56, 64, 73, 77, 85

Garfield, Charles A., 288, 401-10
Garrity, T. F., 356, 379
Gassman, M., 154
Gengerelli, J. A., 154
Gerber, I., 352, 379
Gertler, R., 81, 87
Gertner, Caren, 435n
Getty, C., 81, 82, 86
Gibbs, J. P., 65
Gillerman, G., 275
Gilmore, Gary, 67
Girardin, P., 234
Glaser, B. G., 181, 184, 187, 266
Glasgow, L. A., 153
Glass, G. V., 222, 223
Glover, E., 124, 129
Glueck, E., 64
Glueck, S., 64
Goffman, Erving, 160, 161, 191, 191n, 192, 193, 193n, 194, 195, 196, 202
Goldfarb, A. I., 352, 361, 362, 366, 367, 368, 369, 379
González, Anna Marie, 427n, 466n
Good, Robert A., 397, 398
Goodman, L., 79, 85
Gordon, G., 303, 308
Gordon, T., 108, 112
Gotlieb, J. K., 155
Gottman, J. M., 222, 223
Gould, J., 312, 320, 322
Grace, W. J., 155
Grad, B., 369, 379
Granick, S., 380
Greaves, C., 246, 249
Greenacre, P., 128
Greene, W. A., Jr., 154
Grumet, J., 79, 86
Gustafson, J. M., 325, 335

Habenstein, Robert W., 192n, 198, 202
Hagnell, O., 154
Halikes, J. A., 65, 112, 353, 378
Hall, G. S., 75, 85
Hamilton, Gordon, 140, 141
Handal, P. J., 73, 80, 85

Hanson, S., 187
Harris, Louis, 326
Hart, J., 242, 249
Hays, J. E., 75, 85, 235
Hedge, A. R., 154
Heller, J., 187
Henry, W., 303, 308
Hermann, L., 77, 78, 80, 85
Hersh, S. P., 161, 212-24
Hilgard, J. R., 64
Hinton, J. M., 185, 186, 189
Hochet, T. P., 155
Hoefer-Janker, Dr. Hans, 384, 386, 390, 391, 395, 396
Hoerr, S. O., 181, 188
Hofer, M., 104, 112
Hoffman, F. C., 154
Holleb, Dr. Arthur, 397
Hollenbeck, A. R., 161, 212-24
Hollender, M. H., 306, 308
Hollingshead, A. B., 59, 65, 90, 97
Holmes, T., 100, 112
Howe, Leland W., 470n
Hughes, C. H., 154
Hughes, Everett C., 199n
Hutschnecker, Dr. Arnold, 151, 154
Huxley, Aldous, 401

Iammarino, N. K., 74, 81, 86
Ibarra, I. D., 188
Iker, H., 155
Illich, I., 423, 424
Imbus, Sharon, 163, 269-75

Jackson, D. M., 275
Jasnau, K. F., 363, 364, 379
Jeffers, F. C., 74, 77, 86, 379, 380
Jeffrey, D., 242, 249
Jenkins, C. D., 357, 379
Joesten, Rev. Leroy, 263
Johnson, A. M., 64
Jones, A., 321, 323
Jones, Dr. Chester, 13
Jones, E. E., 73, 86
Jones, H. W., 155
Jones, J., 446n, 470n
Jones, R., 187
Josephy, H., 359, 379
Jung, Carl, 152

Kalish, Richard A., 77, 82, 86, 287, 308, 336-47
Kamisar, Y., 317, 320, 323
Kapp, Frederic, 81, 87, 287, 324-35
Karon, M., 213, 224
Kasl, S. J., 359, 361, 379
Kasper, A., 42, 45, 179, 187
Kass, Leon, 415, 424
Kastenbaum, R., 76, 82, 83, 86, 182, 183, 187, 188, 239, 247, 249, 379
Kavanaugh, R., 2, 33, 37, 45, 106, 112, 271
Kavetsky, R. E., 154
Kelly, Britton, 279
Kelly, Orville E., 163, 164, 276-83
Kelly, Wanda, 277, 279, 283
Kelly, W. D., 186, 188
Kennedy, John F., 35, 103
Kennedy, M., 370, 372, 373, 380
Kennedy, Robert F., 121
Kent, D. P., 379
Kety, S. S., 62, 65
Killian, E. C., 361, 362, 366, 368, 369, 379
Kirkner, F. J., 154
Kirkpatrick, J., 56, 64
Kirschenbaum, Howard, 470n
Kirschner, G., 129, 153
Kissen, D. M., 153, 154
Kissen, M., 154
Kleban, M. H., 356, 378
Klein, D. C., 375, 379
Klein, Melanie, 17, 64
Klein, R. F., 356, 379
Klemchuk, H., 153
Klerman, G. L., 266
Klopfer, B., 154
Kneisl, C., 81, 82, 86
Koff, T. H., 267
Kohl, Marvin, 312, 323, 327, 335
Koocher, Gerald, 4, 88-97, 213, 224
Kopel, K., 234
Kostin, I., 79, 86
Kowal, S. J., 154
Koza, Pamela, 286, 287, 310-22
Kral, V., 369, 375, 379
Kramer, M., 334, 335
Krant, M. J., 254, 267
Kraus, A. S., 60, 65
Krech, D., 334, 335

Subject Index

observation, systematic,
methodology for, in
hospital setting, in-
teractions between
primary caregivers
and children with
cancer and, 213–24
occupation of deceased,
newspaper reporting
and, 345
others, fear of death of,
death anxiety and,
69. *See also* signifi-
cant others
overactivity, without sense
of loss, as distorted
reaction, 12

parents, loss of, during
childhood and
adolescence,
bereavement
research and, 56–57
perception of death as
crisis, 100–102
peripherality, 36
physical health, death anxiety and, 76–77
physical suffering, fear of,
death anxiety and,
68
physicians, attitude and
behavior of, coping
with dying patients
and, 179–82
physiological reaction to
crises, 104
place or location of death
newspaper reporting
and, 341–43
terminal care and,
253–55
planning for living, structured exercise for,
458–62
potential for change, as
characteristic of
death as crisis, 103
prediction
of death for elderly, en-
vironmental events
and, 349–80
conclusion, 375–78
loss of significant
other, 351–58
relocation, 359–70
retirement, 370–75
of grief, model for,
33–44

of unfavorable bereave-
ment outcome,
62–64
preoperational child, talking to, about death,
92, 94, 95
preventability, in model
for prediction and
intervention of
grief, 36
unpreventability, 37
primary caregivers, interactions between
children with cancer
and, 213–24
privacy circles, structured
exercise for, death
education and,
463–65
problem, insoluble, as
characteristic of
death as crisis, 104
professionals, attitudes of,
toward death and
dying, terminal care
and, 253. *See also*
hospital setting;
medical staff;
technology; terminal
care
prognostic evaluation,
symptomatology
and management of
acute grief and, 15
prolonged duration of
grief, 38–39, 40,
41–42
psychological reaction to
crises, 105–106
psychotherapy. *See* re-grief
work; ritual, death
punishment, fear of, death
anxiety and, 69
purpose, sense of, death
anxiety and, 78–79

quality of life, control,
and right to die,
413–24
Natural Death Act of
Texas, 415–20
questionnaire, for attitudes
toward euthanasia,
327–29
results, 329–33

rates, death, attitudes,
ethnic press and,
337–47

reactions
to crises, 104–106
behavioral, 105
physiological, 104
psychological, 105–106
delay or postponement
of, 11–12
distorted, 12–15
realization of death, confronting, structured
exercise for, 435–36
re-grief work, study of,
115–29
applied, 118–23
dreams during, study of,
123–26
investigation of, 126–28
phases of, 116–18, 123
re-grief work, 116–18
relatives, alteration in relationship to, as
distorted reaction,
13
religion of deceased,
newspaper reporting
and, 344
religiosity, death anxiety
and, 77
relocation, as predictor of
death for elderly,
359–70
reorganization phase of re-
grief work, 116
reporting death. *See* ethnic
press
retirement, as predictor of
death for elderly,
370–75
right to die
control, 213–14
Natural Death Act of
Texas, 415–20
quality of life, 414
rite of passage, final,
technology and,
structured exercise
for, 468–70
ritual, death, therapy
through, 131–41
conclusions, 140
customs in Mexico,
134–35
drama, ritual, 137–39
hospital setting, 136–37
mourning, death and,
133–34
reactions and results,
139–40
See also funerals

transition state, 47–52
common factors, 47–48
personal experiences of
death encounters,
48–51
preparing for reality of,
51–52
treatment. *See* re-grief
work; ritual, death
types of death, newspaper
reporting and,
339–41

unexpectancy as
characteristic of
death as crisis, 103

unprecedented survival,
autonomy for burn
patients and, 269–75

values grid, structured exercise for, death
education and,
470–72

warm-up exercise, death
education and,
473–74
widowhood
bereavement research
and, 57–59

crisis of, in family cycle,
167–76
adjustment, death
and, 168–69
child and widowhood,
172–75
conclusions, 175–76
family, 167–68
problems of widow,
169–72
husband sanctification
and, 205–11
See also significant
others
wife, loss of, bereavement
research and, 57–59
workshops. *See* education,
death; exercises,
structured